FIFTH EDITION

NEUROLOGY
for the SPEECH-LANGUAGE PATHOLOGIST

FIFTH EDITION

NEUROLOGY

for the SPEECH-LANGUAGE PATHOLOGIST

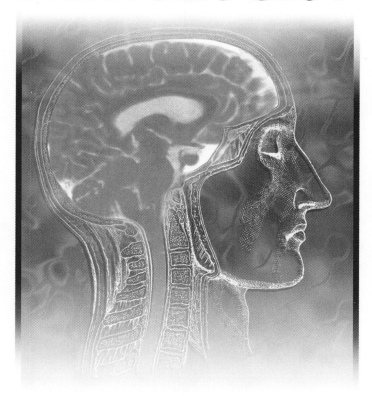

Wanda G. Webb, PhD, CCC-SLP

Assistant Professor
Department of Hearing and Speech Sciences
School of Medicine
Vanderbilt University
Nashville, Tennessee

Richard K. Adler, PhD, CCC-SLP

Professor
Speech/Language/Hearing Sciences
College of Education & Human Services
Minnesota State University—Moorhead
Moorhead, Minnesota

with 232 illustrations

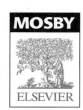

MOSBY

ELSEVIER

MOSBY
ELSEVIER

11830 Westline Industrial Drive
St. Louis, Missouri 63146

NEUROLOGY FOR THE SPEECH-LANGUAGE PATHOLOGIST   ISBN-13: 978-0-7506-7526-0
Copyright © 2008, Mosby, Inc. All rights reserved.   10: 0-7506-7526-8

Previous editions copyrighted 2001, 1996, 1991, 1986.

ISBN-13: 978-0-7506-7526-0
        10: 0-7506-7526-8

Vice President and Publisher: Linda Duncan
Senior Editor: Kathy Falk
Managing Editor: Kristin Hebberd
Associate Developmental Editor: Andrew Grow
Publishing Services Manager: Julie Eddy
Project Manager: Richard Barber
Design Direction: Maggie Reid

Printed in Canada

Last digit is print number: 9 8 7 6 5 4 3 2 1

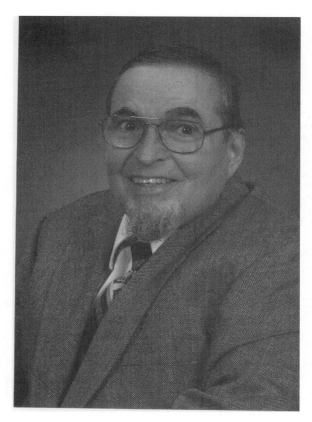

This book is dedicated in loving memory to Dr. Russell J. Love,
former senior author, who passed away in March 2006 at the age of 75.

Russell J. Love was born in Chicago, attended Tulane University, and graduated with his Master's degree and then later his PhD from Northwestern University. As a clinician, he served as a speech-language pathologist at the Moody School for Cerebral Palsied Children in Galveston, Texas; the VA hospital in Coral Gables, Florida; Michael Reese Hospital in Chicago, Illinois; and the Bill Wilkerson Center in Nashville, Tennessee. As a professor, he taught at DePaul University and at Vanderbilt University and retired as professor emeritus from Vanderbilt in 1995. Among other acknowledgments of his contribution, Dr. Love was awarded the Honors of the Tennessee Association of Audiologists and Speech-Language Pathologists and was made a fellow of the American Speech-Language-Hearing Association (ASHA). He was most proud of his work as an advocate for the rights of persons with communication and physical disabilities.

Dr. Love's memory is cherished by his family, his friends, and his colleagues as a man of perseverance, intelligence, compassion, and quick wit. He was a caring and devoted husband, father, grandfather, teacher, collaborator, and friend. My wish for every student reading this text is that you will find a teacher or mentor who will guide you in your studies and your career as carefully and with as much respect and insight as Dr. Love guided me and so many others. He had an enthusiasm and love for our profession and for teaching that enabled him to be a positive influence in the lives of countless patients, students, and young professionals.

Working on research and on the conception of this book with him were some of the best moments of my life. I miss my friend. It is my fervent hope that he would have approved of what Dr. Adler and I have done in this new edition, which also carries his name, as our work was done to honor that name.

Wanda G. Webb

Acknowledgments

For authors primarily trained in the field of speech-language pathology, rather than neurology, a project like this demands reliance on colleagues in neurology to assist in the development of the work. Howard S. Kirshner brought his expertise to bear on the earlier editions, which establish the foundation of the current text. We remain in his debt for that guidance.

Although we have not had the honor of meeting him, we are indeed indebted to Dr. Duane Haines, Professor and Chair of the Department of Anatomy and Professor of Neurology at the University of Mississippi Medical Center in Jackson, Mississippi. Dr. Haines is the editor of the comprehensive text, *Fundamentals of Neuroscience for Basic and Clinical Applications* from which, with his generous permission, we obtained a number of pictures and drawings used in this book. We are most grateful to him, as well as the illustrators and various contributors to his text for sharing their fine work to enhance this text.

We are indebted as well to several members of the editorial staff, past and present, of Butterworth-Heinemann and now Elsevier. In past editions, specific individuals of the Butterworth-Heinemann staff have been named in the acknowledgments, as have various people in Nashville who provided invaluable secretarial support for those earlier editions. We will not reiterate their names here, but that is not to detract from the value of their contributions. They will always be remembered by Dr. Webb as critical to the success this book has enjoyed. For this edition, we are most grateful for the guidance of Andrew Grow and Kristin Hebberd, and the editing expertise of Laura Kudowitz and Rich Barber.

The support and understanding of Kathy Falk, Senior Editor with Elsevier, is greatly appreciated. It has been a difficult and often emotional task to get this edition to completion with the illness and subsequent death of Dr. Love. The sensitivity and patience of Ms. Falk and her editorial staff helped to lessen the burden, and we thank them for that.

Wanda G. Webb
Richard K. Adler

I am especially grateful to Dr. Webb for her patience and understanding during the writing of this edition. It was very difficult to proceed knowing that the senior author of previous editions was one of my mentors – someone to whom I looked up. Dr. Love and Dr. Webb began writing this text more than 20 years ago, and I am extremely grateful to Dr. Webb and to Kathy Falk of Elsevier for giving me the privilege of becoming the second author of this edition.

I am also extremely grateful to my partner, Dave; my family; and many of my colleagues at Minnesota State University Moorhead for their ongoing encouragement that helped me get through the process. And finally, a hearty thank you is in order to my students, past and present, who have inspired me to strive for better lectures, texts, and illustrations. Many of these students actually grew to appreciate my neuroanatomy and physiology course, and I am sure future students will appreciate this new text.

Richard K. Adler

During the best of times, no undertaking as complex as this revision is completed without the support of co-workers, family, and friends. I first want to express my appreciation to Dr. Richard Adler for taking on this project and seeing it through with me. It is a mammoth task to revise and update someone else's writing. His ideas, cooperation, patience, and good humor have made this task easier for me and have contributed greatly to bringing this text to publication. My family and friends have been extremely supportive through the grieving for Dr. Love and the writing of the revision without him. My husband, Joe Luttrell, has been a solace and a cheerleader and has given up personal time to allow me to work on this project. Like Dr. Adler, I am grateful to my students and my colleagues at Vanderbilt University for all they have taught me and continue to teach me. And finally, my thanks go to Barbara Love, Dr. Love's beloved wife, who has supported me and has enabled me to keep the warm memories of Russell and our work together that have carried me through this project.

Wanda G. Webb

Foreword

Speech Pathology and Neurology: Intersecting Specialties

Neurology is the study of the effects of disease in the nervous system—brain, spinal cord, cerebellum, nerves, and muscles—on human behavior. The neurologist examines specific functions—including higher cortical functions; cranial nerve functions; and motor, sensory, and cerebellar functions—all to localize disorders to specific areas of the nervous system. These lesion localizations, along with the clinical history of how the deficit developed, allow for a precise diagnosis of the disease process. Laboratory and brain imaging tests may help to confirm the diagnosis, but the process should always start with localization and disease diagnosis in a clinical neurologic evaluation.

Speech and communication are among the most complicated functions of the human brain, involving myriad interactions between personality, cognitive processes, imagination, language, emotion, and lower sensory and motor systems necessary for articulation and comprehension. These functions involve brain pathways and mechanisms, some well understood and others only beginning to be conceptualized. The brain mechanisms underlying higher functions such as language are known largely through neurologic studies of human patients with acquired brain lesions. Animal models have shed only limited light on these complex disorders.

Stroke has historically been a great source of information because this "experiment of nature" damages one brain area while leaving the rest of the nervous system intact. For more than a century, patients with strokes and other brain diseases have been studied in life, and the clinical syndromes have then been correlated with brain lesions found at autopsy. Recently, new methods of brain imaging have made possible the simultaneous study of a lesion in the brain and a deficit of communication in the same patient. These advances in brain imaging, including computerized tomography, magnetic resonance imaging, and positron emission tomography, have brought about a burgeoning of knowledge in this area. Functional brain imaging modalities such as functional MRI and PET scanning now permit the visualization of brain activation in normal subjects during language tasks, and these studies have contributed further to our knowledge of the organization of language in the brain.

In this book, Drs. Love, Webb, and Adler have laid the factual groundwork for the understanding of the nervous system in terms of the organization of the brain, descending motor and ascending sensory pathways, and cranial nerves and muscles. Understanding these anatomic systems makes possible the understanding and classification of the syndromes of aphasia, alexia, dysarthria, and dysphonia, as well as the effects of specific, localized disease processes on human speech and communication. All these subjects are clearly and accurately reviewed. The speech-language pathologist who studies this book should have a much improved comprehension of the brain mechanisms disrupted in speech-impaired and language-impaired patients, and, thereby, a greater understanding of the disorders of speech and language themselves.

Perhaps the most important by-product of this book should be a closer interaction between neurologists and speech-language pathologists. Neurologists understand the anatomic relationships of the brain and its connections, but they often fail to use speech and language to their full limits in assessing the function of specific parts of the nervous system. A careful analysis of speech and language functions can supplement the more cursory portions of the standard neurologic examination devoted to these functions. Thus, detailed aphasia testing supplements the neurologist's bedside mental-status examination, and close observation of palatal, lingual, and facial motion during articulation supplements the neurologist's cranial nerve examination. The neurologist's diagnosis of the patient's disorder, on the other hand, should aid the speech-language pathologist in understanding the nature and prognosis of the speech and language disorder. The neurologist and speech-language pathologist should ideally function as a team, complementing each other. For this teamwork to occur, however, each specialist must comprehend the other's language. To this end, these authors have made the language of the neurologist understandable to the speech-language pathologist. As a neurologist who has worked closely with two of them, I applaud them for this important accomplishment.

I would like to end with a personal statement about Dr. Russell Love, one of the two original authors of this book. Dr. Love was an inspiring scientist and colleague who personified the relationship between speech-language pathologist and neurologist. In his long career, he taught generations of speech-language pathologists and neurologists. To the end, he was always gracious, optimistic, and informative in all of his interactions.

Howard S. Kirshner
Professor and Vice-Chair
Department of Neurology
Vanderbilt University Medical Center
Nashville, Tennessee

Preface

Introduction

It is indeed rare to find a speech-language pathologist in practice today who does not interact with the medical profession. The person practicing in hospitals, rehabilitation settings, nursing homes, or home health settings obviously will be a part of a medical team, whether formal or informal. The person practicing in the school systems, where the majority of speech-language pathologists and many educational audiologists are employed, also frequently will need to interact in some way with the medical profession, as will persons in private practice. In both of these settings, medically fragile children and adults are treated who have a communication disorder associated with a medical condition. This evolution in patient population has made it critical for the speech-language pathologist and audiologist to be well-versed concerning anatomy and physiology of body systems related to speech, language, and hearing. Arguably the most important system is the nervous system—the foundation of all movement and thought associated with speech and language.

Background

The idea for this text was first conceived by Drs. Love and Webb out of a frustration with the fact that there was, at that time (1986), no textbook written by speech-language pathologists for that profession that was devoted strictly to the neurology of "the human communication nervous system." Over the years, there have been several textbooks published that are devoted to this topic and written by practicing speech-language pathologists. However, most of these texts only emphasize the anatomy and physiology of the nervous system underlying normal communication. *Neurology for the Speech-Language Pathologist* is dedicated not only to the study of the normal system function, but also to the understanding of the disorders that occur when the nervous system is developmentally abnormal or becomes diseased or damaged.

Audience

The targeted audience for this book is, of course, students preparing to become practicing speech-language pathologists. Students intending to enter the profession of audiology frequently will be enrolled in a class on neurology of human communication. Although this text does not go into the depth of the auditory system that students will need later, they will find it useful for their future endeavors. The text is also written to serve as a reference for speech and hearing professionals already in practice who wish to update themselves in neurology or who may not have had a specific curriculum regarding the neurologic foundation of communication and its disorders.

Concept and Importance to the Profession

As Dr. Howard Kirshner states in the foreword to this book, the speech-language pathologist and the neurologist are able to work together more successfully for the patient's benefit when they "speak the same language." This was one of the initial thrusts of the creation of this textbook. Ultimate benefit is also achieved when speech-language pathologists can understand the terminology and the concerns of other professions involved in the habilitation and rehabilitation of patients. Thus the content has evolved over the years to help the speech-language pathologist obtain a better understanding of nervous system function in related systems often treated by other professionals, such as those in physical therapy, occupational therapy, and neuropsychology.

In this new century, there is a demand for evidence-based practice, meaning that there is a demand that the speech-language pathologist design and use diagnostic and treatment methodologies based on sound theory and research-based evidence that supports that theory and practice. Knowledge about nervous system function and how the brain develops, initiates, and maintains movement; learns and remembers; and recovers or changes after injury is critical to successful practice. This book is dedicated to enhancing that knowledge.

Organization

The Fifth Edition is organized in a similar fashion to previous editions. In the introductory chapter, the intertwining histories of the professions of speech-language pathology and neurology are discussed. Chapter 1 also discusses the advances in neuroimaging, which have allowed for the explosion of knowledge concerning brain and behavior relationships as well as facilitated more accurate diagnosis of disease and injury. Chapters 2 and 3 are foundation chapters, providing an overview of the anatomy of the central and peripheral nervous systems, including the development of the nervous system from conception through birth. Chapters 4 through 7 describe anatomy and physiology of neuronal function, the sensory systems of vision, hearing and touch, and the motor system and cranial nerves. Chapters 8 and 9 discuss speech disorders of adults and children, emphasizing the neurologically based motor speech disorders but also discussing neurophysiology related to articulation and fluency. Chapter 10 is new to this textbook and explores the neuroanatomy and neurophysiology underlying language and learning. Chapters 11 and 12 discuss disorders of language and learning in adults and children, respectively.

The first four chapters provide the reader with anatomical terms and location and function of structures in an overview of the entire nervous system without getting too much into the details of the specific systems. The idea is to have a mental concept of the entire nervous system and the structural and functional relationships before studying in depth the systems most relevant to communication and related disorders.

Distinctive Features

- The text combines information concerning both neuroanatomy and neurophysiology with information about speech and language disorders associated with nervous system dysfunction.
- The disorder section of the text includes separate chapters on speech and language and are further divided into pediatric and adult disorders.
- Included in the text is information designed to help the reader understand related disorders – such as disorders of visual processing and hearing and limb movement – that are treated by other members of the habilitation or rehabilitation team.
- The text also includes a description of a neurologist's typical bedside exam and assessment for adults and pediatric patients.

Learning Aids

- There are 232 photos, scans, illustrations, and diagrams – many of them highlighted with the second color for clarity – that depict anatomic structure and function within the nervous system as well as characteristics of neurologic disease or injury.
- Detailed vocabulary listings are provided on the first page of each chapter, highlighted within the chapter discussion, and defined within the back-of-book glossary.
- Chapters 5 through 12 each contain a case history and description of a patient with a condition pertinent to the system or disorder discussed within that chapter. Cases are followed by questions for consideration and discussion.
- Detailed summary and application boxes appear at the end of each chapter and organize the information into bulleted listings for ease of reference; they also double as a handy study tool.

- Appendices provide a listing and brief description of medical conditions related to communication disorders, an outline of a bedside neurologic examination, and a screening neurologic examination – all invaluable references for student clinicians and practitioners.

Ancillary Materials

An Evolve website has been created specifically to accompany *Neurology for the Speech-Language Pathologist,* 5th Edition. Resources are available for free to all students via the URL: http://evolve.elsevier.com/Webb/neurology/. Instructor resources are available to all adopting instructors, who can register for free access via their sales representative. Following is a summary of the resources available online:

For Instructors

- A **test bank** features 350 objective-style questions – multiple-choice, true/false, and fill-in-the-blank – each with an accompanying rationale for the correct answer and a page-number reference to direct the reader to the exact textbook page on which that content is discussed.
- An **image collection** featuring tables and artwork from the textbook – two-color renderings, photographs, and brain-imaging scans – is available for download into PowerPoint or other presentations.
- More than 25 high-quality **animations** are also included, providing three-dimensional views of various neuroanatomy and neurophysiology structures, concepts, and diseases and disorders.

For Students

- **Flashcards** reproduce the book's glossary into a fun and interactive tool that helps readers practice terminology and ensure content mastery. The flashcards are excellent resources for exam preparation.
- **Answers to case study questions** are included to help readers test their knowledge and understand chapter content as it applies to realistic patient situations.
- Chapter reference lists are reproduced in a **bibliography** that contains Medline links, allowing readers to search quickly and easily for relevant literature and connect directly to specific journal articles.

Wanda G. Webb
Richard K. Adler

Contents

FIFTH EDITION

NEUROLOGY
for the SPEECH-LANGUAGE PATHOLOGIST

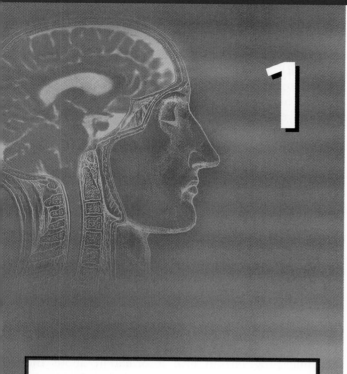

1

Introduction to Speech-Language Neurology

We must admit that the divine banquet of the brain was, and still is, a feast with dishes that remain elusive in their blending, and with sauces whose ingredients are even now a secret.
MacDonald Critchley, *The Divine Banquet of the Brain,* 1979

KEY**TERMS**

CHAPTER**OUTLINE**

Why Neurology?

The 1990s were labeled by the United States Congress as the Decade of the Brain. Likewise, 1990 was the year of the Americans with Disabilities Act (ADA). In 2006, American Speech-Language-Hearing Association (ASHA) members learned about the reauthorization of the IDEA (Individual Disability Education Act). Since the inception of the federal laws to help and protect all Americans who have a variety of disabilities, including communication and hearing disorders, ASHA academic and clinical standards have undergone major changes as well. A tremendous expansion of knowledge has occurred in the neurosciences, including increased complexities of the types and severity of disorders treated by all speech-language pathologists (SLPs), from the school-based SLP and educational audiologist to the hospital-based certified SLP professional. ASHA has recognized these neuroscientific advances by realizing that SLPs and audiologists must have an expanded knowledge of neuroanatomy and physiology to remain a viable member of either the Individual Educational Plan (IEP) or the Interdisciplinary Team (IDT). That is why academic and clinical standards for all SLPs and audiologists underwent a major change in the early twenty-first century.

To the student of speech-language pathology and audiology, these governmental reform acts and advances in neuroscience have played a significant role in forming the current academic and clinical standards used by ASHA. The new certification standards that are required as of July 2004 mandate particular knowledge and skills for students to be prepared to serve a variety of communication and hearing disorders in children and adults. From an undergraduate's general education, which is now required to include biological and physical sciences, to the graduate student wishing for in-depth study of stroke, traumatic brain injury, or tracheoesophageal disorders, academic programs have had to increase neuroscience offerings. Significant research from language and the neurology of speech and language in the 1990s promised a new era of understanding of the age-old problems of speech and language disorders.[36] The work of the linguist, the cognitive psychologist, and the neuroscientist, as well as the SLP and audiologist, has brought to the field of communication sciences and disorders an accelerated knowledge of the specialized brain mechanisms that underlie speech, language, and hearing and their disorders. Specialists now possess the knowledge and skills to understand, implement, analyze, and synthesize the neurologic bases of speech, language, and hearing, as well as the skills required to meet the ADA, IDEA, and new ASHA standards.

Widespread interest in the study of neurogenic issues has increased among speech and language students as opportunities for clinical experiences and employment in schools, hospitals, rehabilitation centers, and other health care agencies continue to increase. Increased longevity of human beings has caused a greater incidence of hearing, speech, and language disorders such as presbycusis, dementia, **aphasia**, dysarthria, and apraxia. With improving medical technology, traumatically brain-injured infants, children, and adults are now saved from death much more frequently than in the past. The speech and language disorders of these survivors present new and greater challenges to the SLP and audiologist.

In 1986, when the first edition of this text appeared, only half of undergraduate and graduate training programs in communication disorders offered specific coursework in neurology with an emphasis on speech and language mechanisms. As of this new edition, 20 years later, the majority of the 296 programs in the field provide such coursework. Adler[2] surveyed all accredited ASHA programs in *Speech-Language Pathology and Audiology*. The survey consisted of questions asking academic programs to give information about the anatomy and physiology (A&P) and neuroanatomy and physiology (N&P) courses required in their undergraduate and master's degree course sequences. Results indicated that the A&P course is offered in every program, and more than 70% of the accredited programs offered N&P courses. Many of these courses in neuroanatomy are on the graduate level, and all respondents made it clear that the N&P course is quite relevant and is required by all students to meet the standards and prepare students for medical SLP positions.

Accompanying a growing interest among neurologists in communication sciences and disorders has been a parallel increase in the number of practicing SLPs. In the past 4 decades, membership in ASHA has risen from 2203 in 1952 to more than 123,000 members and affiliates in 2006 (*www.asha.org*). Although not all of these individuals are interested in neurologic disorders, many are, and for those who wish to study and specialize in neurologic speech and language disorders, a certification body, the Academy of Neurologic Communication Disorders and Sciences, accepts qualified members. Specialization in adult neurologic impairment, child neurologic impairment, or both is possible. In the past 5 to 10 years, ASHA special interest divisions have begun the process of specialization certifications in many areas, including child language and fluency. At the time of this writing, Division 2, Neurological Speech, Language, and Hearing Disorders, was exploring specializations as well.

Most SLPs and audiologists work in schools, hospitals, or medical center or university clinics. All settings currently use an IDT approach and call the team a variety of names, including IDT, IEP team, clinical rounds team, or interdisciplinary management team (IMT). Regardless of name, the main function is to assess the client, discuss results from all disciplines, write a treatment plan that includes goals and objectives, and ensure that all goals and objectives have one outcome—the improvement of speech and language functioning for that client. The client might be a child in school or an adult in a traumatic brain injury, dementia, or Alzheimer's unit; in an aphasia unit cluster; or enrolled in a university clinical speech and hearing program. The SLP is an important contributor to the team efforts by providing test results, as well as insight into a client's speech and language deficits and assets as related to brain functioning; cognitive ability after trauma or assessment; and educational, vocational, subacute, or rehabilitation center placement.

Recent Contributors to the Study of Neurologic Communication Disorders

During the past 4 decades, two towering figures have dominated the field of language and speech. One, a neurologist, was **Norman Geschwind** (1926-1984). He almost single-handedly resurrected the early neurologic literature of Europe focusing on language disorders and related deficits. Geschwind brought this body of knowledge to the attention of the American medical audience when interest in aphasia and related disorders was waning. He particularly highlighted the value of identifying lesions in the connective pathways of the brain, as well as diagnosing lesions in the traditional localized cortical areas of the brain that had been associated with language disorders for more than a century. His masterwork, "Disconnection Syndromes in Animals and Man," was published in *Brain* more than 35 years ago.[21]

Geschwind taught brilliantly at Harvard University Medical School for many years and inspired generations of students to pursue neurology as a specialty and to concentrate on disorders of higher cerebral function. This area is now known as **behavioral neurology**. Aphasic disorders and other related defects, such as agnosia and apraxia, were considered minor aspects of a general neurologic practice until Geschwind highlighted them in neurology and related fields.

Thanks to Geschwind's original and incisive thinking, the study of language and its disorders returned to its rightful place of importance among the vast range of neurologic diseases. His thinking was so innovative that it influenced many other scientific disciplines, particularly linguistics, psychology, and philosophy. Geschwind is one of the few physicians who has been honored by having their scientific papers collected and published before their death.[22]

The second towering figure in the latter half of the twentieth century in the field of neurology of speech and language has been **Noam Chomsky**, a linguist of international renown. Chomsky is credited with creating a scientific revolution in the understanding of syntax and other components of language,[28] and he has been called a major intellectual force, a "modern master" of creative and scientific thought.[46]

Beginning in 1957 with his monograph *Syntactic Structures*,[9] Chomsky developed a theory of grammar, stressing mental processes that replaced the structural analysis of language based on the mechanistic and behavioral viewpoint exemplified by the writings of Bloomfield.[4] Chomsky disputed the traditional idea that language is essentially a system of habits established by training and forcefully argues that every human being has the innate capacity to use language. Innate grammatical processes, he believes, are triggered by external stimuli but function autonomously. The concept of innateness implies a biologic, neurologic, and genetic basis for language.

Chomsky's definition of grammar differs from that of structuralist linguists in that it is concerned with a specific and formal description of language, as well as neurologic language processes as they work in the human brain. The details of these aspects of language, however, are not clearly explained in Chomsky's writings, and it can be difficult, even with knowledge of transformational-generative grammar, to reconcile the details of the newer linguistic theory of Chomsky with the older neurologic theory of Geschwind and his followers. Box 1-1 summarizes the work of both Geschwind and Chomsky in speech-language neurology.

The more recent literature, however, is beginning to synthesize the linguistic and neurologic positions in explaining disordered communication. Steven Pinker, a cognitive psychologist and linguist, wrote that language may be considered an "instinct" in the same sense that Charles Darwin conceived of animal instincts. Pinker asserts that grammar is a perfect example of a biological trait determined by the Darwinian principle of natural selection and that it is genetically based. In addition, Pinker stated that the intricately structured neural circuits that support language and speech are "laid down by a cascade of precisely timed genetic events."[46] A genetic nature of language is supported by cases of inherited disturbance that appear to be accompanied by specific defects of grammar.[25]

Even earlier than Pinker's work, a biological defense of Chomsky's concept of innateness appeared in a

Two Key Leaders in Speech and Language

Norman Geschwind (1926-1984)

- Revitalized early neurologic literature focusing on language disorders and related deficits
- Brought body of knowledge to attention of American medical audience
- Highlighted the value of identification and diagnosis of lesions in areas associated with language disorders
- Published masterwork "Disconnection Syndromes in Animals and Man" (1965) in *Brain*
- Largely founded the field of behavioral neurology
- Influenced other disciplines such as linguistics, psychology, and philosophy

Noam Chomsky (1928-)

- Created scientific revolution in understanding syntax and other components of language
- Published *Syntactic Structures* in 1957, which outlined his theory of grammar
- Argued the revolutionary notion that the capacity for language learning and usage is innate, not learned
- Theorized that grammar includes neurologic language processes that parallel a formal description of language

---

well-known but somewhat controversial book by Eric Lenneberg (1921-1975), *The Biological Foundations of Language*.[37] Lenneberg clearly placed language development in a developmental neurology context. One of the highlights of this book was Lenneberg's attempt to define a critical period for the acquisition of early language. Lenneberg maintained that the acquisition of syntax was paced by the rate of cerebral maturation and the lateralization of language mechanisms. He asserted that the rapid acquisition of language starts at approximately 2 years of age, as the brain begins to grow rapidly, and slows at puberty (at approximately 12 years of age), when cerebral growth reaches a plateau. Although often criticized, the concept of critical periods is consistent with the importance of biologic and neurologic mechanisms for language development, and some have supported Lenneberg's claims.[33]

Although the concepts of Lenneberg, Geschwind, and particularly Chomsky concerning neurologic aspects of language have been widely criticized, they have focused interest on the need to understand brain function in detail when studying speech and language

disorders. The work of these three neurologic theorists is discussed further in later chapters.

Not all biologic and neurologic theories of language have come from linguists or cognitive-behavioral psychologists. Harold Goodglass and Edith Kaplan were neuropsychologists and students of Geschwind who worked together at the Boston Veterans Administration Hospital to develop diagnostic theories of aphasia and assessment protocols for testing aphasic language behaviors,[24] thereby contributing to the SLP's knowledge of language and neuroanatomy and neurology.

SLPs have provided a vast amount of assessment and intervention insights into the field of neurologic communication disorders from the vantage point of the therapy room. Although many SLPs have collaborated with neurologists to make extremely important contributions, the work of Nancy Helm-Estabrooks serves as a focal model for clinicians. Helm-Estabrooks was employed at the Boston Veterans Administration Hospital for much of her career as an SLP. There she was strongly affected by the excitement generated by Norman Geschwind and his students as they developed the field of behavioral neurology. Helm-Estabrooks has worked closely with various neurologists and neuropsychologists and is recognized worldwide for her innovative contributions, particularly in testing and therapy techniques for patients with neurogenic disorders. An example of her work is the *Manual of Aphasia Therapy*,[30] written with the internationally known neurologist Martin L. Albert.

The SLP must understand the results of speech and language assessment in terms of the underlying neurologic mechanisms. Further, the SLP should be able to be conversant with current methods of neurologic diagnosis and treatment as they apply to persons with communication disorders. The neurologist's point of view toward speech and language disorders should be familiar to every clinician. In turn, neurologists must be knowledgeable about the assessment methods and therapy procedures of the communication disorders specialist. The understanding of each other's work is particularly crucial because neurology and the study of speech and language disorders have developed independently for many years and are only now beginning to interact more closely. This increased interaction will certainly result in additional benefits for members of both professions and those they serve.

The clinical neurologist must work closely with the SLP in evaluating the communication disorders of the neurologic client. The SLP is clearly not responsible for making the final diagnosis of a neurologic disorder. Nevertheless, the SLP is responsible for assessing all relevant aspects of speech, language, and related disorders in clients with a known or suspected neurologic disorder.

Historic Roots: Development of Speech-Language Pathology as a Brain Science

Speech-language pathology traces many of its roots to clinical neurology. In 1861, the French physician **Pierre Paul Broca** (1824-1880) studied the brains of two patients who had sustained language loss and motor speech disorders.[5] This study allowed him to localize human language to a definite circumscribed area of the left hemisphere, thereby laying the foundation for a brain science of speech and language. Broca's discovery went far beyond the now-classic description of an interesting brain disorder called aphasia. Possibly foremost among his conclusions were the assertions that the two hemispheres of the brain are asymmetric in function and that the left cerebral hemisphere contains the language center in most human beings. Important implications of brain **asymmetry** are even now coming to light some 130 years later. Asymmetry of function is more pervasive than originally thought. It extends well beyond language to other brain areas and their functions.

Another conclusion that has had lasting importance for neurology since Broca's death is that specific behavioral functions appear to be associated with clearly localized sites in the brain. The corollary of this observation is that behavioral dysfunction can point to lesions at specific sites in the nervous system. The concept of **localization of function** in the nervous system has been repeatedly demonstrated by clinical and research methods since Broca first articulated it more than a century ago. This observation was so profound that it became a significant historic force in the establishment of the medical discipline of **clinical neurology**. Much of clinical neurology depends on the physician's ability to lateralize and localize a lesion in the nervous system.

An important fact for speech-language pathology was that Broca's discovery stimulated a period of intensive search for a workable explanation of the brain mechanisms of speech and language. Probably no period in the history of neurologic science has so advanced the understanding of communication and its disorders as those years between Broca's discovery and World War I. An overview of Broca's life work can be found in Box 1-2.

One of the first and foremost outcomes of this intensive study of speech-language brain mechanisms was the establishment of neurologic substrata for modalities of language deficit other than the expressive oral language described by Broca. In 1867 William Ogle published a case that demonstrated that a cerebral

---

BOX 1-2

The Work of Pierre Paul Broca (1824-1880)

- Touchstone study in 1861 allowed Broca to localize human language to a specific region of the left hemisphere, suggesting that the two hemispheres of the brain are asymmetric in function
- First to identify the brain disorder aphasia
- Articulated localization of function, leading to the establishment of the medical discipline of clinical neurology
- Stimulated intensive research into a workable explanation of the brain mechanisms of speech and language

---

writing center was independent of Broca's center for oral language.[41] In 1874 **Carl Wernicke** (1848-1905) identified an auditory speech center in the temporal lobe associated with comprehension of speech, as opposed to Broca's area in the frontal lobe that was an expressive speech center.[54] Lesions in Broca's area produced a motor aphasia, and one in Wernicke's area produced a sensory aphasia. In 1892 Joseph Dejerine identified mechanisms underlying reading disorders.[16] Disorders of cortical sensory recognition, or the **agnosias**, were named by Sigmund Freud in 1891,[19] and in 1900 Hugo Liepmann comprehensively analyzed the **apraxias**, disorders of executing motor acts resulting from brain lesions.[38]

EARLY LANGUAGE MODELS

Of the many neurologic models of the cerebral language mechanisms generated soon after Broca's great discovery, Wernicke's 1874 model has best withstood the test of time. Wernicke stressed the importance of cortical language centers associated with the various language modalities, but he also emphasized the importance of **association fiber tracts** connecting areas or centers. Like his teacher Theodore Meynert (1833-1892), he understood that the connections in the brain were just as important as the centers for a complete picture of language performance.[40] In addition, Wernicke organized the symptoms of language disturbance in such a way that they could be used diagnostically to predict the lesion site in either connective pathways or centers in the language system. Ironically, the Wernicke model was eclipsed until the last half of the twentieth century, when it was revitalized and expanded by Norman Geschwind and his followers.[22]

Wernicke's model came under criticism by the English neurologist Henry Head in 1926.[29] He lumped Wernicke with a cadre of early neurologists he considered the more flagrant of the "diagram makers," implying that they constructed language models that were highly speculative and not supported by empirical evidence. Current methods of neurologic investigation, including electrical cortical stimulation, isotope localization of lesions, **computed tomography (CT)**, and regional blood flow studies in the brain, have generally vindicated Wernicke's model of language.

Neurologic speech mechanisms, as opposed to language mechanisms, also received attention in the late nineteenth century. In 1871, the famous French neurologist Jean Charcot (1825-1893) described the "scanning speech" that he associated with "disseminated sclerosis," now known as multiple sclerosis.[8] The term scanning, probably inappropriate, has also been widely used to describe speech with cerebellar or cerebellar pathway lesions (see Chapter 8). In 1888 an English neurologist, William Gowers (1846-1915), surveyed the neurologic speech disorders, known as dysarthrias, in a well-known book titled *A Manual of Diseases of the Nervous System.*[26]

WORLD WAR I

World War I had a profound influence on the study of speech and language mechanisms resulting from neurologic insult. With a large population of head-injured young men with penetrating skull wounds, some neurologists felt an urgency for treatment. A handful of dedicated neurologists provided therapy for these traumatic language disorders because the profession of speech pathology was not yet born. Not until the next decade did the profession really begin. Lee Edward Travis has the distinction of being the first individual in the United States to specialize in the field of speech and language disorders at the doctoral level. In 1927 he became the first director of the speech clinic at the University of Iowa. His special interest was in stuttering, which he began to study in a neurologic context. Influenced by the neuropsychiatrist Samuel Terry Orton (1879-1948), Travis researched the hypothesis that stuttering was the result of brain dysfunction,[52] specifically an imbalance or competition between the two cerebral hemispheres to control the normal bilateral functioning of the speech musculature. Orton's hypothesis of dysfunctioning neural control of the speech musculature[42] has generally been discredited, but his hemisphere competition theory of stuttering still surfaces from time to time in different guises to explain certain communication disorders.

Although several of the founders of **speech pathology** in the United States believed that psychologic explanations were more rewarding for understanding speech and language problems, notable exceptions existed. In particular, Harold Westlake of Northwestern University; Robert West of the University of Wisconsin; Jon Eisenson, formerly of California State University; and Joseph Wepman of the University of Chicago were all advocates of neurologic principles in communication disorders.

MODERN TIMES

During World War II, which brought in its wake thousands of injured soldiers and other military personnel with traumatic aphasia, neurologists, psychologists, and SLPs were used in treatment programs for the first time. This effort produced a series of books and articles on aphasia rehabilitation; perhaps the most notable for the neurologically oriented SLP was Wepman's *Recovery from Aphasia* (1951). It served as a textbook of language disorders for the growing number of students in the field and often served as their first introduction to the study of a major neurologic communication disorder.

The study of neurologic speech mechanisms was greatly advanced after World War II by the work of Wilder G. Penfield (1891-1976) and his colleagues in Canada. Penfield, a neurosurgeon, used the technique of electrical cortical stimulation to map cortical areas directly, particularly speech and language centers. In 1950 in *The Cerebral Cortex of Man*[43] (written with Theodore Rasmussen) and in 1959 in *Speech and Brain Mechanisms*[44] (written with Lamar Roberts), he documented his observations on cerebral control of speech and language function and wrote on the concepts of subcortical speech mechanisms and infantile cerebral **plasticity**.

The 1960s and 1970s were marked by several advances of neurologic concepts in communication and its disorders. As already mentioned, newer linguistic theory, particularly that proposed by Noam Chomsky,[10,11] emphasized the universal features and innate mechanisms reflected in language. The biologic aspects of language and speech were highlighted by the linguist and psychologist Eric Lenneberg, who specifically placed language acquisition in the context of developmental neurology.[37] The split-brain studies reported by Roger Sperry and his colleagues,[49] in which the commissural tracts between the hemispheres were severed, indicated specific functions of the right hemisphere were different from the left.

Major anatomic differences in the right and left language centers were also demonstrated in the human brain. Most significant for SLPs and audiologists are larger areas in the left temporal lobe in the fetus, infant, and adult.[23,53,55] These differences suggest an anatomic basis for cerebral dominance for language and appear to contradict a theory of progressive lateralization of speech centers.

Throughout the 1960s and 1970s considerable attention was paid to neurologic speech disorders. Neurologists and SLPs in the Mayo Clinic Neurology Department[13-15] documented the acoustic-perceptual characteristics of the major **dysarthrias** in a viable classification scheme. This work has stimulated widespread study of the various adult dysarthrias in speech science laboratories around the country.

The 1960s and 1970s were also marked by the development of three psychometrically sound and widely used aphasia tests: the *Minnesota Test of Differential Diagnosis of Aphasia*,[48] the *Porch Index of Communicative Ability*,[47] and the *Boston Diagnostic Aphasia Examination*.[24]

The 1980s brought further advances in aphasia. The *Western Aphasia Battery*[34] and the first edition of the *Communication Activities in Daily Living*[31] were published. By the 1990s, further advances in assessment for aphasia, traumatic brain injury and, for the first time, language and communication problems caused by dementia produced the *Scales of Cognitive Abilities for Traumatic Brain Injury*,[1] the *Arizona Battery for Communication Disorders of Dementia*,[3] the third edition of *Examining for Aphasia*,[17] the *Burns Brief Inventory of Communication and Cognition*,[6] the second edition of the *Communication Activities in Daily Living*,[32] the *Comprehensive Aphasia Test*,[50] and the second edition of the *Frenchay Aphasia Screening Test*.[18]

NEURODIAGNOSTIC STUDIES IN SPEECH AND LANGUAGE

Brain Imaging

The cortical areas believed to be critical for language function have been established by what is called the clinicopathologic method in neurology. Developed into a powerful technique by the great French neurologist Jean Charcot, this method establishes a relation between the site of a lesion and the behavioral functions that are lost or modified. The underlying assumption is that the area of lesion is related to the lost or disordered function. This simple logic is important in clinical neurology; it forms the basis of neurologic diagnosis and is the foundation of the historically traditional neurologic examination.

In the mid-1970s, the clinicopathologic technique of diagnosis of the site of neurologic lesions was revolutionized by modern technology that, through relatively noninvasive means, vastly clarified the actual sites of

lesions and made diagnoses more valid and reliable. Objective neurodiagnostic tests, such as CT scans, **positron emission tomography (PET)** scans, **single-photon emission tomography (SPECT)** scans, and **magnetic resonance imaging (MRI)** scans, as well as other clinical neurodiagnostic tests, have established the value of the clinicopathologic method in medicine. The four scanning techniques are the most widely used in clinical neurodiagnosis.

CT and MRI scans permit study of the structure of the human brain with a degree of detail that is occasionally comparable with the detail revealed by postmortem examination. In fact, MRI, which generates fine cross sections of brain structure without penetrating radiation, may even go beyond postmortem examination because it allows views of multiple slices of the brain.

The CT scan yields a three-dimensional representation of the brain (Fig. 1-1), unlike the conventional **radiograph**, which provides a two-dimensional projection of a three-dimensional object. On a radiograph, the body appears on x-ray films as overlapping structures that are sometimes difficult to distinguish. The CT scanner uses an **x-ray** beam that is passed through the brain from one side of the head, and the radiation not absorbed by the intervening tissue is absorbed by a series of detectors revolving around the subject's head. The data from the radiation detectors allow a calculation of the density of tissue in a particular slice of brain. A computer then reconstructs a two-dimensional cross-sectional picture of the brain observed by the camera. Several cross sections may be printed corresponding to different planes through the head. Contrast substances are sometimes injected in the patient to increase the density of damaged tissue. This enhancement technique allows clearer visualization and more accurate diagnosis.

MRI, probably the most widely used diagnostic imaging technique in neurology, generates cross-sectional images by using radio waves and a strong magnetic field to detect the distribution of water molecules in living tissue (Figs. 1-2 and 1-3). The technique allows accurate assessment of brain tissue densities, and an excellent pictorial image can be generated by the computer. An MRI scan of the spinal trigeminal tract (Fig. 1-4) gives the SLP and audiologist insight into representative levels of the pons, medulla, and midbrain. Another example of imaging that helps students and clinicians understand the benefits of imaging for neuroscience is an image of the major tracts interrupted in a spinal cord hemisection, as in Brown-Séquard syndrome (Fig. 1-5).

Generally, MRI is more sensitive to abnormalities than CT. However, it is significantly more expensive to generate the image. Damasio and Damasio[12] pointed out that the analysis of CT and MRI images is sometimes

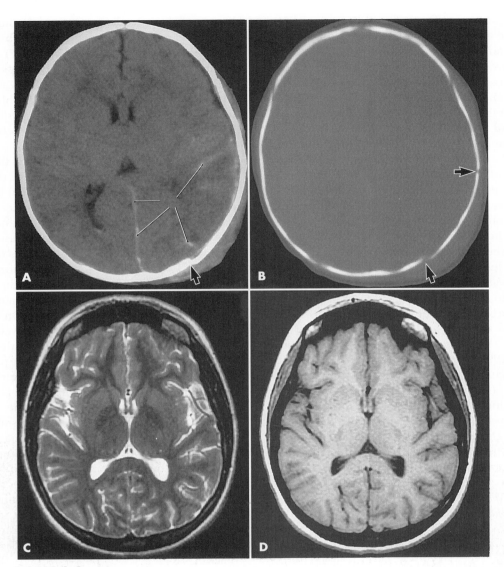

FIGURE **1-1**

CT scans of a 2-month-old infant with shaken baby syndrome (**A** and **B**) and MR images of a normal 20-year-old woman (**C** and **D**). On the CT study, note that the brain detail is less than on the MR images but that the presence of blood (**A**, in the interhemispheric fissure between the hemisphere and the brain substance) is obvious. In the same patient, the bone window (**B**) clearly illustrates the outline of the skull but also clearly shows skull fractures (*arrows* in **A** and **B**). In this infant, the ventricles on the left are largely compressed and the gyri have largely disappeared because of pressure from bleeding into the hemisphere. The pressure results in the effacement of the sulci and gyri on the left side. In the T2-weighted image (**C**), cerebrospinal fluid is white, internal brain structures are seen in excellent detail, and vessels are obvious. In the T1-weighted image (**D**), cerebrospinal fluid is dark and internal structures of the brain are somewhat less obvious. (Reprinted from Haines, D. [2006]. *Fundamental neuroscience* [3rd ed.]. Philadelphia: Churchill Livingstone.)

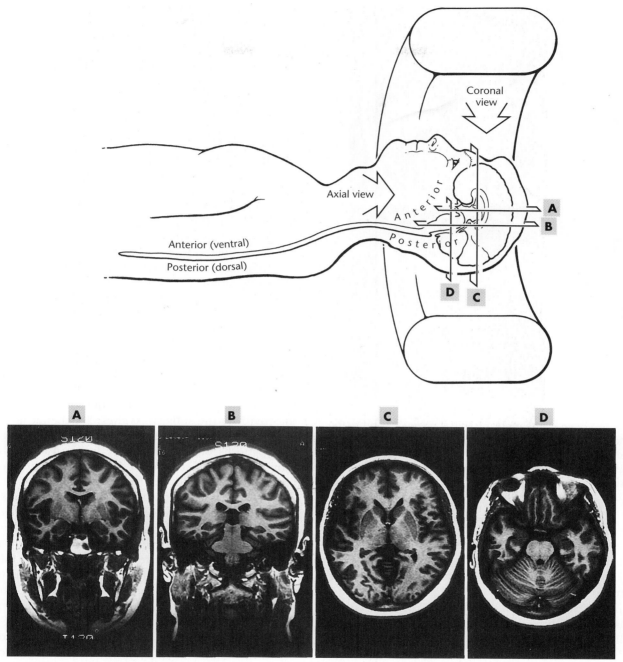

FIGURE 1-2
The relation of imaging planes to the brain. The diagram shows the usual orientation of a patient in an MRI machine and the planes of the four scans (T1-weighted images) that are shown. **A** and **B**, Coronal scans; **C** and **D**, axial scans. (Reprinted from Haines, D. [2006]. *Fundamental neuroscience* [3rd ed.]. Philadelphia: Churchill Livingstone.)

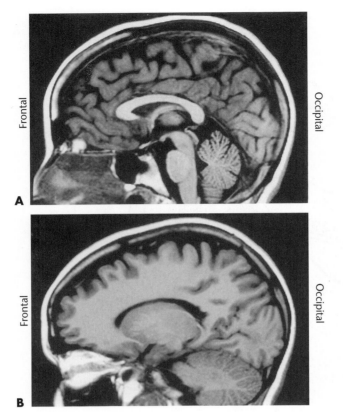

Frontal

Occipital

A

Frontal

Occipital

B

FIGURE **1-3**

MRI of the brain in the median sagittal plane (**A**) and in the sagittal plane but off the midline (**B**). The frontal lobe is to the left, and the occipital lobe is to the right. Other directions within the brain in this plane are noted in Figure 1-7. (Reprinted from Haines, D. [2006]. *Fundamental neuroscience* [3rd ed.]. Philadelphia: Churchill Livingstone.)

difficult in that the number of brain slices provided for viewing may vary from institution to institution and from patient to patient. The number of slices may even vary in the same patient as scanning devices are improved over time.

These factors sometimes lead to difficulty in accurate localization of lesions. Although precise accuracy in localization may not be critical to the clinician who needs only to know the nature of a lesion and its rough extent, it may be vital to the neuroscientist who wants to correlate lesion with dysfunction. To improve such correlations, brain templates have been developed to increase the accuracy of reading and comparing various types of **brain scans**.

CT and MRI are unable to detect certain forms of cellular and subcellular brain pathology directly. Dynamic neuroimaging procedures that use emission tomography (PET and SPECT) are helpful in cases in which imaging of brain structures alone is not decisive. For instance, in some cases of early dementia CT and

MRI scans appear normal, but language and neuropsychologic testing reveals serious cerebral dysfunction.

The PET scan is a visual technique in which the subject is given a radioactively labeled form of glucose, which is metabolized by the brain. The radioactivity is later recorded by a special detector. Unlike CT and MRI scans, a PET scan measures metabolic activity in different brain areas. More active areas metabolize more glucose, and more radioactivity is focused in these areas. Thus regional three-dimensional quantification of glucose and oxygen metabolism or blood flow in the human brain is achieved. This technique is advantageous in that glucose metabolism is a more direct measure of the function of neural tissue than is cerebral blood flow, particularly in patients whose regulatory vascular mechanisms are affected by cerebral injury or disease. PET scan studies have been used to research higher mental functions during different cognitive and language tasks and appear to offer an excellent tool for the study of language in the human brain. This technology is expensive because it requires a cyclotron or atomic accelerator. To date, only major medical centers use this technology.

SPECT uses the mechanism of CT scan reconstruction, but instead of detecting x-rays the instrument detects single photons emitted from an external tracer. Radioactive compounds that emit gamma rays are injected into the subject. As these biochemicals reach the brain, emissions are picked up that are converted into patterns of metabolism or blood flow in three-dimensional cross sections of the brain. The picture resolution of SPECT is less than that of PET, but the equipment is less expensive because a cyclotron is not required. This technology is used at small medical centers.

Other neuroimaging techniques often used in neurologic assessments include the **functional MRI (fMRI)**, **regional cerebral blood flow (rCBF)**, and **magnetoencephalography (MEG)**. They are often used in studies of the somatosensory pathways. These studies are able to demonstrate the functional organization of the somatosensory areas that are activated by various touch stimuli. Imaging studies including **electroencephalography (EEG)**, MEG, and fMRI have also provided insight into the localization of brain regions responsible for processing pain.[20,35] EEG, in fact, shows patterns of increased brain activity after the application of painful stimuli. fMRI is capable of revealing increased thalamic and cortical activation in response to the application of innocuous (touch, cool, warm) and nociceptive (cold and hot) stimuli.

Thus in only a century and a quarter, dramatic gains have been realized in knowledge about brain function as it relates to speech and language. Also in this time, a

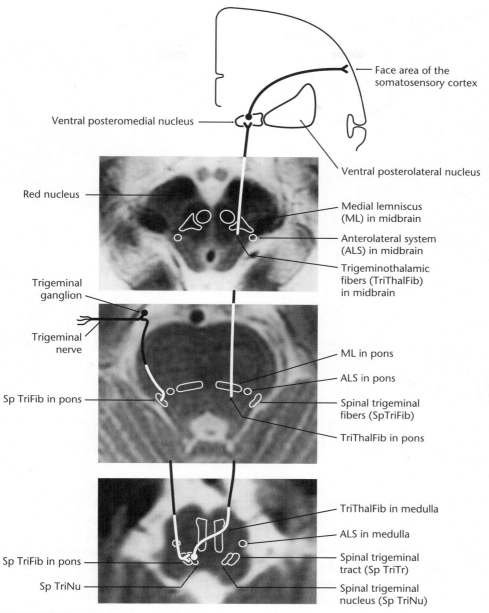

Face area of the somatosensory cortex

Ventral posteromedial nucleus

Red nucleus

Trigeminal ganglion

Trigeminal nerve

Sp TriFib in pons

Sp TriFib in pons

Sp TriNu

Ventral posterolateral nucleus

Medial lemniscus (ML) in midbrain

Anterolateral system (ALS) in midbrain

Trigeminothalamic fibers (TriThalFib) in midbrain

ML in pons

ALS in pons

Spinal trigeminal fibers (SpTriFib)

TriThalFib in pons

TriThalFib in medulla

ALS in medulla

Spinal trigeminal tract (Sp TriTr)

Spinal trigeminal nucleus (Sp TriNu)

FIGURE 1-4

The location of the spinal trigeminal tract and nucleus and anterior trigeminothalamic fibers in MR images at representative levels of the medulla, pons, and midbrain. This illustrates the location of these fibers when viewed in images routinely used in the clinical setting. Remember that the face is represented right side up when the spinal trigeminal tract and nucleus are viewed in the clinical orientation. (Reprinted from Haines, D. [2006]. *Fundamental neuroscience* [3rd ed.]. Philadelphia: Churchill Livingstone.)

new discipline, **speech-language pathology**, was born, experienced tremendous growth, and earned respect as a profession. Today's SLP is obligated to continue to advance the profession by being knowledgeable in neuroanatomy and neurologic disease as they affect human communication (Fig. 1-3).

Box 1-3 lists the various types of brain imaging. As more advances into neuroimaging are developed from research by neurologists, radiologists, imaging technicians, and others, the SLP and audiologist will be able to understand more about a patient's deficits. Treatment planning has become more evidenced based

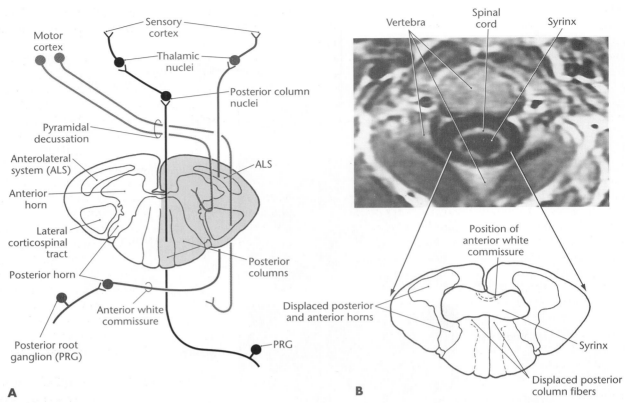

FIGURE 1-5

Major tracts interrupted in a spinal cord hemisection (**A**, Brown-Séquard syndrome) that account for the characteristic sensory and motor losses. MR images of a cervical syringomyelia (**B**) with resultant expansion of the lesion into fibers of the anterior white commissure. In both **A** and **B**, the cross section of the spinal cord is shown in an orientation identical to that seen in the clinical setting. (Reprinted from Haines, D. [2006]. *Fundamental neuroscience* [3rd ed.]. Philadelphia: Churchill Livingstone.)

as well as the chosen technique to compensate for or teach the individual with communication disorders.

Evoked Potentials

Neurodiagnostic advances such as CT, MRI, PET, and SPECT have increased the ability to understand the contribution of neuronal transmission to speech and

language behavior. Another older diagnostic technique, the EEG, has been used for decades to diagnose lesions of the brain and help clarify their nature. EEGs measure the electronic neuronal transmission in the brain with the use of noninvasive scalp electrodes. The EEG has been particularly helpful in diagnosing epilepsy and its subtypes. Epileptic syndromes range from mild abnormal electrical disturbances (petit mal seizures) to more serious abnormalities (grand mal seizures). Single (febrile) convulsions or a series of convulsions or seizures may occur.

The EEG has also been used to study what has been called specific event–related electrical potential. The method uses an averaging computer to separate the electrical activity surrounding the specific event from the ongoing electrical background activity of the brain. If a stimulus is repeated enough times and each repetition produces a circumscribed electrical response, computer averaging can establish the onset of a response and its termination. This is called an event-related potential. It may be a response to internal or external stimulation of the nervous system.

Although this technique has been used widely by some speech and psychological researchers, it is not without problems.[7] Both its validity and reliability can be questioned. Whether an electrical potential that occurs after a stimulus is of cerebral origin or is brought about by a motor act is not always certain. When a language stimulus evokes a cerebral potential, brain activity is not always present, and the absence of an electrical potential to a language stimulus does not mean no electrical activity occurred. Many electrical currents simply do not reach the surface electrodes; some are too small and erratic. In addition, the waveforms derived from stimulation are highly complex, and which section of the waveform that was generated in response to the language stimulus has psychological meaning is sometimes difficult to determine.

Despite these limitations, event-related potential has the capacity to measure events in the brain millisecond by millisecond. A research paradigm frequently used in language studies yields a readiness potential. The subject is asked to repeat a word or phrase or speak freely with pauses of 3 or 4 seconds between portions of an utterance. The continuous EEG recording that precedes the onset of speech is analyzed by averaging waveforms across several utterances to discover the readiness potential.

Another measure that can be derived is called the **contingent negative variation (CNV)**, or expectancy waveform. The subject is shown two separate visual stimuli. The interval between the stimuli is set, and the subject is required to say a particular word or phrase when the second visual stimulus arises. Under these conditions an electrical expectancy waveform occurs after the first stimulus.

Even with its many limitations, measurement of cerebral-evoked potentials offers the hope of finding physiologic correlates of psycholinguistic brain processes that occur so rapidly that they cannot be measured by other existing neurodiagnostic techniques. For instance, several attempts have been made to study the cerebral potential preceding speech, known as the readiness potential.

In 1971, McAdam and Whitaker reported that a late negative potential occurred at Broca's area approximately 150 ms before a subject uttered a polysyllabic word.[39] As a control, the authors reported potentials from nonspeech acts, such as coughing. They found that nonspeaking activities produced negative potentials in a symmetric way over both hemispheres, and they interpreted their findings to indicate that Broca's area on the left was involved in speech planning. Grozinger et al[27] argued that McAdam and Whitaker's methodology was faulty; in addition, Grozinger et al. reported asymmetric potentials over the two hemispheres as early as 2 to 3 seconds before the onset of

speech, not just a few hundred milliseconds.[27] They also reported early potentials related to respiration rather than onset of speech.

Other investigators[51] argued that scalp electrodes were not free of contamination from sources of noncerebral origin and advocated direct cortical recordings from speech and language areas as the best approach to solving these technical problems. CNV studies claiming to find potentials that were larger over the dominant hemisphere were criticized on the grounds that hemispheric differences in CNV were not related to preparation in speech. Szirtes and Vaughan[51] suggested that asymmetrical CNVs in which a word is used as the first stimulus may be invalid.

In summary, the studies of electrical stimulation preceding speech are not conclusive, only suggestive, and certainly require a series of controlled studies to be considered valid. These studies do, however, suggest that very small electrical events occur within milliseconds after an auditory or visual event and that event-related potentials are one experimental method with which to measure language events as rapid as language. However, valid and reliable experimental paradigms need to be worked out.

More recent research with PET and SPECT scanning has answered some of the questions raised by evoked potential research with better reliability.[45] Evoked potentials are used in audiologic testing.

Directions and Planes

Several terms are used to designate direction in neuroanatomy. Some of these terms are used synonymously. **Anterior** means toward the front, and **posterior** indicates toward the back. **Superior** refers to upper; **inferior** means lower. The terms cranial and **cephalic** can be used in place of superior. The word **rostral**, meaning near the mouth or front end, is sometimes substituted for cranial or cephalic.

Medial means toward the medial plane, and **lateral** means further from the median plane. **Ventral** means toward the belly or front; **dorsal** is toward the back. Ventral is sometimes used to indicate structures lying at the base of the brain. Table 1-1 describes terms used for the connective pathways in the nervous system, and Figure 1-6 provides visualization of the planes and directions as seen in neurologic imaging.

Anatomic Orientation

This text uses many drawings and photographs to aid in visualization. When viewing drawings in texts or creating

TABLE 1-1
Connective Pathways in the Nervous System

TERM	DEFINITION
Bundle	A group of fibers; a fasciculus
Column	A pillar of fibers
Fasciculus	A small bundle
Funiculus	A cord of nerve fibers in a nerve trunk
Lemniscus	A ribbon of fibers
Tract	A large group of nerve fibers; a pathway

BOX 1-4
Standard Anatomic Positions and Planes

- The median plane, or section, passes longitudinally through the brain and divides the right hemisphere from the left hemisphere.
- The sagittal plane divides the brain vertically at any point and parallels the medial plane.
- A coronal, or frontal, section is any vertical cut that separates the brain into front and back halves.
- A horizontal plane divides the brain into upper and lower halves and is at right angles to the median and coronal planes.
- A transverse cut is any section that is at right angles to the longitudinal axis of the structure.

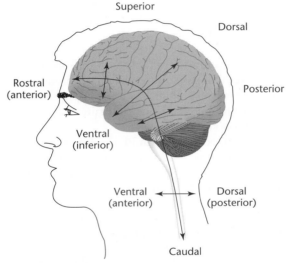

FIGURE 1-6
Axes of the human central nervous system. (Reprinted from Martin, J. G. [1989]. *Neuroanatomy.* New York: Elsevier.)

anatomic sketches, constantly orient yourself in terms of the standard anatomic positions and planes. The human body itself may be defined in terms of an anatomic position, one in which the body is erect and the head, eyes, and toes pointed forward. The limbs are at the side of the body and the palms face forward. From this fundamental position other positions, planes, and directions are defined. These positions, planes, and directions apply to the brain as well as other sections of the body. The planes and sections in Box 1-4 are traditionally defined (Fig. 1-7; see Fig. 1-2).

How to Study

Most students in speech-language pathology receive a limited introduction to the neurosciences in their undergraduate careers. The majority of students are enrolled in courses designed to acquaint them with the anatomy and physiology of speech, but these courses usually focus on speech musculature. Students often do not receive an adequate introduction to neuroanatomy and neurophysiology of speech and language. It is assumed that students will learn these details in courses in aphasia, adult dysarthria, and rehabilitation of speech in cerebral palsy. Students find that neuroscience courses taken as advanced undergraduates or beginning graduate students are difficult.

Students often say that neurology courses are difficult because they believe they must learn the technical term for each hill and valley in the complex anatomy of the brain. In addition, the technical terms are unfamiliar, usually derived from Greek and Roman word roots. This text concentrates on crucial terminology for an understanding of speech and language and the diseases and conditions that result in communication disorders. The number of terms believed to be important has increased over the various editions of this text as the scope of practice for SLPs has expanded. Because of the crucial role that SLPs now play on many medical, rehabilitation, and educational teams, they also must be familiar with terminology used by other health professionals when discussing the client's condition. A glossary is provided at the end of the text.

Part of the strategy in mastering any text in the biological sciences is to give the study of drawings, diagrams, and tables in the text as much time as the narrative sections. If the reader can come away from a study of this text with a set of working mental images of the structures and pathways of the nervous system that are important to communication and can recall them at critical times, then one of the purposes of the authors will be realized. With an emphasis on imagery

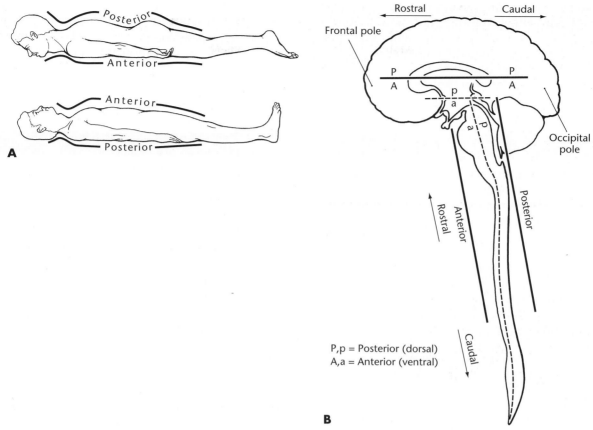

FIGURE **1-7**
A, The anatomic directions of the body are absolute with respect to the axes of the body, not with respect to the position of the body in space. **B**, The central axis and anatomic directions of the central nervous system. The *dashed line* shows the long (rostrocaudal) axis of the central nervous system. The long axis of the spinal cord and brainstem forms a sharp angle with the long axis of the forebrain. Posterior (dorsal) and anterior (ventral) orientations are also shown. (Reprinted from Haines, D. [2006]. *Fundamental neuroscience* [3rd ed.]. Philadelphia: Churchill Livingstone.)

as one of the better ways to learn neurology, it should be no surprise that the authors urge readers to use as a teaching aid their own drawings of structures and pathways. Even crude sketches, carefully labeled, teach the necessary anatomic relations and fix pathways, structures, and names in the mind.

Chapters 2 and 3 provide an overview of the nervous system in total. Subsequent chapters often refer back to certain sections of these chapters to review the written information and the illustrations that provide a beginning foundation of knowledge regarding the neurologic characteristics of the communicative nervous system. Chapters 4, 5, and 6 expand teaching on the structure and physiology of neurons, the sensory systems of touch, vision and hearing, and the motor system.

Chapters 7, 8, and 9 discuss cranial nerves and the disorders of speech production that SLPs commonly assess and treat in children and adults. Chapters 10, 11, and 12 deal with the anatomy and physiology of the parts of the nervous system primarily concerned with language and learning. Disorders of language and learning that affect children and adults are discussed after the section on the neuroanatomy of these areas. A synopsis of facts and clinical applications important to the SLP are presented at the end of each chapter. Chapters 4 through 11 also provide case studies, that is, a description of a patient and the signs and symptoms of his or her disorder. Questions are provided to consider regarding the patient's symptoms. Answers can be found on the Evolve website.

The reader is encouraged to attempt to integrate verbal material with eidetic imagery, as well as with thoughtful consideration of what patients with these conditions experience. Students must call on all their brainpower, bringing into play the special capacities of both the right and left hemispheres of the brain.

The left hemisphere is specialized for its capacities of verbal analysis and reasoning, whereas the right hemisphere is specialized for its imagery functions. Both hemispheres use subcortical areas to retrieve memories and empathize with others. So readers will use their whole brain to learn about the whole brain.

Synopsis of Clinical Information and Applications for the Speech-Language Pathologist

- The source of all speech and language behavior is the brain
- 1990: Americans with Disability Act
- 2004: New ASHA clinical and academic standards
- 2005: IDEA was reauthorized
- 2008: Revised ASHA clinical and academic standards
- ASHA membership, 1952 = 2203
- ASHA membership, 2006 = more than 123,000
- All employment settings use an interdisciplinary approach, including an IEP team in schools
- Norman Geschwind: First neurologist to outline the literature focusing on language disorders and related deficits
- Geschwind influenced linguistics, psychology, and philosophy
- Noam Chomsky: First international linguist to correlate language and speech with brain functioning
- Chomsky: Language is innate and implies a biologic, neurologic, and genetic basis for language
- Pinker: Synthesized the linguistic and neurologic bases of language
- Lenneberg: Wrote *The Biological Foundations of Language*
- Goodglass and Kaplan: Neuropsychologists and students of Geschwind
- Broca: First to localize human language to the left hemisphere
- Behavioral functions are attributed to specific sites in the brain
- Ogle: Identified a writing center in the brain independent of Broca's area
- Carl Wernicke: Identified an auditory center for speech associated with comprehension of speech, opposing Broca, who identified the expressive center
- The temporal lobe has become identified with language and speech comprehension and the frontal lobe with language and speech expression
- Broca's area lesions produce a motor aphasia
- Wernicke's area lesions produce a sensory aphasia
- Freud: First to identify cortical sensory areas or agnosias
- Liepmann: First to identify the apraxias of motor execution
- Travis: First identified stuttering to be the result of brain dysfunction, specifically the imbalance between the two hemispheres
- Neurologic aspects of communication disorders by Harold Westlake, Joseph Wepman, Robert West, and Jon Eisenson
- Wepman's *Recovery from Aphasia* served as first textbook of language disorders in the field of speech pathology
- Penfield: First to use cortical mapping for identifying areas of language and speech functions in the brain
- In the 1960s and 1970s, the first recognized tests for aphasia: Schuell, *Minnesota Test of the Differential Diagnosis of Aphasia*; Porch, *Porch Index of Communicative Ability*; Goodglass and Kaplan, *Boston Diagnostic Aphasia Examination*
- 1990s: Testing for neurogenic speech and language disorders advances especially for communication disorders associated with traumatic brain injury, and dementia
- Brain imaging: Clinicopathologic method of neurology
- CT, PET, MRI, and SPECT scans: Neurodiagnostic imaging
- Other techniques: fMRI, rCBF, MEG, EEG
- Specific terms describe the connective pathways in the nervous system
- Directions and planes identify sites of lesions and injuries
- Epileptic syndromes and seizure activities are measured by EEG

REFERENCES

1. Adamovich, B., & Henderson, J. (1992). *Scales of cognitive abilities for traumatic brain injury.* Austin, TX: Pro Ed.

2. Adler, R. K. (2004). *The anatomy and physiology of speech and the neuroanatomy and physiology of speech courses: State of the art.* Chicago: ASHA Convention.

3. Bayles, K., & Tomoeda, C. (1993). *Arizona battery for communication disorders of dementia.* Austin, TX: Pro-Ed.

4. Bloomfield, L. (1933). *Language.* New York: Holt, Rinehart and Winston.

5. Broca, P. (1861). *Remarques sur le siége de la faculté du langage articulé, suivies d'une observation d'aphémie (perte de la parole).* Bulletin, Société

6. Burns, M. (1997). *Burns brief inventory of communication and cognition.* San Antonio, TX: Psych Corp.

7. Caplan, D. (1987). Cerebral evoked potentials and language. In Caplan, D. (Ed.). *Neurolinguistics and linguistic aphasiology: An introduction.* New York: Cambridge University Press.

8. Charcot, J. M. (1890). *Oeuvres compléte de J. M. Charcot.* Paris: Lecrosnier et Babe.

9. Chomsky, N. (1957). *Syntactic structures.* The Hague: Mouton.

10. Chomsky, N. (1972). *Language and mind.* New York: Harcourt and Brace.

11. Chomsky, N. (1975). *Reflections on language.* New York: Pantheon Books.

12. Damasio, H., & Damasio, A. R. (1989). *Lesion analysis in neuropsychology.* New York: Oxford University Press.

13. Darley, F. L., Aronson, A. E., & Brown, J. R. (1969a). Differential diagnostic patterns of dysarthria. *Journal of Speech and Hearing Research, 12,* 246-249.

14. Darley, F. L., Aronson, A. E., & Brown, J. R. (1969b). Clusters of deviant speech dimensions in the dysarthrias. *Journal of Speech and Hearing Research, 12,* 462-469.

15. Darley, F. L., Aronson, A. E., & Brown, J. R. (1975). *Motor speech disorders.* Philadelphia: W. B. Saunders.

16. Dejerine, J. (1892). Contribution a etude anatomopathologique et clinique des differentes varietes de cectie verbal. *Mémoires de la Société de Biologie, 27,* 1-330.

17. Eisenson, J. (1994). *Examining for aphasia* (3rd ed.). Austin, TX: Pro Ed.

18. Enderby, P., Wood, V., & Wade, D. (2006). *Frenchay aphasia screening test.* Hoboken, NJ: Wiley Publishers.

19. Freud, S. (1953). *On aphasia: A critical study.* Translated by F. Stengel. New York: International Universities Press.

20. Gaillard, W. D., Balsamo, L., Xu, B., McKinney, C. Papero, P. H., Weinstein, S., Conry, J., Pearl, P. L., Sachs, B., Sato, S., Vezina, L. G., Frattali, C., & Theodore, W. H. (2004). fMRI language tasks panel improves determination of language dominance. *Neurology, 63,* 1403-1408.

21. Geschwind, N. (1965). Disconnection syndromes in animals and man. *Brain, 88,* 237-294, 585-644.

22. Geschwind, N. (1974). *Selected papers on language and the brain.* Boston: D. Reidel.

23. Geschwind, N., & Levitsky, W. (1968). Human brain: Right-left asymmetries in temporal speech region. *Science, 168,* 186-187.

24. Goodglass, H., & Kaplan, E. (1972). *Assessment of aphasia and related disorders.* Philadelphia: Lea & Febiger.

25. Gopnik, M., & Crago, M. (1991). Family aggregation of developmental language disorder. *Cognition, 39,* 1-50.

26. Gowers, W. R. (1888). *A manual of diseases of the nervous system.* Philadelphia: Blakiston.

27. Grozinger, B., Kornhuber, H., Kriebel, J. (1977). Human cerebral potentials preceding speech production, phonation and movements of the mouth and tongue, with reference to respiratory, and extracerebral potentials. In Desmidt, J. E. (Ed.), *Language and hemispheric specialization.* Basel: Krager.

28. Harris, R. A. (1993). *The linguistics wars.* New York: Oxford University Press.

29. Head, H. (1926). *Aphasia and kindred disorders* (2 Vols.). London: Cambridge University Press.

30. Helm-Estabrooks, N., & Albert, M. L. (1991). *Manual of aphasia therapy.* Austin, TX: Pro-Ed.

31. Holland, A. (1980). *Communication activities in daily living.* Austin, TX: Pro-Ed.

32. Holland A., Frattali, C., & Fromm, D. (1999). *Communication activities in daily living* (2nd ed.). Austin, TX: Pro Ed.

33. Hurford, J. R. (1991). The evolution of the critical period of language acquisition. *Cognition, 40,* 159-201.

34. Kertesz, A. (1982). *Western aphasia battery.* Austin, TX: Pro Ed.

35. Kirshner, H. S. (Ed.). (1995). *Handbook of neurological speech and language disorders.* New York: Marcel Dekker.

36. Koeda, M., Takahashi, H., Yahata, N., Asai, K., Okubo, Y., & Tanaka, H. (2006). A functional MRI study: Cerebral laterality for lexical-semantic processing and human voice perception. *American Journal of Neuroradiology, 27,* 1472-1479.

37. Lenneberg, E. (1967). *Biological foundations of language.* New York: Wiley.

38. Liepmann, H. (1900). Das Krankheitbild der apraxie ("motorischen asymbolie"). *Monatsschrift fur Pyschiatrie und Neurologie, 8,* 15-40.

39. McAdam, D. W., & Whitaker, H. A. (1971). Electrocortical localization of language production: Reply to Morrell and Huntington. *Science, 174,* 1360-1361.

40. Meynert, T. (1885). *Psychiatry.* Translated by B. Sachs. New York: Putnam.

41. Ogle, W. (1867). Aphasia and agraphia. *St. George's Hospital Reports, 2,* 83-122.

42. Orton, S. T. (1937). *Reading, writing and speech problems in children.* New York: W. W. Norton.

43. Penfield, W., & Rasmussen, T. (1950). *The cerebral cortex of man.* New York: Macmillan.

44. Penfield, W., & Roberts, L. (1959). *Speech and brain mechanisms.* Princeton, NJ: Princeton University Press.

45. Peterson, S.E., Fox, P.T., Snyder, A.Z. and Raichle, M.E. (1990). Activation of extrastriate and frontal cortical areas by visual words and word-like stimuli. *Science, 149,* 1041-1044.

46. Pinker, S. (1994). *The language instinct.* New York: William Morrow.

47. Porch, B. (1967, 1971). *The Porch index of communicative ability.* Palo Alto, CA: Consulting Psychologists Press.

48. Schuell, H. (1965). *The Minnesota test for differential diagnosis of aphasia.* Minneapolis: University of Minnesota Press.

49. Sperry, R. W., Gazzaniga, M. S., & Bogen, J. E. (1969). Interhemispheric relationships: The neocortical commissures; syndromes of hemispheric disconnection. In Vinken, P. J., & Bruyn, G. W. (Eds.), *Handbook of clinical neurology* (Vol. 4). Amsterdam: North Holland.

50. Swinburn, K., Porter, G., & Howard, D. (2004). *Comprehensive aphasia test.* New York: Psychology Press.

51. Szirtes, J., & Vaughan, H. G. (1977). Characteristics of cranial and facial potential associated with speech production. In Desmidt, J. E. (Ed.). *Language and hemispheric specialization.* Basel: Karger.

52. Travis, L. E. (1931). *Speech pathology.* New York: Appleton-Century-Crofts.

53. Wada, J. A., Clark, R., & Hamm, A. (1975). Cerebral asymmetry in humans. *Archives of Neurology, 2,* 239-246.

54. Wernicke, C. (1874). Der aphasische Symptomenkomplex. Breslau: Cohn and Weigert. Translated in Eggert, G. H. (1977). *Wernicke's works on aphasia. A sourcebook and review.* The Hague: Mouton.

55. Witelson, S. F., & Pallie, W. (1973). Left hemisphere specialization for language in the newborn: Neuroanatomical evidence of asymmetry. *Brain, 96,* 641-647.

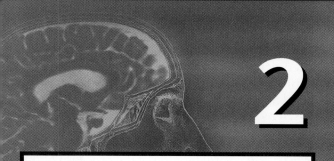

2

Organization of the Nervous System I

The brain is the organ of destiny. It holds within its humming mechanism secrets that will determine the future of the human race.

Wilder Graves Penfield, *The Second Career*, 1963

KEY**TERMS**

allocortex	neocortex (isocortex)
anesthesia	neuroglial cells
angular gyrus	neurons
anomia	occipital lobe
arcuate fasciculus	oligodendrocytes
astrocytes	parahippocampal gyrus
axon	paralimbic areas
basal ganglia	paresthesia
boutons	parietal lobe
brainstem	perisylvian zone
Broca's area	pons
caudal	premotor area
central nervous system	primary auditory
cerebellum	receptor cortex
cerebrum	primary motor
cingulate gyrus	projection cortex
colliculi	primary olfactory
corpus callosum	receptor cortex
corpus striatum	primary somatosensory
diencephalon	cortex
encephalon	primary visual receptor
ependymal cells	cortex
epithalamus	putamen
fissure	reflex arc
frontal lobe	reflexes
ganglia	secondary association
gray matter	areas
gyrus	soma (perikaryon)
homunculus	somatic
hyperkinesia	somesthetic
hypokinesia	substantia nigra
hypothalamus	subthalamus
innervate	sulcus
Island of Reil	supplementary
limbic system	(secondary) motor area
(limbic lobe)	synapse
magnum foramen	tectum
medulla oblongata	temporal lobe
microglia	thalamus
midbrain	uncus
(mesencephalon)	Wernicke's area
motor association areas	white matter (fimbria)

CHAPTER**OUTLINE**

Human Communication Nervous System
  Foundations of the Nervous System
    Nerve cell
    Structure and function of neurons
    Neuroglia
    Gray matter
  Organization
Central Nervous System
  Cortical Divisions
    Cortical localization maps
    Cerebral lobes
      Frontal lobe
      Parietal lobe
      Temporal lobe
      Occipital lobe
    Perisylvian zone
  Cerebral connections
    Corpus callosum
    Split-brain research
  Specific Cortical Areas
    Primary motor projection cortex
    Primary somatosensory cortex
    Primary auditory receptor cortex
    Primary visual receptor cortex
    Primary olfactory receptor cortex
    Association cortex
      Specific association areas
        Cortical motor speech association areas
        Sensory association areas
        Categories of association cortex
  The Limbic System
    Structures below the Cortex
      Diencephalon

Human Communication Nervous System

The nervous system is the source of all communication in human beings. Only human beings can express novel utterances to each other through oral or gestural language. Our highly advanced system of oral and gestural language identifies us as unique in the animal kingdom. This facility is the result of an aggregate of intricate nervous system mechanisms that have developed in the human brain through a series of dramatic evolutionary changes. Over a period of thousands of years, a novel representation and organization of neural structures and processes has been created in the human brain that results in what may be called the human communication nervous system. How does this nervous system differ from the communication nervous system of other animals? A clear answer to this question is beginning to emerge from attempts to teach the great apes, particularly chimpanzees, different types of communication systems. Attempts to teach oral speech to chimpanzees have been notably unsuccessful. Only human beings have the specialized vocal tract enabling the potential for producing the complex acoustic signal known as speech or oral language. On the other hand, attempts to teach chimpanzees by using visual and gestural representations of human language have been somewhat successful. Chimpanzees have been taught to use colored plastic chips to represent morphemes and in other cases have learned to use some signs taken from American Sign Language to the extent that they can communicate adequately, and even creatively, in a rudimentary manner. Whether these nonverbal languages are characteristically human is open to question, but human beings and chimpanzees do share some characteristics of communication. The chimpanzee most likely uses cortical structures of the brain to master visual and gestural components of human language.

Some have suggested that overall brain size, which reflects the total volume of the cerebral cortex, the total number of nerve cells in the brain, and the degree of dendrite growth or proliferation of the processes of the nerve cell, is crucial to information processing and communication processing. Considering these factors, what are the differences between the human brain and that of the chimpanzee?

The chimpanzee's impressive but limited gestural language is reflected by its average brain weight of 450 g compared with an average weight of 1350 g for the human brain. Generally, a lack of uniqueness has been found in the parietal, occipital, and temporal lobes of both chimpanzees and human beings. In the frontal lobe of the brain, however, human beings are distinguished by Broca's area, which has been associated with the control of expressive language. With the exception of Broca's area, the primary difference between the human and chimpanzee cortex is quantitative, with the temporal lobe, inferior parietal lobe, and frontal lobe anterior to Broca's area being larger in human beings. These areas, as detailed in later chapters, are portions of the cerebral cortex that make an advanced language system possible. These particular species-specific brain structures, plus the human being's special vocal tract and the significant increase in the size of the information- and communication-processing cortex, account for the exceptional capability for communication.[10]

FOUNDATIONS OF THE NERVOUS SYSTEM

Anatomically, the human nervous system has two major divisions: the **central nervous system** (CNS) and the peripheral nervous system (PNS). The CNS, also called the neuraxis, consists of the brain and spinal cord. The PNS consists of two types of nerves, the cranial and the spinal nerves, and their **ganglia**. The nerves of the PNS connect the brain and spinal cord with peripheral structures such as muscles, glands, and organs. Both divisions of the nervous system contain **somatic** parts that control bodily movements and **innervate** sensory organs as well as autonomic parts that innervate visceral organs. Chapters 2 and 3 discuss in depth the anatomy and physiology of the two divisions of the nervous system.

Before that, however, a study of the microstructure and foundation of the nervous system will be helpful for understanding the complex function of the larger structures.

Nerve Cell

As taught in elementary science classes, all living things are composed of cells, the building blocks of life. The nervous system is no exception. It is a collection of two different types of cells: nerve cells, also called **neurons**, and **neuroglial cells**. The human nervous system contains approximately 100 billion nerve cells. Neuroglial cells are found in an even higher number.

Cells of the nervous system are no different in their basic cell structure than any other cell. Both neurons and neuroglial cells consist of a cell body, also known as a **soma** or **perikaryon**. They also can be seen microscopically to have processes extending from them, with the neuron's many dendrites and one axon being critical to communication between different parts of the nervous system. Also, as with other cells in the body, cells of the nervous system maintain their defined structure with a cytoskeleton. A cytoskeleton is composed of microtubules, intermediate filaments (neurofilaments), and microfilaments. The cytoskeleton of the cell's appendages, the dendrites and axon, provide scaffolding for transport of molecules along these structures (Fig. 2-1). Cytoskeleton dysfunction has been linked to disorders affecting the human nervous system, such as neurofibromatosis and type 2 and Duchenne muscular dystrophy.

Although cells are the building blocks on which the human body is structured, they also are composed of smaller units. These units are organelles, which are composed of molecules. As in all living matter, nerve cells have four major classes of molecules: lipids, proteins, carbohydrates, and nucleic acid (DNA and RNA).

All cells contain an organelle called the nucleus. The nucleus is bound by a bilipid membrane that has several openings or pores in it. The nucleus contains the DNA of the cell. DNA carries the genetic code of each living organism. In human beings, the human genome (the entire genetic set) is found in the 46 chromosomes duplicated in each cell of the body. Each chromosome is composed of proteins and one long, continuous strand of DNA. The genetic information contained in the DNA is encoded into proteins, which carry out the various cellular reactions that constitute life. The nucleus of the cell contains at least one prominent nucleolus where RNA is synthesized. RNA serves both storage and transcoder functions as an intermediary between the DNA and the targeted proteins.

Surrounding the nucleus is a mass of cytoplasm containing organelles that serve to synthesize proteins and maintain cellular metabolic balance. Found in this cytoplasm are rough and smooth endoplasmic reticulum, free ribosomes, Golgi apparatus, lysosomes, and mitochondria. The endoplasmic reticulum and the ribosomes are in abundance in neuronal cell bodies because of their key participation in protein synthesis, which is constantly needed for optimal nervous system function. The Golgi apparatus organelles help with delivery of the proteins and other substances and "bud" vesicles for secretion of these substances. Mitochondria are membrane-bound organelles that provide the energy cells need to function. This power center of the cell produces adenosine triphosphate, the cell's main energy source. Cells in the nervous system have the highest metabolic rate of any cells in the human body and therefore must continually renew their energy source.

Because lipids do not dissolve in water, the bilipid membrane surrounding the nerve cell body forms a barrier between what is inside the cell (the intracellular material) and what surrounds it on the outside (the extracellular material). This membrane is also studded with globular proteins that serve as channels that allow molecules of certain chemicals (neurotransmitters) to pass through when the membrane is appropriately stimulated. These channels are usually specific to one type of molecule, barring others from entering the cell.

Structure and Function of Neurons

Figure 2-1 shows a multipolar neuron or nerve cell. Neurons are specialized to receive, conduct, and transmit nerve impulses. This transmission may be to a muscle, gland, or another nerve cell. Although nerve cells vary widely in terms of size and shape, they all have certain characteristics in common. They all have two types of processes extending from the cell body. The processes specialized to receive the impulses moving toward the cell are dendrites. They have a broad base, taper away from the cell body, and branch somewhere in the vicinity of the cell body. Most neurons are multipolar and have several dendrites extending from the cell body. Effectively, these dendrites expand the area of the neuron available for contact by other neurons. The presence of many dendritic spines expands the area of contact even farther. These dendritic spines appear as small hairlike or bulbous structures on the dendrite's membrane.

The other type of process extending from a neuron conducts the impulse away from the cell and is called the **axon**. Each neuron has only one axon. Collateral branches, however, can be found coming off most axons.

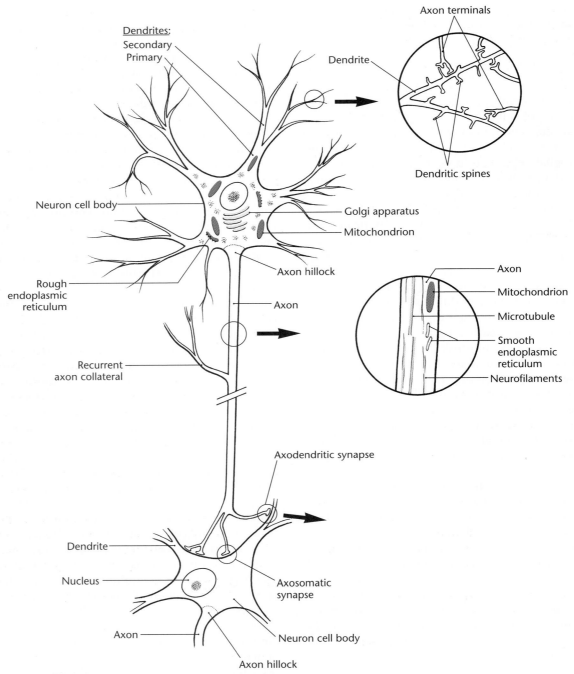

FIGURE **2-1**
A simple nerve cell (neuron). (Reprinted from Haines, D. [2006]. *Fundamental neuroscience* [3rd ed.]. Philadelphia: Churchill Livingstone.)

The cytoplasm of an axon contains structural elements called microtubules and neurofilaments that help maintain its cytoskeleton. These elements also help transport organelles and metabolic substances along the axon. Axons come in different diameters and lengths.

The thicker axons conduct impulses more rapidly than thinner ones because they are usually myelinated (i.e., covered by a white, glistening lipoprotein sheath called the myelin sheath). This fatty sheath of myelin insulates the axon and allows more rapid propagation of the

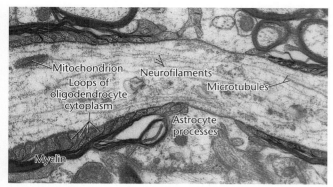

FIGURE **2-2**
Longitudinal view of a myelinated axon in the CNS. (Reprinted from Haines, D. [2006]. *Fundamental neuroscience* [3rd ed.]. Philadelphia: Churchill Livingstone.)

impulse along the axon. Most axons (and some dendrites) are well myelinated, although some thinner axons are either unmyelinated or thinly myelinated. Figure 2-2 shows a longitudinal cut of a myelinated axon.

The axon loses any myelin sheath at its destination and divides into several small terminal branches. At the end of these branches usually are swellings referred to as axon terminals or **boutons**. The bouton establishes contact with another neuron or the cells of a muscle or gland. The site of this contact is a **synapse** or a synaptic junction. The synapse is the primary means by which the neuron elicits responses in target cells, typically by a release of a chemical known as a neurotransmitter. Chapter 4 provides a more in-depth discussion of the synapse.

Aside from the movement of neural impulses down an axon, proteins and other organelles move along the axon in a process called axoplasmic transport. This helps maintain the structural and functional integrity of the axon. This transport may be anterograde from the cell body distally and retrograde back toward the cell body from the axon terminal. The retrograde transport mediates the movement of substances providing trophic support, or nourishment, for the neuron. An example of trophic support are substances known as nerve growth factors.

Neuroglia

Composing the majority of cells in the nervous system are the glial, or neuroglial, cells. The CNS contains four types of neuroglial cells: astrocytes, oligodendrocytes (called Schwann cells in the PNS), microglia, and ependyma.

Glial cells do not propagate neural impulses but provide extremely important supportive functions to the nervous system. **Astrocytes** provide the structural matrix surrounding and supporting neuron cell bodies in the CNS. In many tissues of the body, solutes can pass rather freely from the blood into the cells of that tissue by diffusing through gaps between the endothelial cells. In the CNS, the astrocytes cause the walls of the capillaries to form tight endothelial junctions so that most solutes passing into neural tissue must go through the endothelial cells themselves. Water, gases, and small lipid-soluble molecules may pass easily across the endothelial cells, but most other substances must be carried across by transport systems. Thus the passage of substances into neural tissue from the blood is not always easily accomplished. Astrocytes of the CNS also play a major role in maintaining the appropriate environment for neuronal function. Because astrocytes produce neural growth factor substances, they may play a vital role in neural plasticity and the brain's adaptation after injury.

Oligodendrocytes form and maintain myelin, the fatty sheath covering on axons. In the PNS, Schwann cells perform this function for nerves and nerve roots. **Microglia** are numerous and perform "scavenger" functions. They may migrate to the site of injury in the brain, multiply, and become brain macrophages, cleaning out debris after neural cell death. They are sometimes referred to as the brain's immune system because the microglia mediate immune response to injury or infection. **Ependymal cells** line the cavities (ventricles) in the brain as well as the central canal of the spinal cord. Specialized ependymal cells form structures called choroid plexus, which are found in each ventricle and manufacture cerebrospinal fluid. Glial cells called satellite cells are found in both the CNS and the PNS. These cells surround the neuron cell bodies; their specific function is not known.

Beyond the functions stated previously for glial cells, they are also important in the early development of the CNS. Study of the embryology of the nervous system indicates that glia serve to guide developing neurons in their migration to the correct location. Box 2-1 outlines the basic structure of neuroglial cells in the human nervous system.

Gray Matter

Some areas of the brain and spinal cord appear gray and others appear white. The white areas, called white matter, contain many myelinated axons, with the pearly white myelin covering responsible for the color of the area. **Gray matter** contains aggregations of nerve cell bodies embedded in delicate nerve processes. The cortex is the superficial covering of gray matter found over the cerebral hemispheres and in the cerebellum. The gray matter seen in the interior of the brain consists of large groups of nerve cell bodies; these are called subcortical nuclei. The thalamus and the structures making up the basal ganglia are composed of subcortical nuclei.

BOX 2-1

Summary of Glial (Neuroglial) Cells

- Provide supportive functions in the nervous system
- Do not propagate neural impulses
- Serve in early development of CNS, guiding developing neurons to their correct locations

Astrocytes

- Provide structural matrix for cell bodies in the CNS
- Cause capillary walls to form tight endothelial junctions to ensure that most solutes must pass through endothelial cells
- Help maintain appropriate environment for neuronal function
- Allow for neural plasticity and help brain adapt to injury

Oligodendrocytes

- Form and maintain myelin

Microglia

- Perform scavenger functions such as cleaning out debris after neural cell damage and forming brain macrophages
- Mediate immune response after injury or infection to the brain

Ependyma

- Line ventricles in the brain and spinal cord
- Specialized types form choroid plexus, which manufactures cerebrospinal fluid

Satellite Cells

- Found in CNS and PNS
- Surround neuron bodies but function unknown

The cortex is horizontally organized into six cell layers. The organization of these layers is known as the cytoarchitecture of the brain. Each layer contains a different type of cell, with the pyramidal cells, the largest cells in the brain, found in layer 5. The cortex is organized vertically as well as horizontally. Vertical columns of interconnected neurons each hold a functional unit of cells that share a related purpose and a related location of the stimulus that drives their function. For example, the visual cortex has visual orientation columns. Cell bodies also aggregate as columns in the spinal cord and form the H-shaped mid-portion of the cord.

ORGANIZATION

To comprehend the human communicative nervous system thoroughly, a basic understanding of the organization of the system as a whole is required. The nervous system should be thought of as separate from the other tissues and structures of the body. Imagine the major parts of the nervous system as if they were displayed on a dissection table spread out for study. On the table would be an oval-shaped brain with a tail-like appendage, called the spinal cord, hanging from its base. The cranial nerves are attached to the base of the brain. Another set of nerves, the spinal nerves, project from both sides of the spinal cord (Fig. 2-3). Of all these parts—the brain, cord, and nerves—the brain is by far the most important for communication. Within the brain, evolutionary neural mechanisms of the communication nervous system are developed.

The nerves that exit the brain merely transmit sensory or motor information to and from the brain to control the speech, language, and hearing mechanisms. The nerves attached to the spinal cord innervate, or send nerve impulses to, muscles of the neck, trunk, and limbs and bring sensation from these parts to the brain.

From this oversimplified first mental image of the structure and function of the communication nervous system, a more precise and complex picture will be developed of the aspects of anatomy, physiology, and

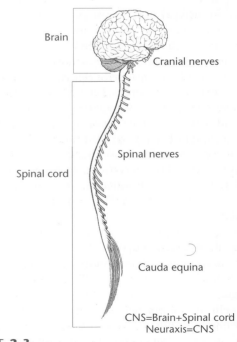

Brain

Cranial nerves

Spinal nerves

Spinal cord

Cauda equina

CNS=Brain+Spinal cord
Neuraxis=CNS

FIGURE **2-3**
The CNS, including the brain and spinal cord. The CNS is synonymous with the term neuraxis.

diagnosis of neurogenic speech, language, and hearing disorders. This chapter takes an in-depth look at the two divisions, beginning with the CNS. Chapter 3 deals with the anatomy of the PNS and autonomic nervous system.

Central Nervous System

The brain is gray, shaped like an oval, and slightly soft to the touch. The average brain weighs approximately 1350 g, or roughly 3 pounds. The brain normally is housed in the part of the bony skull called the cranium. A synonym for brain is **encephalon**. The largest mass of brain tissue is identified as the **cerebrum**. The human cerebrum has evolved to include three parts: the cerebral hemispheres, basal ganglia, and limbic lobe (in earlier terminology, rhinencephalon).

The cerebral hemispheres are the two readily discernible large halves of the brain. The cerebral hemispheres are connected by a mass of white matter called the **corpus callosum**. During development the cerebral hemispheres become enormously enlarged and overhang the structures deep in the brain called the diencephalon and brainstem. The cerebral hemispheres are crucial for communication, particularly the left hemisphere, where the major neurologic mechanisms of speech and language are found.

CORTICAL DIVISIONS

The cerebral hemispheres are identical twins in looks, but the functions of their parts dramatically differ. Each cortical mantle of a hemisphere is anatomically divided into four different principal lobes: frontal, temporal, parietal, and occipital. These lobes can be located on the brain surface by using certain landmarks, the gyri and sulci. A **gyrus** is formed from the enfolding of the cortex during development. A **sulcus** is a groovelike depression that separates the gyri. Another name for a sulcus is **fissure**. The gyri and sulci seen on the surface of the brain serve as boundaries for the lobes (Figs. 2-4 and 2-5).

Cortical Localization Maps
For more than a century, neuroanatomists have divided and classified the human cortex into different areas. These tireless attempts to fractionate the cortex followed the unparalleled achievement of Paul Broca. In 1861 Broca demonstrated that different cortical regions were associated with different mental functions, one of which was expression of speech.[2] The localization systems that followed have most frequently been based on

cell study of the cortex made by histologic methods. They allow the development of cytoarchitectural diagrams or maps based on the varied cell structures of the cortex. The most popular map, developed by the German neurologist Korbinian Brodmann (1868-1918), is represented in Figures 2-4 and 2-5. Note that each area of the cortex is numbered, providing a much more convenient way to specify a cortical site than by a complex description of gyri and sulci. Brodmann's map is open to criticism on the grounds that it chops the cortex into innumerable specific centers, implying that cortical areas have sharply defined limits, but it is a convenient tool in clinical practice for indicating cortical localization. Brodmann's classification numbers are sometimes provided in this text to orient the reader to Figures 2-4 and 2-5.

Cerebral Lobes
Frontal Lobe
The **frontal lobe** is bounded anteriorly by the lateral sulcus, or sylvian fissure, and posteriorly by the central sulcus, or rolandic fissure. The frontal lobe accounts for approximately one third of the surface of the hemisphere. In the frontal lobe is a long gyrus immediately anterior to the central sulcus. This prominent gyrus is called the precentral gyrus, and it comprises the majority of what is known as the primary motor cortex (area 4). The term "motor strip" is also used for this area. Nerve fibers composing a large motor pathway called the pyramidal tract descend into the brain and spinal cord from starting points in the primary motor area. The cells in this area are responsible for voluntary control of skeletal muscles on the opposite, or contralateral, side of the body. This fact has important clinical significance, which is discussed later in the chapter.

The connections between the controlling area on the primary motor cortex and the voluntary muscles served are arranged so that a map of motor control can be drawn on the cerebral cortex to show how the muscles are innervated from the cortex. This map is referred to as a **homunculus**, which is Latin for "little man" (Fig. 2-6). The areas are represented in an almost upside-down or inverted fashion. The area of cortical representation given to a particular part does not appear to be strongly related to the size of that part of the body, because the leg and arm are given smaller areas than the hand or mouth. Rather, the body parts that require the most precision in motor control are apportioned the larger cortical areas. Also shown in Figure 2-6 is the cortical sensory map, which is a mirror image of the motor map.

Immediately anterior to the primary motor area are the premotor cortex and another area with motor assignment, the supplementary motor area. These ancillary

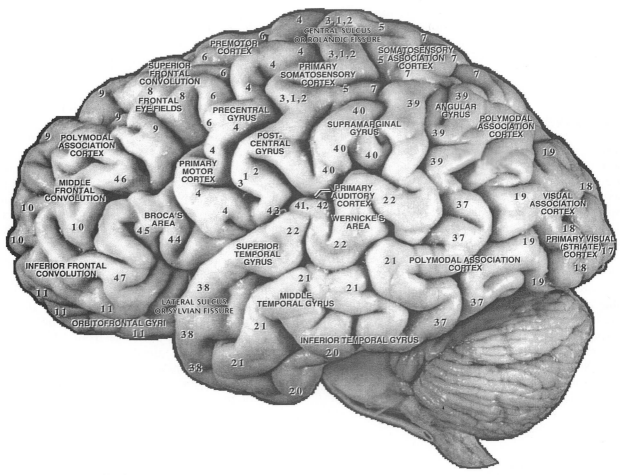

FIGURE **2-4**
Superior view of the cerebral hemispheres with cortical binding, according to Brodmann.
(Reprinted from Werner, J. J. [2001]. *Atlas of neuroanatomy.* Boston: Butterworth-Heinemann.)

motor areas (area 6) are important in motor learning and in the performance of routine and less-practiced motor sequences.

In the frontal lobe of the left hemisphere is an important region known as **Broca's area** (areas 44 and 45). Located in the inferior (third) frontal gyrus of the lobe (Fig. 2-7), Broca's area in most people appears to be important for the production of fluent, well-articulated speech. The left hemisphere is the dominant hemisphere in most persons, meaning that this hemisphere controls language functions. Approximately 90% of the population is right handed with left dominance for language. Even the majority of persons who are left handed show left dominance for language. If damage to Broca's area occurs in adults who are left hemisphere–dominant for language, a characteristic breakdown occurs in the normally fluent production of verbal language. Broca's aphasia, which is one of the classic syndromes of acquired language disorders or aphasias, may be diagnosed. Ablation of the area in the nondominant hemisphere corresponding to Broca's area has an effect on speech in only a small percentage of the population.

Another part of the frontal lobe also concerned with initiation of movement are the areas devoted to control of the eyes. The frontal eye fields (area 8) lie just anterior to the premotor cortical area. These areas are involved in initiating rapid eye movements and directing attention.

The rest of the frontal lobe is composed of association cortex, a different type of cortical tissue with less-defined functional assignment. This frontal association area is often referred to as the prefrontal cortex (areas 9, 10, 11, 46, and 47) and contains the frontal association areas. Frontal association areas are vital to successful executive functioning. Appropriate and well-developed executive functioning allows the execution of nonroutine processes that require planning, analysis, feedback, self-regulation, and so forth. The ability to participate successfully in school, work, family, and social settings depends on these frontal association areas.

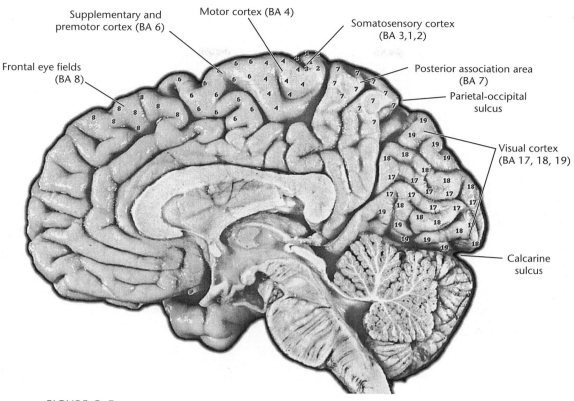

FIGURE **2-5**
Medial view of the right hemisphere. (Reprinted from Werner, J. J. [2001]. *Atlas of neuroanatomy*. Boston: Butterworth-Heinemann.)

Parietal Lobe

The **parietal lobe** is bounded anteriorly by the central sulcus, inferiorly by the posterior end of the lateral sulcus, and posteriorly by an imaginary border line. The primary sensory, also known as somatosensory or **somesthetic**, cortex is found in the parietal lobe (areas 1, 2, and 3), the major portion of which is the postcentral gyrus (see Fig. 2-4). This gyrus lies directly posterior to the central sulcus, or rolandic fissure. On this sensory cortex can be mapped the sensory control of various parts of the body. Somesthetic sensations (e.g., pain, temperature, touch) are sent to the sensory cortex from the opposite side of the body. This arrangement is a mirror image of the motor strip and is sometimes called the sensory strip (see Fig. 2-6).

Two gyri in the parietal lobe are important to locate and become familiar with in regard to language. The first is the supramarginal gyrus (area 40), which curves around the posterior end of the lateral sylvian fissure. The second, the **angular gyrus** (area 39), lies directly posterior to the supramarginal gyrus. It curves around the end of a prominent sulcus in the temporal lobe, the superior temporal sulcus (see Fig. 2-4). Damage in the area of the angular gyrus in the dominant left hemisphere may cause word-finding problems (**anomia**), reading and writing deficits (alexia with agraphia), as well as left-right disorientation, finger agnosia (inability to identify the fingers), and difficulty with arithmetic (acalculia).

The postcentral gyrus is a primary cortical area, whereas the majority of the remaining parietal lobe cortex is composed of association cortex, mostly concerned with somatosensory and visual association function. The parietal lobe has been characterized as the "association area of association areas" because of the multimodal processing that takes place there. As a whole, the parietal lobes may be the most lateralized in function of all the lobes in the cerebrum, although the specialization is not complete. Language functions tend to be concentrated in the left parietal lobe around the gyri just discussed. In the nondominant hemisphere, the parietal lobe association cortex primarily processes spatial information and related selective attention. Damage here may result in difficulty attending to or a complete neglect of the contralateral side of space. Visuospatial and constructional deficits (such as

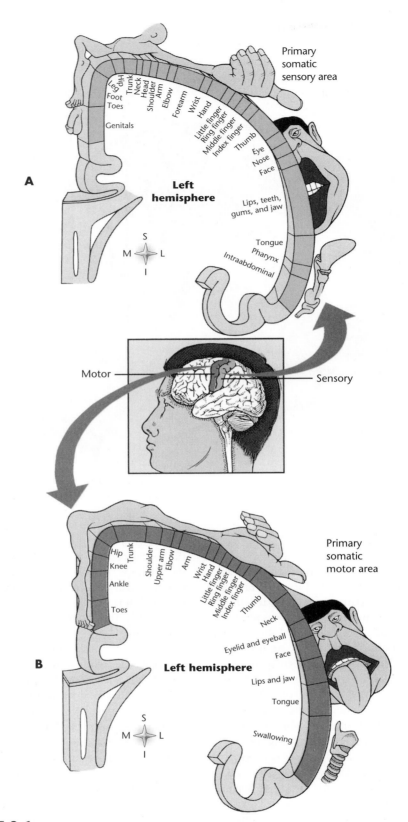

FIGURE 2-6
Primary somatic sensory and motor areas of the cortex. The body parts illustrated show which parts of the body are mapped to specific areas of each cortical area. The exaggerated face indicates that more cortical area is devoted to processing more information to and from the many receptors and motor units of the face than for the leg or arm, for example. (Reprinted from Thibodeau, G., & Patton, K. [2006]. *Anatomy & physiology* [6th ed.]. St. Louis: Mosby.)

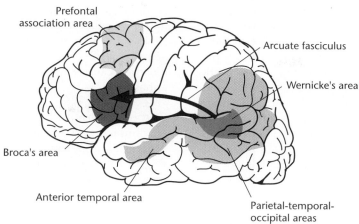

FIGURE **2-7**
Primary language and association areas of the cortex.

in drawing, building small models, and so on) may be found on testing the patient with right-hemisphere parietal lobe damage.

Temporal Lobe

The **temporal lobe** is the seat of auditory processing in the brain. It is bounded superiorly by the sylvian fissure and posteriorly by an imaginary line that forms the anterior border of the occipital lobe. Three prominent gyri of the temporal lobe may be seen on the lateral surface of the brain: the superior, middle, and inferior temporal gyri (see Fig. 2-4). Less visible are the transverse temporal gyri (areas 41 and 42), which can be found on the upper edge of the temporal lobe, extending deep in the medial surface of the brain. The transverse gyrus of Heschl (most commonly called Heschl's gyrus) forms the primary auditory cortex, representing the cortical center for hearing in each hemisphere. Unilateral damage in the auditory cortex does not cause deafness in one ear, but rather may result in difficulty interpreting a sound or locating a sound in space. Bilateral lesions in the auditory cortex cause cortical deafness (see Chapter 5).

The posterior part of the superior temporal gyrus in the left temporal lobe is the auditory association area, best known as **Wernicke's area** (area 22), which is important to the development and use of language. Damage to Wernicke's area results in a particular classification of acquired language disorder called Wernicke's aphasia (see Chapter 10).

If the two borders of the lateral fissure are pulled apart, a cortical structure called the insula, or the **Island of Reil**, may be seen hidden under the area where the temporal, parietal, and frontal lobes come together. The insula is not part of any of the four major lobes but is considered a lobe unto itself. Fiber connections to the insula are not well defined

and the functions are not well understood, but the insula is thought to receive input regarding pain and viscerosensory input. As discussed in Chapter 10, lesions involving the insula in the dominant hemisphere may also contribute to difficulty producing well-articulated, fluent speech.

Occipital Lobe

The **occipital lobe** occupies the small area behind the parietal lobe and is marked on the lateral surface by imaginary lines rather than prominent sulci. Two sulci that can be found on the medial surface of the brain that help locate the occipital lobe are the parietal-occipital sulcus and the calcarine sulcus (see Fig. 2-5). The occipital lobe is concerned with vision, with the primary visual area (area 17) located in gyri that border the calcarine sulcus.

Perisylvian Zone

The cortex surrounding the sylvian fissure in the dominant temporal lobe (left for the majority of the population) is identified as the **perisylvian zone**, where the major neurologic components for understanding and producing language are found. These components include Broca's area, Wernicke's area, the supramarginal and angular gyri, as well as major long association tracts that connect the components (see Fig. 2-7). The central language mechanism and its disorders are discussed in depth in Chapter 9.

CEREBRAL CONNECTIONS

Knowledge of the cerebral hemispheres should also include the types of fibers found in these areas. Projection fibers are long axons of neurons that send impulses to a distant structure in the CNS. The most notable projection fibers are those exiting the primary motor cortex, targeting cranial or spinal nerve nuclei. Commissural fibers connect an area in one hemisphere with an area in the opposite hemisphere. The corpus callosum is the largest set of commissural fibers in the brain. Association fibers form association tracts, connecting areas within the hemisphere. Short association tracts are within lobes, and long tracts are between lobes. One important association tract is the **arcuate fasciculus**, a bundle of nerve fibers within the CNS. (Fasciculus means "little bundle.") It travels from the posterior temporal lobe forward by way of another set of fibers, the superior longitudinal fasciculus, to the motor association cortex in the frontal lobe (Fig. 2-8). Lesions in the area of the arcuate fasciculus may cause a major syndrome of aphasia (an acquired language disorder caused by brain damage) called conduction aphasia.

Corpus Callosum

A commissural pathway called the corpus callosum is of crucial importance to speech-language functions (Fig. 2-9). This pathway serves as the major connection between the hemispheres and conveys neural information

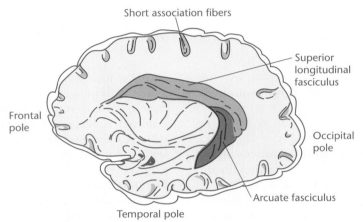

FIGURE **2-8**
Association fiber tracts of the left cerebral hemisphere.

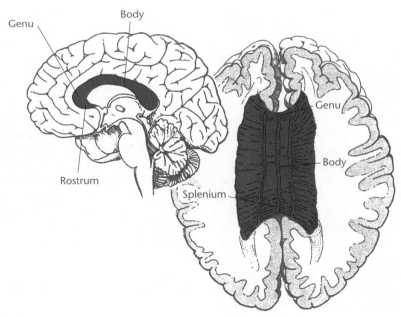

FIGURE **2-9**
The corpus callosum in a medial view and transverse section. It is the largest of the commissures connecting the two hemispheres.

from one hemisphere to the other. The corpus callosum is the largest of the side-to-side interconnections between the two hemispheres. In general, the corpus callosum connects analogous areas in the two hemispheres. The anterior and posterior commissures are small bundles of interhemispheric fibers located anteriorly and posteriorly to the corpus callosum. The anterior commissure connects the olfactory bulbs, amygdaloid nuclei, and the medial and inferior temporal lobes. The posterior commissure fibers connect areas in the occipital lobes, primarily areas concerned with pupillary response and eye movement control.

Split-Brain Research

The corpus callosum and its role in the transfer of information from one hemisphere to another attracted wide attention when split-brain operations were first performed on human beings in the 1960s. This large bundle of commissural fibers may be cleanly and completely severed surgically without damage to other tissue. This operation, called a commissurotomy, has been performed on patients plagued by chronic and severe epileptic seizures that could not be controlled by massive doses of anticonvulsive medication. A seizure that begins in one cerebral hemisphere may easily travel across the corpus callosum to the other hemisphere, producing a bilateral generalized seizure. Neurosurgeons reasoned that sectioning the corpus callosum would contain the seizure to one hemisphere.

Results of the early commissurotomies were even more beneficial than had been anticipated. Not only did the surgery contain seizures to a single hemisphere, but it also reduced seizures overall because of the severing of apparent reciprocal actions between the hemispheres.

The surgery also provided information on the differing psychologic functions of each hemisphere and on the role of the corpus callosum in the brain mechanisms for speech and language. The split-brain patients clearly showed asymmetry for speech and language functions, indicating that the corpus callosum plays a decisive role in transmitting language heard in the right ear (and received at the right primary auditory area) to the left hemisphere, where it is processed by the major mechanisms for speech and language.

Experiments on patients who underwent the split-brain procedure suggested that the right hemisphere was responsible for spatial, tactile, and constructional tasks. These experiments led to speculations that the two hemispheres function in different ways, each having its own cognitive style. The left hemisphere is characterized as logical, analytical, and verbal, the right as intuitive, holistic, and perceptual/spatial. However, they are unquestionably integrated in intact brain function.

SPECIFIC CORTICAL AREAS

The cortical areas can be divided into three major divisions: primary motor projection areas, primary sensory reception areas, and association areas. Association areas comprise the majority of the cortex, making up approximately 86% of it.

The primary motor projection cortices are found in the frontal lobes on the precentral gyri, the bilateral cortical strips from which voluntary movement patterns are initiated. The motor strip serves as a source of descending motor pathways, projecting to lower levels of the nervous system.

The primary sensory reception areas register sensory impulses relayed from the periphery to the thalamus and upward to the cortex. The pathways from thalamus to cortex are called thalamic radiations. The primary reception areas of the cortex are (1) the primary auditory cortex (areas 41 and 42) located in Heschl's gyrus in the temporal lobes, (2) the primary somatosensory cortex in the postcentral gyri of the parietal lobes (areas 1, 2, and 3), and (3) the primary visual cortex (area 17) in the occipital lobes.

Primary Motor Projection Cortex

The **primary motor projection cortex** is known as the motor area, or motor strip. In Brodmann's system, it is area 4. The motor area is located on the anterior wall of the central sulcus and the adjacent precentral gyrus. Figure 2-6 shows the areas devoted to the motor control of the different parts of the body. Recall that this area allows contralateral motor control of the limbs. The inverted arrangement of motor control areas on the bilateral motor cortices reveals that cortical control for the muscles and functions of the speech mechanism is represented at the lower end of the motor area on the lateral wall of the cerebrum. The large areas given over to motor control of the oral mechanism contribute to the coordination of its rapid and precise movements during talking, singing, and changing facial expression.

Anterior to the motor area is the **premotor area** (area 6), considered a supplement to the primary motor projection cortex and related to the extrapyramidal system. If areas 4 and 6 are ablated, spasticity in the limbs results. A third motor area, discovered by Wilder G. Penfield, is found on the ventral surface of the precentral and postcentral gyri. It is called the **supplementary**, or **secondary**, **motor area**.

In more recent years the supplementary motor area has received considerable attention. Its primary function appears to be control of sequential movements, and speech production is a prime example of sequential movement. The supplementary area now appears to be the principal cortical structure in a neural network that initiates speech.

Primary Somatosensory Cortex

The **primary somatosensory cortex** (areas 1, 2, and 3) is on the postcentral gyrus and is a primary receptor of general bodily sensation. Thalamic radiations relay sensory data from skin, muscles, tendons, and joints of the body to the primary somatosensory cortex. Lesions of this cortex produce partial sensory loss (**paresthesia**); rarely does complete sensory loss occur (**anesthesia**). A lesion causes numbness and tingling in the opposite side of the body. Widespread destructive lesions produce gross sensory loss with an inability to localize sensation.

Primary Auditory Receptor Cortex

Heschl's gyrus (areas 41 and 42), as previously described, is the **primary auditory receptor cortex**. The area is found in each temporal lobe, but the left Heschl's area appears to be somewhat larger in most individuals. The significance of this neuroanatomic difference is not completely clear, but it may be related to language dominance.

Primary Visual Receptor Cortex

The **primary visual receptor cortex** is in the occipital lobe along the calcarine fissure, which can be seen from the medial surface of the hemisphere and is not obvious on the outside of the brain. The area, 17 in the Brodmann scheme, is also known as the striate area. It receives fibers from the optic tract. Lesions of the optic pathways cause various degrees of blindness. This partial blindness is considered a visual field defect.

Primary Olfactory Receptor Cortex

The cortical area that allows appreciation of smell is deep in the temporal lobe and is called the **primary olfactory receptor cortex** (area 28, medial surface). It includes an area called the **uncus** and the nearby parts of the parahippocampal gyri of the temporal lobe. The olfactory nerves, the end organs for smell, lie in a bony structure in the nose. The nerves end in the olfactory bulb, which is an extension of brain tissue in the nasal area. The bulbs are supported by an olfactory stalk. Destruction of the olfactory system causes anosmia, or lack of smell. Irritative lesions produce olfactory hallucinations or uncinate fits.

Association Cortex

Specific Association Areas

Cortical Motor Speech Association Areas. Surrounding the foot of the motor and premotor cortices are areas considered **motor association areas**. These areas are numbered 44, 45, 46, and 47 in the Brodmann system. They are called the opercular gyri. Areas 44 and 45

include the pars opercularis, the pars triangularis, and the pars orbitalis. Areas 44 and 45 in the left hemisphere are sometimes called the frontal operculum. Area 44 is known best as Broca's area. Although its function is controversial, Broca's area usually is associated with the formation of motor speech plans for oral expression. The cytoarchitecture of the area is similar in both right and left hemispheres, but traditional theory maintains that only the left is involved with verbal formulation. Regional cerebral blood flow and metabolic rate studies have suggested that right cortical areas may also be activated during some speech and language activities.

Sensory Association Areas. The sensory association areas, where elaboration of sensation occurs, can best be considered as extensions of the primary sensory receptor areas. They are also known as **secondary association areas** or unimodal association areas because only one type of sensory input is processed there. Their margins are necessarily vague, and what the exact functions of certain areas are is controversial. The sensory association areas are richly connected to the receptor areas by a host of association fibers, but these association fibers are often difficult to follow because of the vast number of relays in the cortical association system. Areas 5 and 7 in the parietal lobe are related to general somesthetic sensation. Areas 42 (part of Heschl's gyrus) and 22 (Wernicke's area) are related to language comprehension. Areas 18 and 19 in the occipital lobe are visual association areas, important for visual perception and for some visual reflexes such as visual fixation. Lesions in this area may cause visual hallucinatory symptoms.

The function of the sensory association areas was that of gnosis, or knowing. A deficit in the sensory association function is known as agnosia, a perceptual-cognitive deficit presumed to follow a destructive cerebral lesion; agnosia means lack of recognition. Lesions in auditory association areas affecting the appreciation of incoming sound produce language disorders. Areas surrounding Heschl's gyrus are involved in adding meaning to sound and providing comprehension of language. Lesions in area 42 destroy the ability to appreciate the meaning of sound, and lesions in area 22 compromise the ability to understand spoken language. Lesions of visual association areas may cause different types of visual agnosia in which the patient cannot, through the visual modality alone, recognize certain visual patterns (e.g., objects or faces).

Categories of Association Cortex. The cytoarchitecture of association cortex is different for different areas and determines what kind of neural information can be processed by those cells. Generally, the association areas adjacent to primary motor and sensory areas are unimodal; that is, only one type of information is processed by those cells. These association areas elaborate on the information received at the specific primary motor and sensory areas to which they are adjacent.

Further removed from the primary motor or sensory cortical areas, other types of association cortex are found, termed polymodal and supramodal. Polymodal is sometimes referred to as multimodal, and supramodal may be referred to as heteromodal in some texts.

Polymodal association areas are found somewhat close to the unimodal areas near the primary reception cortex. Polymodal association cortex is linked to processing of two or more sensory modalities. For example, polymodal association cortex, processing both auditory and visual information, can be found in the temporal lobe and in the occipital lobe. The **parahippocampal gyrus** receives input from all areas of the cerebral cortex, processing several different types of sensory information.

The association areas add meaning and significance to the sensory or motor information received in the primary motor or sensory areas. The matching of present sensory information with past sensory information drawn from memory probably takes place in the polymodal association areas, which are linked to several sensory modalities. Motor association areas are sites where motor plans, programs, and commands are formulated with input from auditory and somatosensory processing, particularly touch, and other modalities.

Certain sensory association areas blend and mingle sensory information from several association areas to establish a higher level of cortical sensory information. This type of processing results in a complex level of awareness that is above and beyond mere recognition of sensory data. This level of sensory awareness is known as perception. For example, if someone places a door key in your hand in the dark, you must recognize its shape and judge its size, weight, texture, and metallic surface to match this information with memories and concepts of keys. Only when you can identify your perception of the key can you name the key and relate its function if asked. The everyday sensory recognition of objects relies on complex sensory integration of multiple sensations enhanced by memory and conceptual knowledge of objects with similar qualities. This complex activity of knowing is called gnosis.

The highest level of processing is carried on in association areas best described as supramodal, meaning that these cortical areas are concerned with neural processing that is not directly linked to sensory or motor functions. This kind of association cortex and cortical function can be found primarily in the following areas:

- The prefrontal area, for higher executive function
- Perisylvian cortex, subserving language
- Limbic lobe, subserving emotion and motivation

> **BOX 2-2**
>
> ### Categories of Association Cortex
>
> **Unimodal**
>
> - Only one type of information is processed by the cells in these areas
> - Areas elaborate on information received at adjacent primary motor and sensory areas
> - Information can be related to either motor or sensory input
>
> **Polymodal**
>
> - Found in close proximity to unimodal areas, near the primary reception cortex
> - Linked to processing two or more kinds of sensory information (e.g., auditory and visual information)
> - Matches present sensory information with past sensory information
>
> **Supramodal**
>
> - Highest level of processing
> - Areas concerned with neural processing not linked directly with sensory or motor functions
> - Found primarily in prefrontal area, perisylvian cortex, and limbic lobe

The prefrontal cortex and the perisylvian cortical area and function were previously outlined and are discussed in depth in Chapter 9. The limbic lobe, its structures, and probable association functions are examined below. A summary of categories of the association cortex is provided in Box 2-2.

THE LIMBIC SYSTEM

Mesulam[7] and Benson[1] provided support for the associative function of other areas of the brain that are architecturally considered cortical areas, although not named as part of the cortex in most instances. As most other anatomists do, these authors include in their overviews of association cortex what Mesulam calls heteromodal cortex, which is composed of the six-layer formation accepted as cortical tissue. These associative areas include the supramodal cortex previously discussed. This cortex has the six-layer formation found in 90% of cortex, including the primary motor and sensory areas as well as the multimodal and supramodal association areas. The six-cell-layer cortex is called **neocortex** or **isocortex**.

Cortical regions with tissue composed of fewer than six cell layers are functionally associated with the limbic system and are classified as **allocortex**. Allocortex can also be broken down into different types or regions. Cortical structures with three to five cellular layers are classified as paleocortex, whereas structures with only three cellular layers are classified as archicortex.

Mesulam's and Benson's discussions of other types of associative cortex focus on patterns formed by regions sharing common functions. Beyond the primary association areas and the secondary motor and sensory association areas previously discussed, neuroanatomists of this school point to the higher level associative functions of the more primitive cortex found on the medial surface of the brain. The cytoarchitecture of these structures reveals a composition of primarily three layers, rather than six layers, with some structures showing transition between the six- and three-layer formation. Thus these structures are cortical-like in nature because true cortex has six layers.

The parahippocampal gyrus is a transitional architecture representing a six-layer formation laterally with a change to a three-layer formation more medially. Folded within the parahippocampal gyrus is the hippocampus. The hippocampal gyrus is actually part of the hippocampal formation, which is a curved, rolled-in-and-under area of cortex bulging into the floor of the temporal (inferior) horn of the lateral ventricle. The hippocampal formation consists of the dentate gyrus, hippocampal gyrus, and **white matter**, called **fimbria**, that issues from this area and eventually forms the crus (or leg) of the fornix. Traditionally included as

part of the limbic system, most anatomists now separate these structures from the limbic system because of their involvement in encoding new memories.[9]

The **limbic system** or **limbic lobe** (Fig. 2-10) was named by Pierre Paul Broca, who thought of it as the fifth lobe of the brain. It is occasionally referred to as Broca's lobe because of this. The "lobe" is on the medial surfaces of the two hemispheres. An archlike pattern of cortex surrounding the nonconvoluted central portions of the brain can be observed on the medial surfaces of the hemispheres with the brainstem removed. This internal circular arch is called the limbic lobe (or limbic system or formation). The limbic system includes the oldest (phylogenetically) or most primitive cortex, the rhinencephalon, also called the "smell brain." The prefix *rhino* means nose; the functions of the old animal brain dealt primarily with the sense of olfaction, or smell. Because smell is a much more crucial sense for animals in their adaptation to the environment than it is to human beings, the old brain is relatively large in animals and the cerebral hemispheres are less well developed.

The histologic makeup of the rest of the limbic system is phylogenetically old in relation to the cerebral hemispheres (neocortex) but not as old as the olfactory brain tissue. The limbic system structures have many connections among themselves as well as connections to the hypothalamus (see "Diencephalon" later in this chapter) and to neocortical structures. In the evolution of the human brain, the older parts have come under

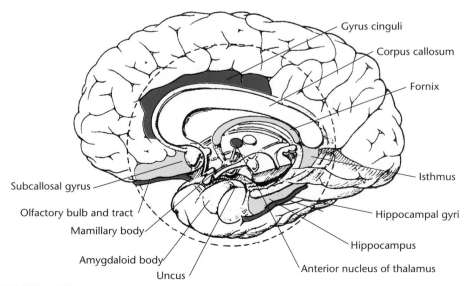

FIGURE **2-10**
The limbic lobe; medial view of the left cerebral hemisphere. The *circled area* is the limbic lobe or Broca's lobe.

the direction of the newer cortical systems, creating a hierarchy. Autonomic and hormonal responses caused by hypothalamic action are under the direction of the limbic structures, which in turn are under the direction of the higher cortical structures. Through these connections, the limbic area helps shape behavioral reaction to sensory input through analysis, reaction, and remembrance of stimuli, situations, reactions, and results.[8] Heimer[6] asserts that the anatomic and functional characteristics of some of the structures of this area are distinct enough to be considered apart from the others, and he questions the concept of a limbic system. For example, the amygdala is the key structure in emotional behavior and the hippocampus and related structures are of primary importance when discussing memory (see Chapter 9).

Mesulam[7] conceives of the limbic system as being formed by several smaller structures, including the subcallosal gyrus, gyrus cinguli, isthmus, hippocampal gyrus, and uncus. A medial view of the left hemisphere indicates some of these structures (see Fig. 2-10). Figure 2-11 shows the subcortical nuclei and fiber bundles that combine with the lobe to form the limbic system. The **cingulate gyrus** (gyrus cinguli) arches over the corpus callosum, beginning at the anterior subcallosal area and arching back to the junction with the parahippocampal gyrus. This juncture is called the isthmus. The uncus is the knob or hooklike area of the parahippocampal gyrus. Mesulam includes in the limbic system structures that are cortical-like in archetype. Cortical-like refers to the fact that their formations are part cortical and part subcortical nuclear in architecture. These structures are the amygdala, substantia innominata, and septal area. They are formed by the simplest and most undifferentiated type of cortex in the forebrain.

A second associative area of cortex is composed of the **paralimbic areas.** Although some neuroanatomists include these areas as part of the limbic system rather than refer to them as paralimbic,[8] Mesulam[7] points out that gradual increases in complexity of the cortex can be found in these areas when compared with the previously mentioned limbic system formations. These structures form an uninterrupted girdle around the medial and basal aspects of the cerebral hemispheres. The paralimbic areas include the **caudal** orbitofrontal cortex, insula, temporal pole, parahippocampal gyrus (proper), and cingulate complex. The parahippocampal gyrus completes the C shape of the limbic lobe. Most of the rostral part of the parahippocampal gyrus is occupied by an area known as the entorhinal area, which can be identified by its irregular surface (similar to an orange peel). The entorhinal cortex is closely related to the hippocampus. The medial view in Figure 2-12 shows the cingulate gyrus and sulcus, the parahippocampal gyrus, and the temporal pole in relation to other medial structures, sulci, and gyri.

If the premise is accepted that cortical functioning is hierarchical and a vast network of interrelated functional systems have different, but similar, neuroanatomic substrates, then the study of the functional systems (such as language, memory, emotion) and their disorders must be tempered with the knowledge that brain function is highly complex, with interdependent systems throughout, and only partially understood. While functional subunits of brain operations are studied, attempts to analyze and synthesize the integration of the neural systems that control human behavior continue at a rapid pace.

Structures below the Cortex

Cell bodies of other structures are amassed below the level of the cortex and appear gray in fresh dissection, although a large number of white matter tracts pass through these areas. The structures or areas of the CNS discussed in this section are the diencephalon (thalamus and related structures), basal ganglia, brainstem, cerebellum, and spinal cord. The cytoarchitecture of these structures differentiates them from cortical tissue, and their functions are primarily associated with sensory and motor processing rather than information processing. As discussion of these structures continues in this text, however, connections with cortical and limbic areas that contribute to cognitive and emotional processing are noted. Discussion of these subcortical structures begins with the diencephalon and works down to the spinal cord.

Diencephalon

Buried deep within the cerebral hemispheres is a group of structures known collectively as the **diencephalon**. This region is almost completely hidden from the surface of the brain and is composed of the following four primary structures:

- Thalamus
- Hypothalamus
- Epithalamus
- Subthalamus

The pituitary gland is also considered part of the diencephalon.

Thalamus. The **thalamus** is located ventrally (toward the belly), and the hypothalamus is located dorsally (toward the back). The thalamus is a large, rounded structure consisting of gray matter. It is made up of two egglike masses that lie on either side of the third ventricle, one of the large openings in the brain through which cerebrospinal fluid flows (Fig. 2-13). The posterior end of

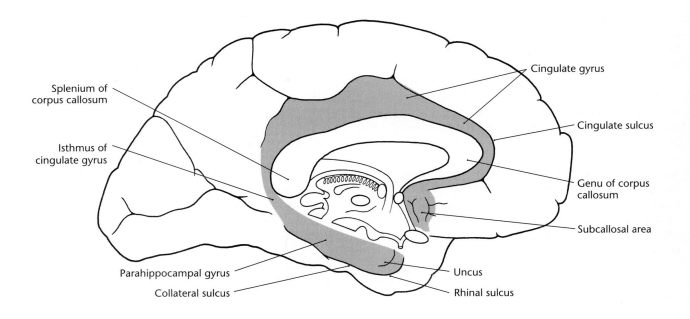

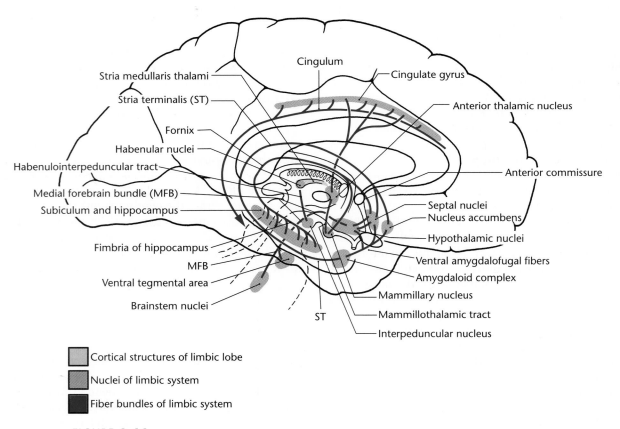

FIGURE **2-11**
Subcortical structures composing the limbic system. (Reprinted from Haines, D. [2006]. *Fundamental neuroscience* [3rd ed.]. Philadelphia: Churchill Livingstone.)

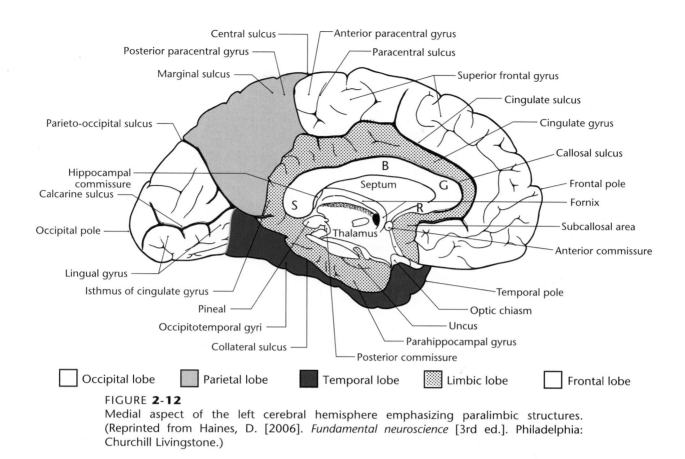

| Occipital lobe | Parietal lobe | Temporal lobe | Limbic lobe | Frontal lobe |

FIGURE **2-12**

Medial aspect of the left cerebral hemisphere emphasizing paralimbic structures. (Reprinted from Haines, D. [2006]. *Fundamental neuroscience* [3rd ed.]. Philadelphia: Churchill Livingstone.)

the thalamus expands in a large swelling, the pulvinar. Wilder G. Penfield, a famous twentieth-century neurosurgeon, was the first to ascribe special subcortical speech and language functions to this structure.

The thalamus integrates sensation in the nervous system. It brings together and organizes sensation from all the classic sensory systems except olfaction. Anatomists usually divide the thalamus into regions and discuss the important nuclei in a particular region. These nuclei act as thalamic relays, sending sensory information upward to sensory areas of the cerebral cortex. The to-and-fro sensory pathways between the thalamus and cerebral cortex are so numerous, and the two structures so interdependent, that assigning a sensory deficit to the thalamus versus the sensory cortical areas of the cerebrum is sometimes difficult. Relays from the cerebellar, limbic, and basal ganglia pathways are also found in the thalamus, subserving motor and autonomic functions as well. The thalamus in the left hemisphere may also play a role in speech and language (see Chapters 6 and 9).

Hypothalamus. The lower part of the lateral wall and the floor of the third ventricle make up the **hypothalamus** (Fig. 2-14). Also on the floor of the third ventricle are two nipple-shaped protuberances called the mammillary bodies, containing nuclei important to hypothalamic function. The hypothalamus is a critical structure to autonomic and endocrine function (see Chapter 3). It controls several aspects of emotional behavior, such as rage and aggression, as well as escape behavior. In addition, it helps regulate body temperature, food and water intake, and sexual and sleep behavior. The hypothalamus exerts neural control over the pituitary gland, which releases hormones involved in many bodily functions.

Epithalamus and Subthalamus. The **epithalamus** is a small region of the diencephalon consisting of the pineal gland, habenular nuclei, and stria medullaris thalami (see Fig. 2-11). The pineal gland contains no true neurons, only glial cells. Through a complicated process involving the hormone melatonin, it participates in regulation of the body's circadian

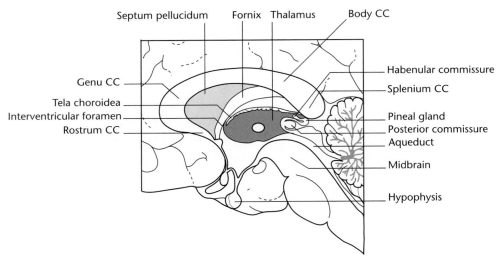

FIGURE **2-13**
The diencephalon and its boundaries. (Reprinted from FitzGerald, M. J. T., & Folan-Curran, J. [2002]. *Clinical neuroanatomy and related neuroscience* [4th ed.]. Philadelphia: W. B. Saunders.)

(24-hour) rhythms. The stria medullaris connects fibers from the habenular nuclei with the limbic system. The specific function of the habenular nuclei in human beings is unclear.

The **subthalamus** consists of a large subthalamic nucleus that is functionally considered a part of the basal ganglia. The subthalamus also consists of a caudal area called the zona incerta. Fibers from neurons in the zona incerta project to many areas, including the cerebral cortex, and may exert an inhibitory effect on the motor pathways.

Basal Ganglia

The **basal ganglia**, or basal nuclei as some texts use, are large masses of gray matter deep within the cerebrum, below its outer surface or cerebral cortex. The division of the structures known as basal ganglia has been confusing in the literature because various anatomists have categorized the structures differently. A review of current literature indicates that most neuroanatomists include the following structures as basal ganglia (or basal nuclei):

- Caudate nucleus
- Putamen
- Globus pallidus
- Substantia nigra
- Subthalamic nucleus

The **putamen** and globus pallidus are sometimes grouped and called the lentiform or lenticular nucleus. The caudate and the putamen grouped together are

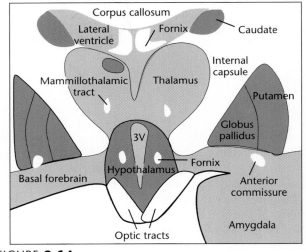

FIGURE **2-14**
Cross-sectional view of the hypothalamus and related structures. (Reprinted from Castro, A., Merchut, M.P., Neafsey, E.J. & Wurster, R.D. [2002]. *Neuroscience: an outline approach.* Philadelphia: Mosby.)

called the striatum (or neostriatum in some texts). These three main parts—caudate, putamen, and globus pallidus—when grouped together are referred to as the **corpus striatum**. Figures 2-15 and 2-16 depict the basal ganglia that include these primary structures.

Input to the basal ganglia is generally considered to be through the caudate nucleus and the putamen, that

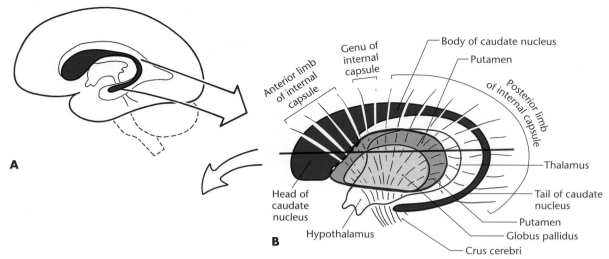

FIGURE **2-15**
Three-dimensional drawing depicting the relationship (**B**) between **A**, the internal capsule (**A**), and **B**, the thalamus, with the three primary structures of the basal ganglia: caudate, putamen, and globus pallidus. (Reprinted from Haines, D. [2006]. *Fundamental neuroscience* [3rd ed.]. Philadelphia: Churchill Livingstone.)

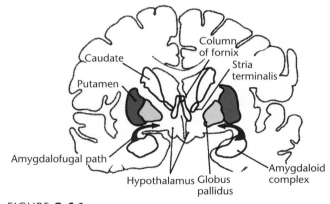

FIGURE **2-16**
Coronal section through body of the caudate nucleus. (Reprinted from Haines, D. [2006]. *Fundamental neuroscience* [3rd ed.]. Philadelphia: Churchill Livingstone.)

is, the striatum. Received here are afferents from all four lobes of the cortex, thalamic nuclei, and part of the substantia nigra (the pars compacta). The output fibers of the basal ganglia usually are from the globus pallidus and another part of the substantia nigra (the pars reticulata). The output of these structures usually is projected to certain thalamic nuclei, the brainstem reticular formation, the superior colliculus, and cortical motor areas in the frontal lobe.

Substantia Nigra
The **substantia nigra** ("black substance" in Latin) is a long nucleus located in the midbrain but considered functionally a part of the basal ganglia because of its reciprocal connections with other brainstem nuclei. It consists of two components, the pars compacta and the pars reticulata, which have different connections and use different neurotransmitters. Degeneration of the pars compacta of the substantia nigra results in the reduction of the availability of the neurotransmitter dopamine. This lack of dopaminergic innervation to the striatum results in disorders associated with hypokinesia or reduced motor movements. Parkinson's disease is a result of reduced functioning of the substantia nigra.

Subthalamic Nucleus
The subthalamic nucleus is the large nucleus of the subthalamus, which is anatomically a part of the diencephalon. The subthalamic nucleus itself, however, is functionally considered a part of the basal ganglia. It receives projections from the globus pallidus, the cerebral cortex, the substantia nigra, and the reticular formation of the pons. The subthalamic nucleus sends projections to the globus pallidus and the substantia nigra. The neurons of this nucleus use an excitatory neurotransmitter, glutamate. The neurons of the subthalamic nucleus are, in normal motor function, usually inhibited from firing by thalamic override. When damage occurs to the basal ganglia pathways and subthalamic or related neurons are not inhibited from firing (i.e., disinhibition occurs), an abnormal increase in involuntary motor movements is seen. This results in disorders associated with hyperkinesia or increased motor movements such as Huntington's chorea.

BASAL GANGLIA CIRCUITS

At least four basic functional circuits have been identified as associated with basal ganglia structures.[4] These neural circuits begin in the cerebrum, go through basal ganglia structures, and then return to various areas in the cortex. Because they begin and end in the cortex, they are often referred to as loops. The circuits traveling through the basal ganglia are identified as a the motor loop, cognitive loop, limbic loop, and oculomotor loop.

The basal ganglia connections with cortical nuclei and subcortical nuclei of structures such as the thalamus and brainstem form what Duffy[3] refers to as the *basal ganglia control circuit* of the motor system. These nuclei and their interconnections are part of the extrapyramidal system. They function in regulating and controlling motor movements and muscle tone, planning for movement, and giving expression to motor movements. Damage affecting basal ganglia function may result in movement disorders resulting in either **hypokinesia** (underactivity of the muscles) or **hyperkinesia** (overactivity of the muscles). Hypokinesia is associated with Parkinson's disease or with parkinsonism. Hyperkinesia is associated with such neurologic disorders as chorea and dystonia. Hypokinetic and hyperkinetic disorders are, in turn, associated with particular patterns of disturbance to the motor speech system. These patterns can be identified as types of a large classification of motor speech disorders called dysarthrias. Damage to other parts of the motor system may result in a different pattern and a different type of dysarthria. These motor speech disorders are further elucidated in Chapter 8.

CEREBELLUM AND BRAINSTEM

The brain contains two other quickly identifiable parts in addition to the large cerebrum: the cerebellum and the brainstem. Both structures are extremely important to an understanding of the neurology of speech.

Cerebellum

The word **cerebellum** means "little brain," and the cerebellum is indeed a much smaller structure than the cerebrum, weighing approximately one eighth as much. The cerebellum is located at the rear of the brain, below and at the base of the cerebrum (Fig. 2-17). It resembles a small orange wedged in the juncture of the attachment of the spinal cord to the melon-shaped cerebrum. The cerebellum as it is understood is a relatively recent evolutionary addition to the nervous system. Initially it was found in fish and was almost solely related to vestibular functioning. As movement

on four legs evolved, the cerebellum developed a rich mass of connections to the spinal cord. As upright posture developed and human beings continued to learn new physical skills, the cerebellum, particularly the posterior lobes, developed many linkages with the cerebrum.

Similar to the cerebrum, the cerebellum consists of two hemispheres. Each is primarily concerned with coordination of movements ipsilaterally, providing fine coordination of movement. The cerebellum plays an important role in postural stability and fixation, as well as in learning a novel motor act. Coordination of the extremely rapid and precise movements of normal articulation of speech also depends on intact cerebellar functioning. Damage may result in a particular type of motor speech disorder, one of the classic dysarthria types called ataxic dysarthria (see Chapter 8). The cerebellum may also have a role in cognitive processing with linkages found with the lateral prefrontal cortex. Cerebellar anatomy and function are discussed in Chapter 6.

Brainstem

The fourth major part of the brain is the **brainstem** (Fig. 2-18). The brainstem and its subdivisions cannot be directly viewed unless the cerebral hemispheres are cut away to reveal the internal structures of the brain. The brainstem appears as a series of structures that seem to be an upward extension of the spinal cord, thrust upward into the brain between the cerebral hemispheres. Often the parts of the brainstem are depicted as extending as vertical segments one above the other, but the parts of the brainstem actually do not sit in a vertical plane. The upper structures are crowded together to fit

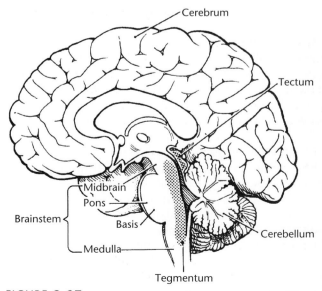

FIGURE **2-17**
Medial view of the right cerebrum, brainstem, and cerebellum.

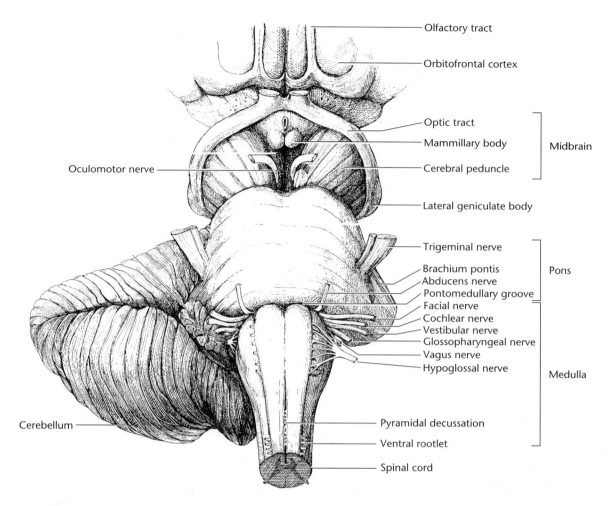

FIGURE **2-18**
Ventral view of the brainstem. (Reprinted from Nauta W. J. H., & Freitag, M. [1986]. *Fundamental neuroanatomy.* New York: W. H. Freeman.)

within the cranium. In some texts and, in fact, previous editions of this text, the diencephalon is included as part of the brainstem. Contemporary neuroanatomy teaching separates the diencephalon and includes only three structures. Moving from the rostral (head) to the caudal (tail) segments, the three brainstem structures are as follows:

- Mesencephalon (midbrain)
- Pons
- Medulla oblongata

Internal Anatomy of the Brainstem

The brainstem also has internal regions, with the presence and function of these regions depending on which structure is being examined. The midbrain has three regions: the **tectum**, tegmentum, and basis. The pons has a tegmentum and a basis. The tegmental regions are always

found in the dorsal (posterior) aspect of the structures, whereas the basilar areas are on the anterior (ventral) aspect. The medulla is not considered to have a tegmental or basilar region as such, but the function of the areas of the medulla that are continuous with the tegmentum and the basis of the other two structures are quite similar in nature. Thus they are referred to as being contiguous areas with the tegmentum and the basilar regions of the midbrain and pons. Basically, the tegmental areas of the brainstem contain cranial nerve nuclei from which the axons of the cranial nerves exit the brain and become part of the PNS. The basilar areas of the brainstem structures all contain ascending and descending sensory and motor fibers. These regions are illustrated in Figure 2-19.

Midbrain. The **midbrain** (see Fig. 2-19), located immediately below the thalamus and hypothalamus, is also called the **mesencephalon**. The midbrain is the narrowest part of the brainstem and contains the tectum, or roof, one of the three longitudinal divisions of the brainstem. On the tectum are four swellings called **colliculi** ("little hills"): two inferior colliculi and two superior colliculi. The tectum and the four colliculi are known collectively as the corpus quadrigemina. The inferior colliculi serve as way stations in the central auditory nervous system, and the superior colliculi are way stations in the visual nervous system.

The crus cerebri is a massive fiber bundle found at the base of the midbrain. It includes fibers descending to the spine (corticospinal), the medulla (corticobulbar), and the pons (corticopontine). The tegmentum of the midbrain contains all the ascending and many of the descending systems of the spinal cord or lower brainstem. The term cerebral peduncles is often used interchangeably with the term crus cerebri, but according to Haines,[5] cerebral peduncle should be used to represent the area of the entire midbrain below the tectum. The base of the midbrain also contains the substantia nigra, which, as explained earlier, is a basal ganglia structure.

Pons. Just below the midbrain in the neuraxis is the **pons**, a massive rounded structure that serves in part as a connection to the hemispheres of the cerebellum (see Fig. 2-19). The connections to the cerebellum are made by a number of transverse fibers on the anterior surface of the pons, forming the cerebellar peduncles. The pons is aptly named; the Latin word for bridge is pons, and the pons is a bridge to the cerebellum. Several cranial nerves exit the brain from the pons, including three that are important to speech and hearing, cranial nerves V (trigeminal), VII (facial), and VIII (vestibulocochlear).

Medulla Oblongata. The **medulla oblongata** is the most caudal brainstem structure. Older terminology identified it as the bulb. It is a rounded bulge that is an enlargement of the upper spinal cord (see Fig. 2-19). A median fissure (furrow) is present on the anterior surface. On either side of this fissure are landmark swellings called pyramids. The pyramids arise from the basilar pons and extend caudally to an area known as the pyramidal decussation. This area is formed by the decussation (crossing to the opposite side) of motor fibers traveling from the precentral gyrus in the frontal lobe to the spinal cord (corticospinal fibers of the pyramidal tract). Posterior to the pyramids are oval elevations, called olives, produced by the olivary nuclei. The olives are important way stations on the pathways of the auditory nervous system. The inferior cerebellar peduncles are also found on the medulla. The peduncles

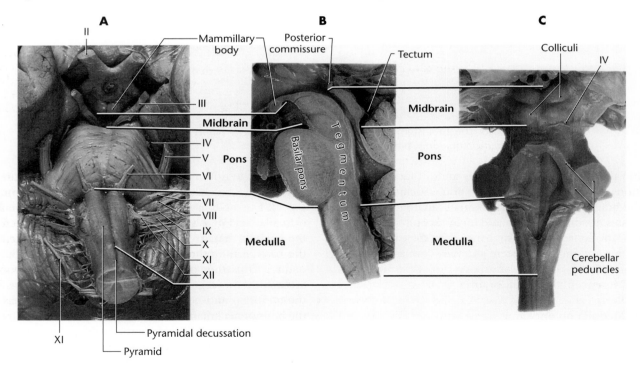

FIGURE **2-19**
Anterior (ventral; **A**), mid-sagittal (**B**), and posterior (dorsal; **C**) views of the brainstem, with cranial nerves referenced by Roman numerals. In **C**, the cerebellum is removed to expose the posterior surface of the brainstem and fourth ventricle. (Reprinted from Haines, D. [2006]. *Fundamental neuroscience* [3rd ed.]. Philadelphia: Churchill Livingstone.)

connect the cerebellum to the brainstem at the level of the medulla. The nuclei of several cranial nerves important to speech production can be found in the medulla, with their axons exiting the brain at this level. Because older terminology for the medulla was bulb, these motor fibers of cranial nerves that terminate in nuclei in brainstem structures are often referred to as corticobulbar fibers. These fibers are also sometimes referred to as corticonuclear fibers because their destination in the brainstem is the nuclei of the cranial nerves.

SPINAL CORD

Recall a mental image of the dissection of the nervous system. Looking at the brain, a long pigtail of flesh is visible hanging from its base; this is the spinal cord. It is normally found in an opening running through the center of the bony vertebral column. The spinal cord is strictly defined. It is caudal to the large opening at the base of the skull called the **magnum foramen**; the nervous tissue encased in the skull proper is the brain.

The spinal cord is divided into five regions. Each of these regions is named for a section of the 31 spinal vertebrae that surround the spinal cord itself. The regions of the cord are cervical, thoracic, lumbar, sacral, and coccygeal. The spinal cord does not extend the complete length of the vertebral column. In the adult it terminates at the level of the lower border of the first lumbar vertebra. In the child it is longer, ending at the upper border of the third lumbar vertebra. Figure 2-20 shows the segmental spinal nerve and the comparable vertebral levels.

A cross section of the spinal cord (Fig. 2-21) reveals an H-shaped mass of gray matter in the center of the spinal segment. As in other parts of the CNS, the gray matter contains neuronal and glial cell bodies, axons, and dendrites. Laminar organization is present in the gray matter, with 10 layers identified. Each layer is composed of neurons that respond to different sensory stimuli or innervate different muscle fibers.

The ventral, or anterior, portion of the cord mediates motor output. The anterior horn cell of the ventral gray matter is the point of synapse of the descending motor tracts (corticospinal) with the ventral roots of the spinal cord. The dorsal, or posterior, portion of the cord mediates sensory input coming into the spinal cord through the dorsal root of the spinal nerves.

Each lateral half of the spinal cord also has white matter columns: a dorsal or posterior column, a ventral or anterior column, and a lateral column. This white matter is composed of myelinated and unmyelinated nerve fibers as well as glial cells. The myelinated fibers

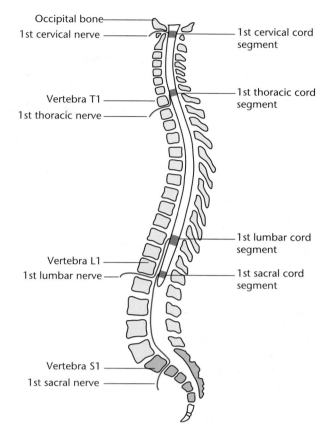

FIGURE **2-20**

Comparison of the level of the vertebral column and spinal cord. Spinal nerves C1-C7 emerge above the corresponding vertebrae, whereas the remaining nerves emerge below. (Reprinted from FitzGerald, M. J. T., & Folan-Curran, J. [2002]. *Clinical neuroanatomy and related neuroscience* [4th ed.]. Philadelphia: Saunders.)

form bundles or fasciculi that rapidly conduct nerve impulses that ascend or descend for varying distances. Bundles of white matter with a common function are called tracts. Major anatomic landmarks of a cross section of the spinal cord are shown in Figure 2-21. Refer often to this drawing when studying sensory and motor pathways.

Close inspection of the form and quantity of gray versus white matter reveals variations at the different levels of the spinal cord. The proportion of gray to white is greatest in the lumbar and cervical regions where the major motor and sensory neurons for the arms and legs are found. In the cervical regions the dorsal column (mediating sensory input) is somewhat narrow and the ventral column (mediating motor output) is broad and expansive. Both columns are broad and expansive in the lumbar region, and in the thoracic region both are narrow.

Combined with a careful sensory examination, testing of muscle functions can be most valuable to the

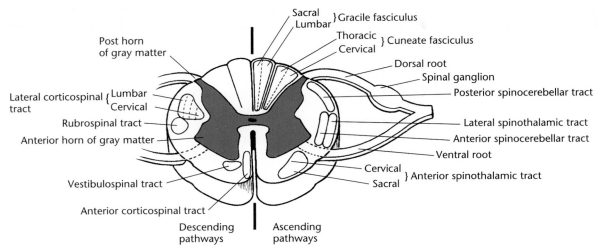

FIGURE **2-21**
Cross section of the spinal cord.

physician in assessing the extent of a lesion. Most muscles are innervated by axons from several adjacent spinal roots. This peripheral nerve innervation pattern is discussed in Chapter 3.

Reflexes

Reflexes are subconscious automatic stimulus response mechanisms. The behavior of lower animals is primarily governed by reflexes. In human beings, reflexes are basic defense mechanisms to painful or potentially damaging sensory stimulation. If, for instance, you accidentally touch a hot stove, the sensation of pain does not need to be sent up the sensory tracts to the cortex. Motor commands from the cortex need not be sent down motor tracts to allow movement. The rapid response to noxious stimuli is processed quickly at the spinal level by a mechanism called the simple **reflex arc**.

The reflex arc contains a receptor and an afferent neuron, which transmits an impulse along the peripheral nerve to the CNS, where the nerve synapses through an intercalated neuron with a lower motor or efferent neuron. From this point an impulse is sent to an efferent nerve, and then an efferent impulse passes outward in the nerve, which moves the effector (i.e., the muscle or gland). A response is then elicited—you simply suddenly withdraw your finger (Fig. 2-22).

There are several types of reflexes: superficial or skin reflexes, deep tendon or myotactic reflexes, visceral reflexes, and pathologic reflexes. Reflexes occur at different levels in the nervous system: spinal level, bulbar level, midbrain level, and cerebellar level. Reflex assessment is a vital tool for assessing the intactness of various sensory motor systems. Reflexes are discussed in more detail in Chapters 6 and 9.

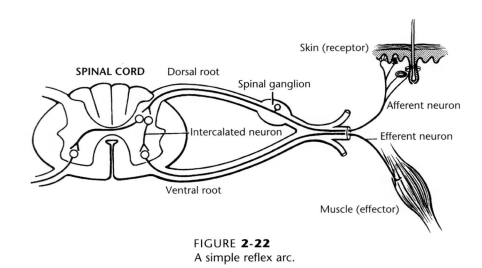

FIGURE **2-22**
A simple reflex arc.

Synopsis of Clinical Information and Applications for the Speech-Language Pathologist

- The uniqueness of Broca's area, a specialized vocal tract, and the expanse of information and communication processing areas give human beings their exceptional ability to communicate.
- The human communication nervous system consists of the CNS and the PNS. The autonomic nervous system is subsumed under both.
- Neurons are composed of organelles, which are composed of molecules. The four major classes of molecules in cells are lipids, proteins, carbohydrates, and nucleic acid.
- A bilipid layer surrounds the cell body of a neuron. The neuron has one axon, which typically carries impulses away from the cell body and may have many dendrites that carry information toward the cell body.
- Retrograde transport up the axon mediates movement of trophic substances, which provide nourishment for the cell.
- Astrocytes, oligodendrocytes, microglia, and ependyma cells are the main types of neuroglial cells. Each has its own specific purpose, primarily providing the structural support and environmental maintenance for the work of the neurons. For example, after cerebral injury, microglia clean up the debris caused by cellular deterioration.
- Gray-appearing areas of the brain contain the nuclei of cell bodies. White-appearing areas signal the presence of myelinated fiber tracts.
- The cortex is organized into six horizontal layers. The most recent (phylogenetically) cortical tissue is called neocortex. Cortical-like tissue with five to three layers is found in paralimbic and limbic system structures.
- The brain is divided into two hemispheres, left and right, with communication between the two primarily occurring through the commissural fiber pathway called the corpus callosum. In most people the left hemisphere is the dominant hemisphere for language.
- Gyri (elevations) and sulci (depressions) on the lateral and medial surfaces of the brain provide important landmarks for delineating the four lobes: frontal, temporal, parietal, and occipital. Particular types of language and other types of neurobehavioral disorders may result from developmental interruption or acquired injury to these areas.
- Important functional areas located in the frontal lobe are primary motor cortex, premotor cortex, supplementary motor area, Broca's area, and the prefrontal association cortex.
- Important functional areas in the temporal lobes are Heschl's gyrus (primary auditory cortex) and Wernicke's area.
- Important functional areas of the parietal lobe are the primary sensory cortex, angular gyrus, and supramarginal gyrus.
- Important functional areas in the occipital lobes are the primary visual cortex and visual association cortex.
- The insula is an older area of cortex located deep to the sylvian fissure. It may have a role in motor programming for speech.
- The perisylvian area in the dominant hemisphere is the major area for understanding and producing language.
- Cerebral connections are made by projection fibers (to distant structures), association fibers (intrahemispheric), and commissural fibers (interhemispheric).
- Approximately 86% of cortex is categorized as association cortex. Some association areas are unimodal (process only one type of information) and some are polymodal (processing two or more types of information). The highest level of processing is carried on in supramodal association areas, which are not associated with any particular type of information. The prefrontal association area, perisylvian area, and the limbic areas have supramodal capability.
- Allocortex is composed of fewer than six layers, is inferior to the cortical mantle, and can be found in paralimbic and limbic system structures. Some of the limbic system structures are the rhinencephalon, cingulate gyrus, isthmus, hippocampal gyrus, and uncus. Paralimbic structures include the temporal pole, parahippocampal gyrus, and the cingulate complex. These paralimbic and limbic areas are primarily involved with emotion and memory.
- The diencephalon is composed of the thalamus, hypothalamus, epithalamus, and subthalamus, as well as the pituitary gland. The thalamus is the main relay structure of the brain. The hypothalamus is concerned with autonomic and endocrine functions.
- The brainstem consists of three divisions: midbrain, pons, and medulla. The tectum, tegmentum, and basis are longitudinal divisions of the three structures. The brainstem contains the nuclei of most of the cranial nerves, which control the sensory input and motor output of the oral and facial musculature.

Continued

Synopsis of Clinical Information and Applications for the Speech-Language Pathologist—cont'd

- The basal ganglia or basal nuclei are groups of subcortical nuclei found deep within the brain. The structures of the basal ganglia are the caudate nucleus, putamen, globus pallidus, and substantia nigra. These function in regulation and control of motor movement, muscle tone, and planning for movement. Damage may result in hypokinesia or hyperkinesia and characteristic motor speech disorders.
- The cerebellum has two hemispheres and is located at the base of the cerebrum, connected through peduncles primarily to the pons. It plays an important part in postural stability and fixation and in learning a novel motor act. A specific motor speech disorder may follow damage to the cerebellum.
- The spinal cord is divided into five regions, each named for a section of the spinal vertebrae surrounding the cord: cervical, thoracic, lumbar, sacral, and coccygeal.
- The center of the spinal cord consists of gray matter. The ventral portion contains motor nuclei, the anterior horn cells. The dorsal part mediates sensation through the dorsal nuclei. White matter tracts ascend from and descend to the spinal cord, mediating motor output and sensation to the limbs and trunk.

REFERENCES

1. Benson, D. F. (1994). *The neurology of thinking*. New York: Oxford University Press.
2. Broca, P. (1861). Remarques sur le siège de la faculté du langage articulé suivis d'une observation d'aphemie. *Bulletin de la Socié*té *d'Anatomie, 6*, 330-364.
3. Duffy, J. R. (2005). *Motor speech disorders: Substrates, differential diagnosis, and management*. St. Louis: Mosby.
4. Fitzgerald, M. J. T., & Folan-Curran, J. (2002). *Clinical neuroanatomy and related neuroscience* (4th ed). Edinburgh: W. B. Saunders.
5. Haines, D. (Ed) (2006). *Fundamental neuroscience for basic and clinical applications* (3rd ed). Philadelphia: Churchill Livingstone.
6. Heimer, L. (1995). *The human brain and spinal cord: Functional neuroanatomy and dissection guide* (2nd ed.). New York: Springer-Verlag.
7. Mesulam, M. M. (1985). *Principles of behavioral neurology*. Boston: F. A. Davis.
8. Mosenthal, W. T. (1995). *A textbook of neuroanatomy with atlas and dissection guide*. New York: The Parthenon Publishing Group.
9. Nadeau, S. E., Ferguson, T.S., Valenstein, E., Vierck, C.J., Petruska, J.C., Streit, W.J. & Ritz, L.A. (2005). *Medical neuroscience*. Philadelphia: Saunders.
10. Wallman, J. (1992). *Aping language*. New York: Cambridge University Press.

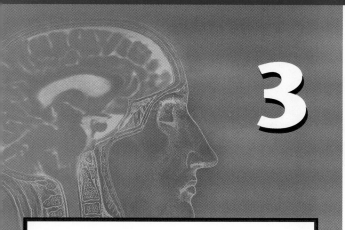

3

Organization of the Nervous System II

The charm of neurology ... lies in the way it forces us into daily contact with principles. A knowledge of the structure and function of the nervous system is necessary to explain the simplest phenomena of disease, and it can only be attained by thinking scientifically.

Henry Head

KEY **TERMS**

afferent
afferent fibers
anterior (ventral) horn
  cells
aqueduct of Sylvius
arachnoid mater
autonomic nervous
  system
bilateral
Broca's (expressive)
  aphasia
cerebrospinal fluid
  (CSF)
choroid plexus
circle of Willis
constructional
  disturbance
contralateral
cortex
cranial nerves
diaphragma sella
dura mater
efferent fibers
embryo
encephalon
endoderm
enteric nervous system
falx cerebri
fetal period
foramen
forebrain
  (prosencephalon)
hemorrhage
hindbrain
  (rhombencephalon)
homeostasis

internal carotid arteries
intervertebral foramina
ipsilateral
lesion
meninges
mesoderm
midbrain
  (mesencephalon)
mitosis
motor fibers
neural tube
notochord
parasympathetic
  division
peripheral nervous
  system (PNS)
phrenic nerves
pia mater
postganglionic
preganglionic
sensory fibers
somites
spina bifida
spinal peripheral
  nerves
subarachnoid space
subdural space
sympathetic division
tentorium cerebelli
teratology
unilateral
ventricular system
vertebral artery
vesicles
Wernicke's (receptive)
  aphasia

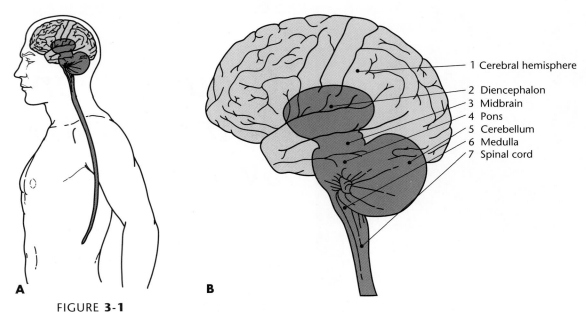

FIGURE **3-1**

A, Location of the CNS in the body. **B**, Seven major divisions of the CNS: (1) cerebral hemisphere, (2) diencephalon, (3) midbrain, (4) pons, (5) cerebellum, (6) medulla, and (7) spinal cord. The midbrain, pons, and medulla comprise the brainstem. (Reprinted from Martin, J.H. [1996]. *Neuroanatomy text and atlas* [2nd ed.]. New York: McGraw-Hill.)

1 Cerebral hemisphere
2 Diencephalon
3 Midbrain
4 Pons
5 Cerebellum
6 Medulla
7 Spinal cord

The central nervous system (CNS) is the controlling influence in the human communication nervous system. Chapter 2 outlined the CNS and it functions. Glial cells provide structure and metabolic support for neurons. However, the CNS would not be functional, or necessary, without the lower level structures reviewed in this chapter. The nervous system consists of separate peripheral and central components organized into two parts—not independent from each other, but interdependent upon each other. This chapter outlines the functions of the peripheral nervous system that allow this interdependence with the CNS (Fig. 3-1).

Peripheral Nervous System

The **peripheral nervous system (PNS)** includes (1) the cranial nerves with their roots and rami (branches), (2) the peripheral nerves, and (3) the peripheral parts of the autonomic nervous system. The peripheral ganglia are groups of nerve cell bodies located outside the CNS forming an enlargement on a nerve or on two or more nerves at their junction. They are primarily sensory in nature although motor ganglia are found particularly in the autonomic nervous system.

The cranial nerves exit from the neuraxis at various levels of the brainstem and the uppermost part of the spinal cord. The peripheral nerves typically include the spinal nerves plus their branches.

Cranial nerves V (the trigeminal nerve), VII (the facial nerve), IX (the glossopharyngeal nerve), and X (the vagus nerve) have their sensory ganglia originating from the neural crest and placode cells and contain pseudounipolar cell bodies. These are classified as the trigeminal or semilunar ganglion (cranial nerve V); the geniculate ganglion of cranial nerve VII; the superior and inferior ganglia of cranial nerve IX, or the glossopharyngeal nerve; and the jugular and nodose ganglia of cranial nerve X, or the vagus nerve. The jugular and nodose ganglia are often referred to as the superior and inferior ganglia of the vagus nerve. Cranial nerve VIII, the vestibulocochlear nerve, primarily arises from the otic placodes. (Placodes are specialized epidermal cells that are found embryologically in the developing head region.) Figure 3-2 illustrates the cranial nerve nuclei and their juxtaposition within the brainstem.

SPINAL NERVES

Spinal peripheral nerves are described as mixed nerves, meaning they carry both sensory and motor fibers. Each spinal nerve is connected to the spinal cord by two roots: the anterior root and the posterior root. The anterior root of the spinal nerve consists of bundles of nerve fibers that transmit nerve impulses away from the CNS. These nerve fibers are called **efferent fibers**.

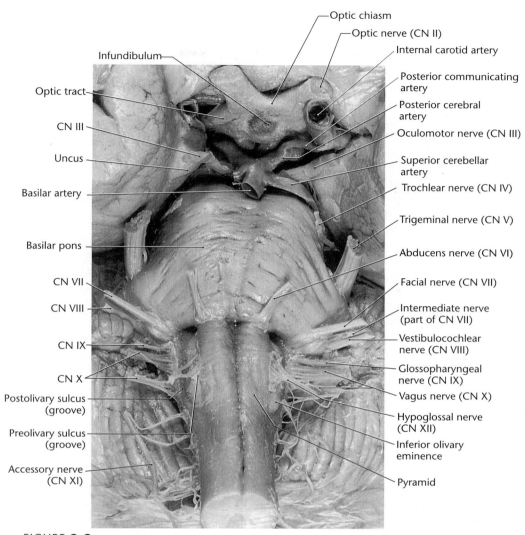

FIGURE **3-2**
An interior (ventral) view of the brainstem with particular emphasis on cranial nerves. (Reprinted from Haines, D. [2006]. *Fundamental neuroscience* [3rd ed.]. Philadelphia: Churchill Livingstone.)

Efferent fibers that go to the muscles and make them contract are called **motor fibers**. The motor fibers of the spinal nerves originate from a group of cells or motor nuclei in the spinal cord called the **anterior (ventral) horn cells**. The anterior horn cells are the point of synapse, or connection, with the spinal nerves as they leave the neuraxis. When nerve impulses have left the neuraxis, they have reached what the great British neurophysiologist Charles Sherrington (1857-1952) called the "final common pathway," or the terminal route of all neural impulses acting on the muscles.

The posterior root of the spinal nerve consists of **afferent fibers** that carry information to the CNS about the sensations of touch, pain, temperature, and vibration. They are called **sensory fibers**. The cell bodies of the sensory fibers are a swelling on the posterior root of the spinal nerve called the posterior root ganglion.

The motor and sensory roots leave the spinal cord at the **intervertebral foramina**, where the roots unite to form a spinal nerve. At this point the motor and sensory fibers mix together.

Clinical principles have been developed based on the organization of the spinal roots that can be used when damage occurs to the spinal cord or spinal nerves. First, recall that a generalization can be made that the anterior, or ventral, half of the spinal cord is devoted to motor or efferent activity, and the posterior, or dorsal, half is devoted to sensory or **afferent** activity. A **lesion**, or damaged area, impairs motor or sensory activities at the cord level depending on the specific site of the lesion. Naturally, large lesions in the spinal cord impair both sensory and motor functions.

As discussed later in this chapter, in early embryologic development paired structures called **somites** are formed on the embryo. These somites differentiate into nonneural tissue (e.g., muscle, bone, and connective tissue). This somitic differentiation results in segmentally distributed zones called dermatomes. The dermatome region of each somite gives rise to a myotome, which is a muscle-forming body, as well as a skin plate for future development of the dermis. The sensory component of each spinal nerve is distributed to a dermatome. Motor axons of the spinal nerves also are distributed along zones determined by the myotome region distribution. Figure 3-3 shows the segmental distribution of underlying muscle innervation. The pattern of cutaneous innervation generally follows the same distribution.

If there is a high spinal cord injury or lesion at the level of the cervical vertebrae, speech production may be affected because the respiratory muscles are controlled by spinal nerves exiting from the intervertebral foramina of the cervical and thoracic regions. If respiration is stopped, death may follow with a lesion above the third, fourth, and fifth cervical nerves. These nerves, called the **phrenic nerves**, innervate some of the breathing muscles, particularly the diaphragm. Spinal cord injuries involving the caudal portion of the cord do not affect speech production but are of interest to the speech-language pathologist, who may work with spinal cord–injured patients on language or other related problems. These injuries are instructive in understanding the effect of lesions at various levels of the nervous system. Injuries in the spinal cord may produce partial or complete loss of function at the level of the lesion. Function is also completely or partially impaired below the level of the lesion. Spinal cord injuries must be considered serious because they impair functions beyond those directly controlled at the lesion point.

CRANIAL NERVES

The **cranial nerves**, in contrast to the spinal nerves, are of more significance to the speech pathologist because all the cranial nerves have some relation to the speech, language, and hearing process, and seven of the 12 nerves are directly related to speech production and hearing. On dissection, the 12 pairs of cranial nerves look like thin, gray-white cords. They consist of nerve fiber bundles surrounded by connective tissue. Like the spinal nerves, they are relatively unprotected and may be damaged by trauma. The cranial nerves leave the brain and pass through the foramina of the skull to reach the sense organs or muscles of the head and neck with which they are associated. Some are associated with special senses such as vision, olfaction, and hearing. Cranial nerves innervate the muscles of the jaw, face, pharynx, larynx, tongue, and neck. Unlike the spinal nerves, which attach to the cord at regular intervals, the cranial nerves are attached to the brain at irregular intervals. They do not all have dorsal (sensory) and ventral (motor) roots. Some have motor functions, some have sensory functions, and some have mixed functions. Their origin, distribution, brain and brainstem connections, functions, and evolution are complicated. (The cranial nerves are discussed in detail in Chapter 7.) They are traditionally designated by Roman numerals: cranial nerve I, olfactory; cranial nerve II, optic; cranial nerve III, oculomotor; cranial nerve IV, trochlear; cranial nerve V, trigeminal; cranial nerve VI, abducens; cranial nerve VII, facial; cranial nerve VIII, acoustic-vestibular; cranial nerve IX, glossopharyngeal; cranial nerve X, vagus; cranial nerve XI, spinal accessory; and cranial nerve XII, hypoglossal (Fig. 3-4).

The cranial nerves from the brainstem are explicitly illustrated in Figure 3-2 and further outlined in Figure 3-5 regarding their location in the anterior (ventral) view and the anterolateral (ventrolateral) view of the brainstem.

Autonomic Nervous System

The innervation of involuntary structures such as the heart, smooth muscles, and glands is accomplished through the **autonomic nervous system**. Although this system has primarily indirect effects on speech, language, and hearing, the speech-language pathology and audiology student must be familiar with its contribution to total body function to understand how involuntary but vital functions such as hormonal secretions, visual reflexes, and blood pressure are controlled within the nervous system.

The autonomic nervous system is distributed throughout both the CNS and the PNS. The **enteric nervous system**, which is formed by neuronal plexus in the gastrointestinal tract, is considered a division of the autonomic nervous system. Enteric functioning has a direct effect on the deglutition and digestion of food. Figure 3-6 illustrates neuronal pathways for the autonomic nervous system as it mediates the peristaltic reflex in the gastrointestinal system.

Aside from the enteric system that deals directly with swallowing and digestion, the major divisions of the autonomic nervous system are the **sympathetic** and **parasympathetic divisions**, which have almost antagonistic functions. The sympathetic system is the body's alerting system, sometimes referred to as the

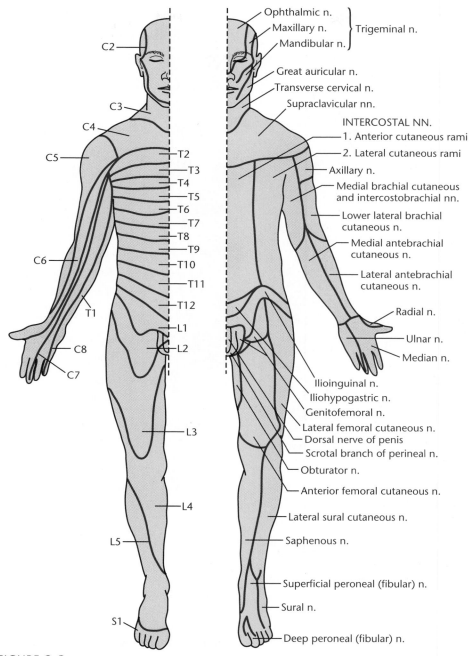

FIGURE **3-3**

Dermatomal patterns *(left)* and peripheral nerve fields *(right)*. (Reprinted from Gilman, S., & Newman, S. W. [1996]. *Manter and Gatz's essentials of clinical neuroanatomy and neurophysiology* [9th ed.]. Philadelphia: F. A. Davis.)

fight-or-flight system. This part of the autonomic nervous system is responsible for such preparatory measures as accelerating the heart rate, causing constriction of the peripheral blood vessels, raising the blood pressure, and redistributing the blood so that it leaves the skin and intestines to be used in the brain, heart, and

skeletal muscles if needed. It serves to raise the eyelids and dilate the pupils. The sympathetic part also decreases peristalsis (the propelling contractions of the intestine) and closes the sphincters.

The parasympathetic part of the autonomic nervous system has an almost opposite calming effect on

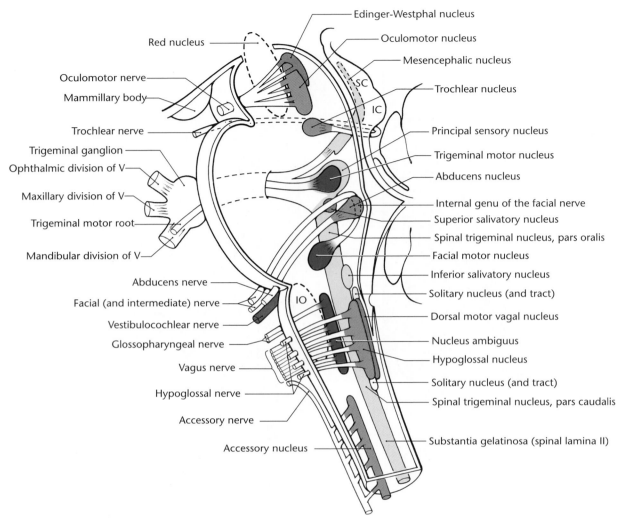

FIGURE **3-4**
The location of cranial nerve nuclei and the course of their fibers within the brainstem.
(Adapted from Carpenter, M. B., & Sutin, J. [1983]. *Human neuroanatomy* [8th ed.]. Baltimore:
Williams & Wilkins.)

bodily function. It serves to conserve and restore energy by slowing the heart rate, increasing intestinal peristalsis, and opening the sphincters. As a result of parasympathetic action, other functions, such as increased salivation and increased secretion of the glands of the gastrointestinal tract, may take place.

The autonomic nervous system is composed of both efferent (conducting away from the CNS) and afferent (conducting toward the CNS) nerve fibers. Several similarities and differences exist between the neural control of skeletal muscle and visceral effectors such as smooth muscle. Lower motor neurons function as the final common pathway linking the CNS to skeletal muscle fibers. Similarly, the sympathetic and parasympathetic outflows serve as the final, but often dual, common neural pathway from the CNS to visceral effectors. However, unlike the somatic nervous system, the peripheral visceral motor pathway consists of two neurons. The first is the **preganglionic** neuron, which has its cell body in either the brainstem or the spinal cord. Its axons project as a thinly myelinated preganglionic fiber to an autonomic ganglion. The second, the **postganglionic** neuron, has its cell body in the ganglion and sends unmyelinated axon (postganglionic fiber) to visceral effector cells such as smooth muscle. Typically, parasympathetic ganglia are close to the

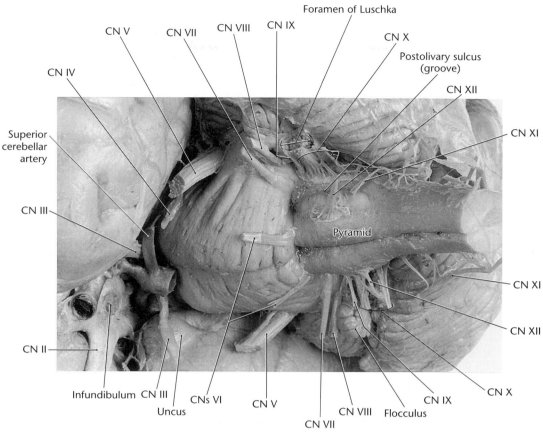

FIGURE **3-5**

An anterolateral (ventrolateral) view of the brainstem with special emphasis on cranial nerves. Note the position and relations of the foramen of Luschka. (Reprinted from Haines, D. [2006]. *Fundamental neuroscience* [3rd ed.]. Philadelphia: Churchill Livingstone.)

effector tissue and sympathetic ganglia are close to the CNS. Consequently, parasympathetic pathways typically have long preganglionic fibers and short postganglionic fibers, whereas sympathetic pathways more often have short preganglionic and long postganglionic fibers. Figure 3-7 illustrates these concepts.

The autonomic system also provides neural control of smooth muscle, cardiac muscle, glandular secretory cells, or a combination of these. For example, the gut wall is composed of smooth muscle and glandular epithelium. The sympathetic and parasympathetic systems have overlapping and, as stated previously, antagonistic influences on those viscera located in body cavities and on some structures of the head such as the iris. Visceral targets are also present in the body wall and limbs. These are found in skeletal muscle (blood vessels) and in the skin (blood vessels and sweat glands). Visceral structures of the body wall and extremities are generally regulated by the sympathetic

division alone. Thus the sympathetic outflow has a global distribution in that it innervates visceral structures in all parts of the body, whereas the parasympathetic outflow serves only the head and body cavities.

Rarely is autonomic activity solely sympathetic or parasympathetic. Both parts work together in the autonomic nervous system along with the endocrine system to maintain the stability of the body's internal environment or **homeostasis**. The endocrine system is a group of glands and other structures that release internal secretions called hormones into the circulatory system. These hormones influence metabolism and other body processes. The endocrine system includes such organs as the pancreas, pineal gland, pituitary gland, gonads, thyroid, and adrenal glands. These work more slowly than the autonomic nervous system.

The integration of the autonomic activity with endocrine and somatic responses, allowing homeostasis to be maintained, is regulated by the hypothalamus.

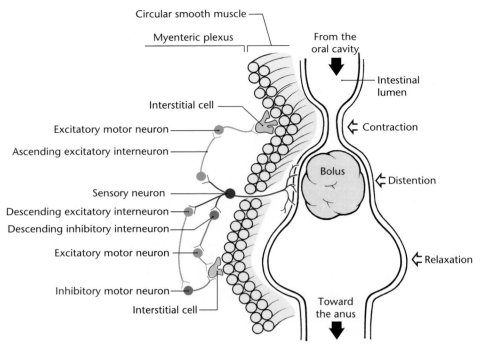

FIGURE **3-6**
Neural pathways mediating the peristaltic reflex. Distention of the intestinal lumen by a bolus of ingested material activates an elaborate intrinsic network that includes sensory neurons, motor neurons, and several types of interneurons. The result is contraction of circular smooth muscle upstream from the bolus and relaxation of circular smooth muscle downstream from the bolus so that it is propelled toward the anus. (Reprinted from Haines, D. [2006]. *Fundamental neuroscience* [3rd ed.]. Philadelphia: Churchill Livingstone.)

Evidence exists for a network of central neuronal circuits that includes the hypothalamus and the insula, the amygdala, and an area in the midbrain called the periaqueductal gray matter. These structures receive input from the nucleus solitarius, a prominent nucleus of the medulla that receives input from all visceral organs. Input is also received from other nuclei in the brainstem and spinal cord. This network is referred to as the central autonomic network and probably is responsible for adjustments to basic cardiovascular and respiratory functions as they relate to a range of body activities such as food intake, emotional behavior, and mental activity.[2]

As stated earlier, the autonomic nervous system is of importance to the speech-language pathologist because of its indirect effect on communication functioning. A good example of the power of the autonomic nervous system is the sweaty palms, dry mouth, blushing, and upset stomach some people experience before delivering a speech. Those indirect effects may make a great deal of difference in how well one communicates.

Protection and Nourishment of the Brain

The brain and the spinal cord, which make up part of the CNS, PNS, and autonomic nervous system and house most of their mechanisms, must be protected and nourished to continue to function. Following is a discussion of the protection and nourishment of these structures.

MENINGES

The spinal cord and brain are the major coordinating and integrating structures for all physical and mental activities of the body and fortunately are well protected. The brain and spinal cord are covered by layers of tissue called the **meninges**. Within certain layers of these meninges is a cushioning layer of fluid called cerebrospinal fluid. The meninges are composed of

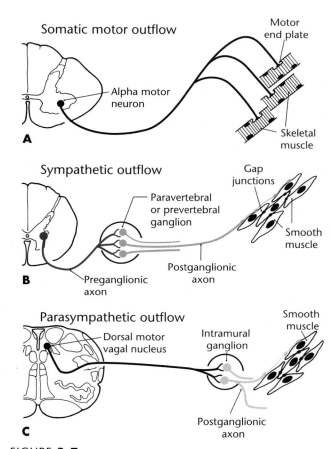

Somatic motor outflow

Sympathetic outflow

Parasympathetic outflow

FIGURE 3-7
Comparison of somatic motor outflow (**A**) with sympathetic (**B**) and parasympathetic (**C**) outflow. (Reprinted from Haines, D. [2006]. *Fundamental neuroscience* [3rd ed.]. Philadelphia: Churchill Livingstone.)

three membranes; moving from the outermost to the innermost covering, they are known as the **dura mater** ("tough mother" in Latin), the **arachnoid mater**, and the **pia mater** (Fig. 3-8).

The dura mater consists of two layers that are closely united except where, in certain spots, they separate to form the venous sinuses. The dura mater of the spinal cord is continuous with that of the brain through the opening in the skull called the **foramen** magnum. In the brain, the dura mater is marked by complex folds that divide the contents of the cranial cavity into different cerebral subdivisions. Around the brain, the inner portions of the dura give rise to infoldings or septa such as the falx cerebri (between the cerebral hemispheres), the tentorium cerebelli (projecting between the cerebellar hemispheres), and the diaphragma sella.

The **tentorium cerebelli** is the second largest of the dural folds (Fig. 3-9). Rostrally, it attaches to the clinoid processes and the petrous portion of the temporal bone and caudolaterally to the inner surface of the occipital bone and a small part of the parietal bone by the transverse sinus. The **falx cerebri** is located below the tentorium cerebelli on the middle of the occipital bone. This small dural infolding extends into the space between the cerebellar hemispheres and usually contains a small occipital sinus that communicates with the confluences of sinuses. The **diaphragma sella**, the smallest of the dural infoldings, forms the roof of the sella turcica, the structure that encloses the pituitary gland. It circles the stalk of the pituitary. The anterior and posterior intercavernous sinuses are found in their respective edges of the diaphragma sella. These infoldings are illustrated in Figure 3-10 as they appear on a magnetic resonance imaging scan.

The major folds of the dura mater brace the brain against rotary displacement (Fig. 3-11). They receive blood from the brain through the cerebral veins and receive cerebrospinal fluid from the subarachnoid space. The blood ultimately drains into the internal jugular veins in the neck. Figure 3-12 illustrates the relation of the three layers, including the dura, arachnoid, and pia maters.

Immediately below the dura is the second membrane covering, the arachnoid mater. This membrane bridges over the sulci or folds of the brain. In some areas it projects into the venous sinuses to form arachnoid villi, which aggregate to form the arachnoid granulations where cerebrospinal fluid diffuses into the bloodstream.

The nerve supply to the dura of the anterior and middle fossae is from branches of the trigeminal nerve. Ethmoidal nerves and branches of the maxillary and mandibular nerves innervate the dura of the anterior fossa, whereas the dura of the middle fossa mainly is served by branches from the maxillary and mandibular nerves. The dura of the posterior fossa receives sensory branches from the dorsal roots C2 and C3 (and C1 when the root is present) and may get some innervation from the vagus nerve. The tentorial nerve, a branch of the ophthalmic nerve, courses caudally to serve the tentorium cerebelli. Autonomic fibers to the vessels of the dura originate from the superior cervical ganglia and gain access to the cranial cavity by simply following the progressive branching patterns of the vessels on which they lie. Nerves to the spinal dura originate as recurrent branches of the spinal nerve located at that level. These delicate strands pass through the intervertebral foramina and distribute to the spinal dura and some adjacent structures.

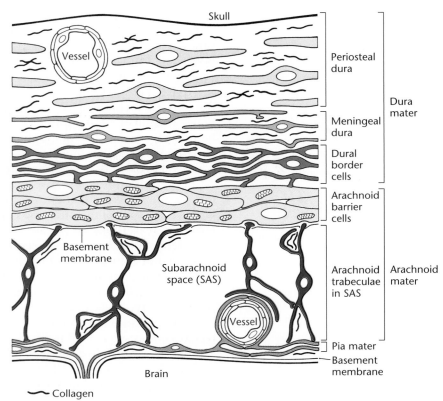

FIGURE **3-8**

The structure of the meninges. Layers of the dura are shown in shades of gray, the arachnoid in shades of dark blue, and the pia in light blue. (Reprinted from Haines, D. E. [1991]. On a question of a subdural space, *Anat Rec 230*, 21.)

Separating the arachnoid and the third membrane, the pia mater, is the **subarachnoid space**, which is filled with cerebrospinal fluid. All cerebral arteries and veins, as well as the cranial nerves, pass through this space. The pia mater closely adheres to the surface of the brain, covering the gyri (ridges) and going down into the sulci. The pia mater also fuses with the ependyma (a cellular membrane lining the ventricles) to form the choroid plexus of the ventricles. Figure 3-11 illustrates the relations of the meninges to the brain and spinal cord and the surrounding bony structures.

VENTRICULAR SYSTEM

The **ventricular system** of the brain has three parts: the lateral ventricles, the third ventricle, and the fourth ventricle. These actually are small cavities within the brain joined to each other by small ducts and canals (Fig. 3-13). Each ventricle contains a tuftlike structure called the **choroid plexus**, which mainly is concerned with the production of cerebrospinal fluid.

Figure 3-14 is an example of a midsagittal view of the brain showing the third and fourth ventricles in relation to the cerebral aqueduct and nearby structures.

The lateral ventricles are paired, one in each hemisphere. Each is a C-shaped cavity and can be divided into a body, located in the parietal lobe, and anterior, posterior, and inferior or temporal horns, extending into the frontal, occipital, and temporal lobes, respectively. The lateral ventricle is connected to the third ventricle by an opening called the intraventricular foramen, or the foramen of Munro. The choroid plexus of the lateral ventricle projects into the cavity on its medial aspect (see Fig. 3-14).

The third ventricle is a small slit between the thalami. It also is connected to the fourth ventricle through the cerebral aqueduct or the **aqueduct of Sylvius.** The choroid plexus is situated above the roof of the ventricle.

The fourth ventricle sits anterior to the cerebellum and posterior to the pons and the superior half of the medulla. It is continuous superiorly with the cerebral aqueduct and the central canal below. The fourth

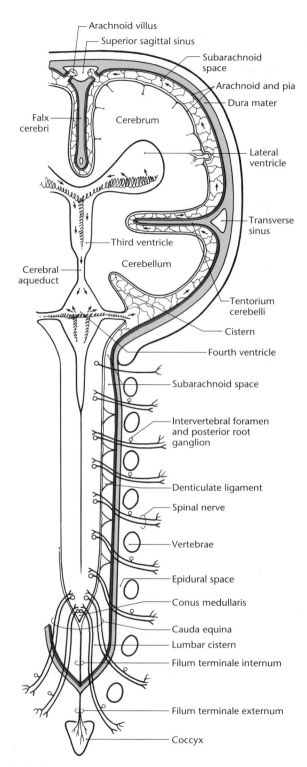

FIGURE **3-9**
The relation of the meninges to the brain and spinal cord and to their surrounding bony structures. The dura is represented in blue, the arachnoid in gray. (Reprinted from Haines, D. E. [2000]. *Neuroanatomy: An atlas of structures, sections, and systems* [5th ed.]. Baltimore: Lippincott Williams & Wilkins.)

ventricle has a tent-shaped roof, two lateral walls, and a floor. The fourth ventricle has three small openings: the two lateral foramina of Luschka and the median foramen of Magendie (Figs. 3-15 and 3-16). Through these openings the cerebrospinal fluid enters the subarachnoid space. The choroid plexus of the fourth ventricle has a T shape. The ventricular system serves as a pathway for the circulation of the cerebrospinal fluid. The choroid plexus of the ventricles appears to secrete cerebrospinal fluid actively, although some of the fluid may originate as tissue fluid formed in the brain substance.

CEREBROSPINAL FLUID

The brain and the spinal cord are suspended in a clear, colorless fluid called **cerebrospinal fluid (CSF)**, which serves as a cushion between the CNS and the surrounding bones, thereby protecting the brain against direct trauma. This fluid aids in regulation of intracranial pressure, nourishment of the nervous tissue, and removal of waste products.

The path of circulation of the CSF is illustrated in Figure 3-17. It flows from the lateral ventricles into the third ventricle, to the fourth ventricle, and into the subarachnoid space. It then travels to reach the inferior surface of the cerebrum and moves superiorly over the lateral aspect of each hemisphere. Some of it moves into the subarachnoid space around the spinal cord.

The CSF produced by the choroid plexus passes through the ventricular system to exit the fourth ventricle through the foramina of Luschka and Magendie (Fig. 3-18). At this point, the CSF enters the subarachnoid space, which is continuous around the brain and spinal cord. The CSF in this subarachnoid space provides the buoyancy necessary to prevent the weight of the brain from crushing nerve roots and blood vessels against the internal surface of the skull. The weight of the brain, approximately 1400 g in air, is reduced to 45 g when it is suspended in CSF. Consequently, the tethers formed by delicate connective tissue strands traversing the subarachnoid space, the arachnoid trabeculae (see Fig. 3-18), are adequate to maintain the brain in a stable position.

The movement of the CSF through the ventricular system and the subarachnoid space is influenced by two major factors. A subtle pressure gradient exists between the points of production of CSF (the choroid plexus in the cerebral ventricles) and the points of transfer into the venous system (arachnoid villi). Because CSF is not compressible, it tends to move along this gradient. It also moves into the subarachnoid space by purely mechanical means, including gentle movements of the

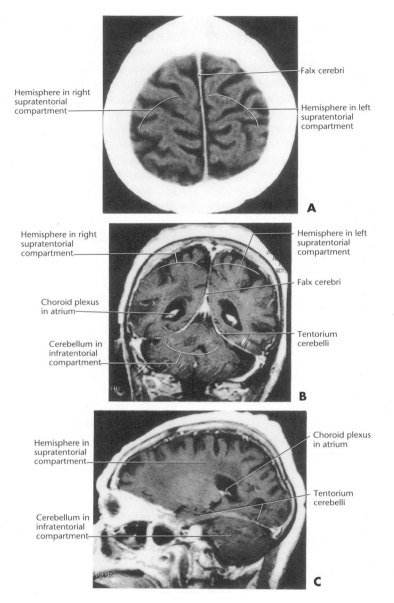

FIGURE 3-10

Axial (**A**), coronal (**B**), and sagittal (**C**) T1-weighted magnetic resonance images showing the relations of the falx cerebri (**A** and **B**) and the tentorium cerebelli (**B** and **C**). Note the positions of the right and left supratentorial compartments and the infratentorial compartment in relation to these large dural reflections in all three planes. (Reprinted from Haines, D. [2006]. *Fundamental neuroscience* [3rd ed.]. Philadelphia: Churchill Livingstone.)

brain on its arachnoid trabecular tethers during normal activities and the pulsations of the numerous arteries found in the subarachnoid space.

Blockage of the CSF movement or a failure of the absorption mechanism results in the accumulation of fluid in the ventricles or around the brain

tissue (Fig. 3-19). This results in hydrocephalus and is characterized by an increase in CSF volume, enlargement of one or more of the ventricles, and usually an increase in CSF pressure.

The CSF is important in medical diagnostic procedures. The pressure of the fluid can be measured; if it

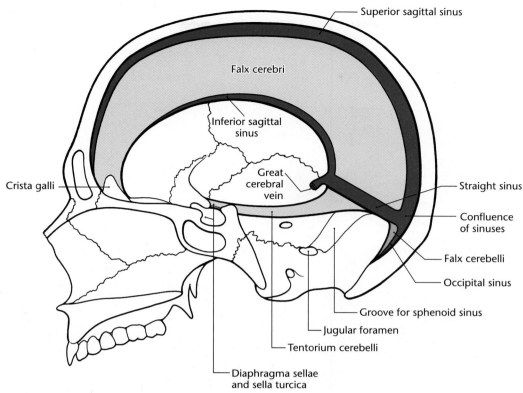

FIGURE 3-11
Mid-sagittal view of the skull showing the dural infolding (reflections) and venous sinuses associated with each. (Reprinted from Haines, D. E., & Fredrickson, R. G. [1991]. The meninges. In Al-Mefty, O. [Ed.]. *Meningiomas.* New York, Raven Press.)

is abnormally high, intracranial tumor, **hemorrhage**, hydrocephalus, meningitis, or **encephalitis** may be suspected. Chemical and cell studies may be made on CSF that is drawn out of the nervous system through a procedure called a lumbar puncture or spinal tap. This route also may be used to inject drugs to combat infection or induce anesthesia. Circulation of the CSF is illustrated in Figure 3-18.

BLOOD SUPPLY OF THE BRAIN

The blood serves the brain much as food serves the body; it nourishes it by supplying its most important element, oxygen. The brain uses approximately 20% of the blood in the body at any given time and requires approximately 25% of the oxygen of the body to function maximally. Initially blood is delivered to the brain through four main arteries. Two large internal carotid arteries are on either side of the neck; these are a result of bifurcation, or splitting, of the common

carotid artery from the heart. The other two main arteries supplying the brain are the vertebral arteries (Fig. 3-20).

Internal Carotid Arteries and Their Branches
The **internal carotid arteries** ascend in the neck and pass through the base of the skull at the carotid canal of the temporal bone. Each artery then runs horizontally forward and perforates the dura mater. After entering the subarachnoid space, the artery turns posteriorly and, at the medial end of the lateral sulcus, divides into the anterior and middle cerebral arteries. Other cerebral arteries are also given off by the internal carotid artery. The ophthalmic artery supplies the eye, the frontal area of the scalp, the dorsum of the nose, and the ethmoid and frontal sinuses. The posterior communicating artery runs posteriorly above the oculomotor nerve and joins the posterior cerebral artery, forming part of the circle of Willis. The anterior communicating artery joins the two anterior cerebral arteries together in the circle of Willis (Fig. 3-21).

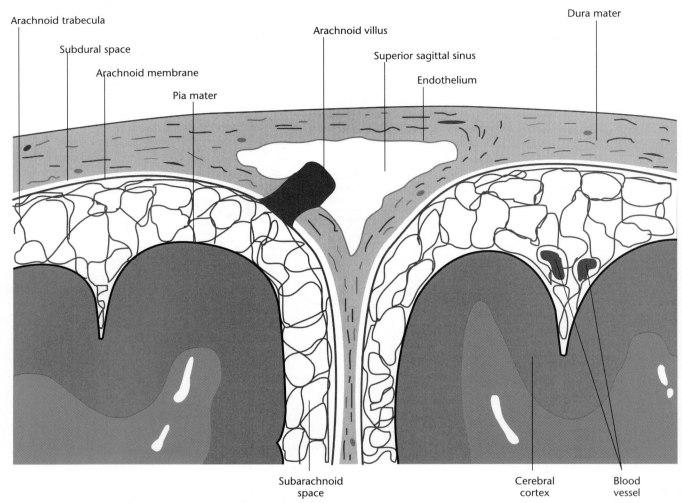

FIGURE **3-12**
Relation of the brain to the dura, arachnoid, and pia maters. (Reprinted from Bullock, T. H., Orkland, R., & Grinnel, A. [1977]. *Introduction to the nervous system*. San Francisco, W. H. Freeman.)

Through these cortical branches, the internal carotid artery provides the blood supply to a large portion of the cerebral hemisphere. The anterior cerebral artery supplies the medial surface of the cortex as far back as the parietal-temporal-occipital sulcus. It also supplies the so-called leg areas of the motor strip. Branches of this artery supply a small portion of the caudate nucleus, lentiform nucleus, and internal capsule. Following is a summary of the internal carotid artery branches (see Fig. 3-20):

- The ophthalmic artery gives rise to the central artery of the retina; damage to this artery (including ophthalmic aneurysms) causes ipsilateral visual loss.
- The posterior communicating artery joins the posterior cerebral artery and the anterior

choroidal artery and follows along the optic tract.
- The anterior cerebral artery passes superiorly over the optic chiasm and is joined by its counterpart the anterior communicating artery; it supplies blood to the hypothalamus and the optic chiasm.
- The middle cerebral artery usually is the larger of the two terminal branches of the internal carotid artery (Fig. 3-22).

The middle cerebral artery is the largest branch of the internal carotid. Its branches supply the entire lateral surface of the hemisphere except for the small area of the motor strip supplied by the anterior cerebral artery, the occipital pole, and the inferolateral surface of the hemisphere, which is supplied by the posterior cerebral artery.

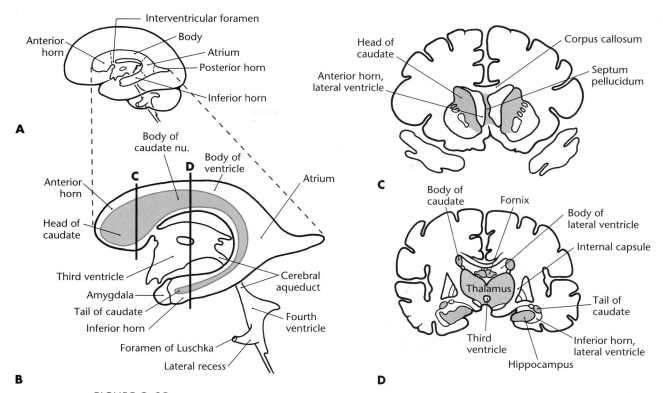

FIGURE 3-13
Lateral view of the ventricles (**A** and **B**) and representative cross sections (**C** and **D**, details from **B**) showing the lateral and third ventricles and the major structures that border on these spaces. (Reprinted from Haines, D. [2006]. *Fundamental neuroscience* [3rd ed.]. Philadelphia: Churchill Livingstone.)

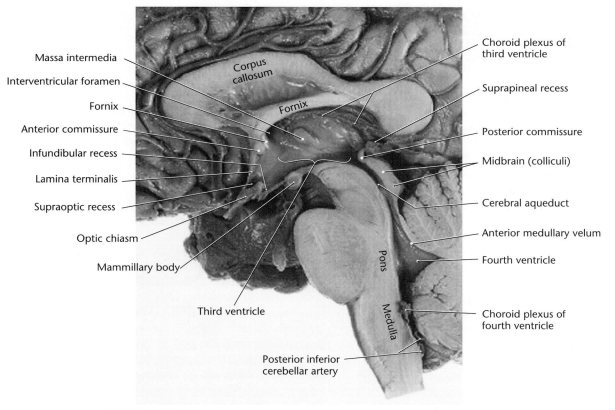

FIGURE 3-14
Mid-sagittal view of the brain showing the third ventricle, cerebral aqueduct, fourth ventricle, and structures closely related to these spaces. (Reprinted from Haines, D. [2006]. *Fundamental neuroscience* [3rd ed.]. Philadelphia: Churchill Livingstone.)

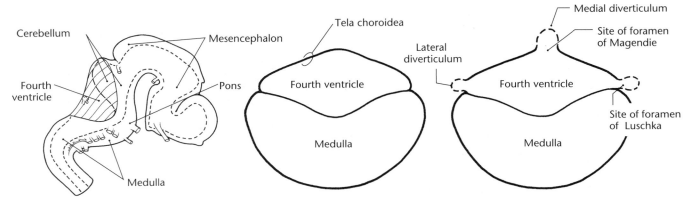

FIGURE **3-15**
Development of the foramina of Luschka and Magendie in the fourth ventricle. (Reprinted from Haines, D. [2006]. *Fundamental neuroscience* [3rd ed.]. Philadelphia: Churchill Livingstone.)

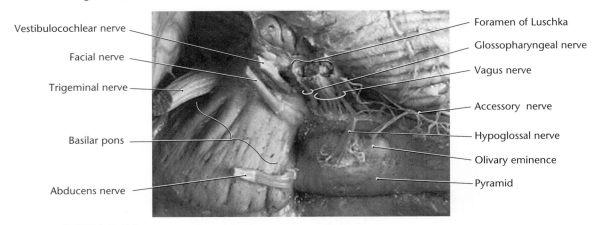

FIGURE **3-16**
Anterolateral view of the brainstem at the pons-medulla junction showing the foramen of Luschka and the principal structures located in this area. Note the tuft of choroid plexus in the foramen. This area of the subarachnoid space, into which the foramen of Luschka opens, is the lateral cerebellomedullary cistern. (Reprinted from Haines, D. [2006]. *Fundamental neuroscience* [3rd ed.]. Philadelphia: Churchill Livingstone.)

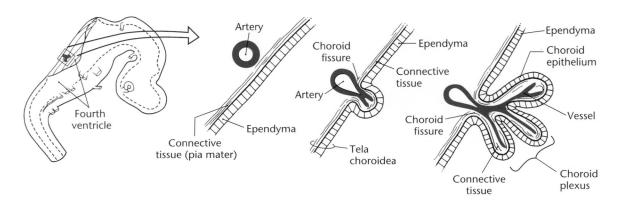

FIGURE **3-17**
Development of the choroid plexus. (Reprinted from Haines, D. [2006]. *Fundamental neuroscience* [3rd ed.]. Philadelphia: Churchill Livingstone.)

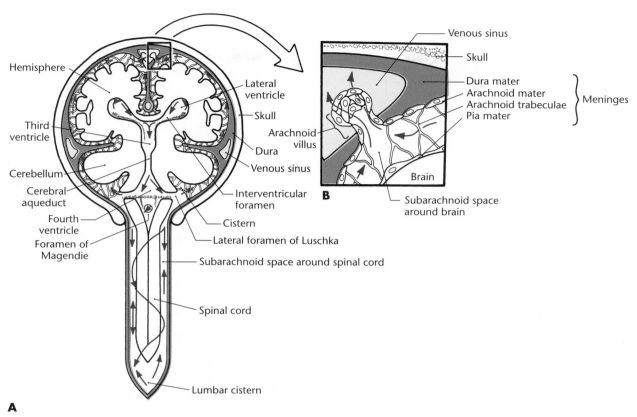

FIGURE **3-18**

Representation of the brain and spinal cord (**A**) showing the locations of choroid plexus (blue) and the routes of flow taken by CSF (gray) through the ventricles and the subarachnoid space around the CNS. The detail (**B**) shows the relation of an arachnoid villus to the subarachnoid space and the venous sinus. Although not shown, the venus sinus is lined by an endothelium. CSF enters the venous system primarily by transport though the cells of the arachnoid villus (**B**, *dashed gray arrows*), although some fluid moves between these cells (**B**, *solid gray arrow*). (Reprinted from Haines, D. [2006]. *Fundamental neuroscience* [3rd ed.]. Philadelphia: Churchill Livingstone.)

The middle cerebral artery's central branches also provide the primary blood supply to the lentiform and caudate nuclei and the internal capsule.

Vertebral Artery and its Branches

The **vertebral artery** passes through the foramina in the upper six cervical vertebrae and enters the skull through the foramen magnum. It passes upward and forward along the medulla and at the lower border of the pons and joins the vertebral artery from the opposite side to form the basilar artery. Before the formulation of the basilar artery, several branches are given off, including the following:

- The meningeal branches, which supply the bone and dura of the posterior cranial fossa

- The posterior spinal artery, which supplies the posterior third of the spinal cord
- The anterior spinal artery, which supplies the anterior two thirds of the spinal cord
- The posterior inferior cerebellar artery, which supplies part of the cerebellum, the medulla, and the choroid plexus of the fourth ventricle
- The medullary arteries, which are distributed to the medulla

After the basilar artery is formed by the union of the opposite vertebral arteries, it ascends and then divides at the upper border of the pons into the two posterior cerebral arteries. These arteries supply the inferolateral surface of the temporal lobe and the lateral and medial surfaces of the occipital lobe (i.e., the visual cortex).

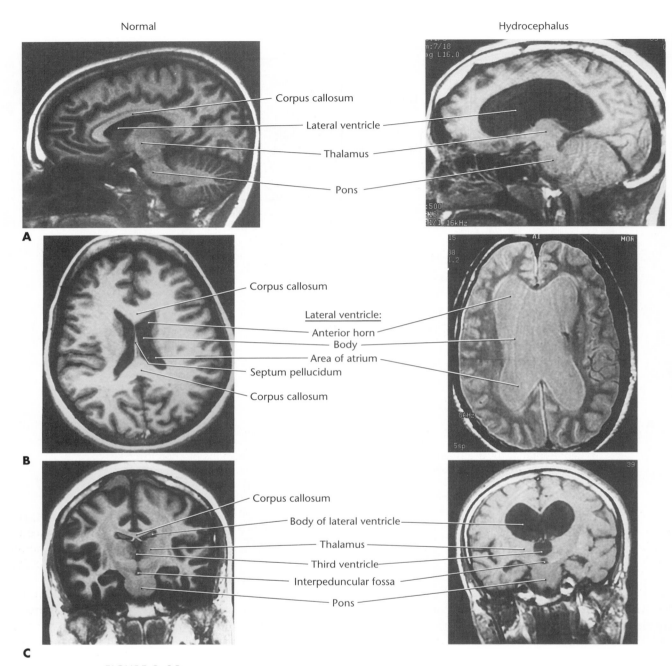

Normal   Hydrocephalus

Corpus callosum

Lateral ventricle

Thalamus

Pons

Corpus callosum

Lateral ventricle:

Anterior horn
Body
Area of atrium
Septum pellucidum
Corpus callosum

Corpus callosum

Body of lateral ventricle

Thalamus

Third ventricle

Interpeduncular fossa

Pons

FIGURE **3-19**
Comparison of normal and hydrocephalic brains in sagittal (**A**), axial (**B**), and coronal (**C**) planes as seen on magnetic resonance images. (Reprinted from Haines, D. [2006]. *Fundamental neuroscience* [3rd ed.]. Philadelphia: Churchill Livingstone.)

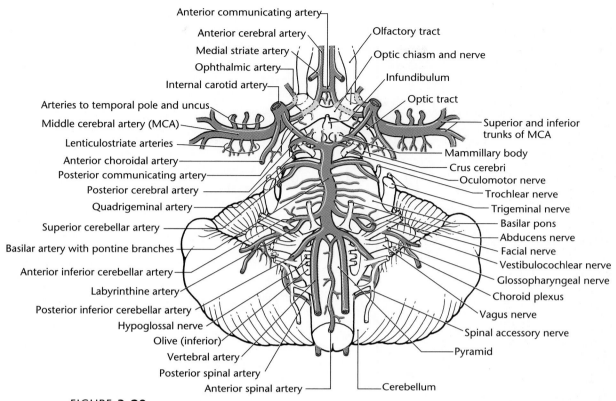

Anterior communicating artery
Anterior cerebral artery
Medial striate artery
Ophthalmic artery
Internal carotid artery
Arteries to temporal pole and uncus
Middle cerebral artery (MCA)
Lenticulostriate arteries
Anterior choroidal artery
Posterior communicating artery
Posterior cerebral artery
Quadrigeminal artery
Superior cerebellar artery
Basilar artery with pontine branches
Anterior inferior cerebellar artery
Labyrinthine artery
Posterior inferior cerebellar artery
Hypoglossal nerve
Olive (inferior)
Vertebral artery
Posterior spinal artery
Anterior spinal artery

Olfactory tract
Optic chiasm and nerve
Infundibulum
Optic tract
Superior and inferior trunks of MCA
Mammillary body
Crus cerebri
Oculomotor nerve
Trochlear nerve
Trigeminal nerve
Basilar pons
Abducens nerve
Facial nerve
Vestibulocochlear nerve
Glossopharyngeal nerve
Choroid plexus
Vagus nerve
Spinal accessory nerve
Pyramid
Cerebellum

FIGURE 3-20

Arteries on the base of the brain showing the relation of vessels to structures and the arrangement of the circle of Willis. (Reprinted from Haines, D. [2006]. *Fundamental neuroscience* [3rd ed.]. Philadelphia: Churchill Livingstone.)

They also supply parts of the thalamus and other internal structures (Figs. 3-21 and 3-23).

Other branches of the basilar artery include the following (see Fig. 3-20):

- The pontine arteries, which enter the pons
- The labyrinthine artery, which supplies the internal ear
- The anterior inferior cerebellar artery, which supplies the anterior and inferior parts of the cerebellum
- The superior cerebellar artery, which supplies the superior portion of the cerebellum

Circle of Willis

The **circle of Willis** (see Fig. 3-21), or the circulus arteriosus, is formed by the anastomosis of the two internal carotid arteries with the two vertebral arteries. The anterior communicating, anterior cerebral, internal carotid, posterior communicating, posterior cerebral, and basilar arteries are all part of the circle of Willis

(see Fig. 3-20). This formation of arteries allows distribution of the blood entering from the internal carotid artery or vertebral artery to any part of both hemispheres. Cortical and central branches arise from the circle and further supply the brain.

The bloodstreams from the internal carotid artery and vertebral artery on both sides come together at a certain point in the posterior communicating artery. At that point the pressure is equal and they do not mix. Should, however, the internal carotid artery or the vertebral artery be occluded or blocked, the blood will pass forward or backward across that point to compensate for the reduced flow. The circle of Willis also allows blood to flow across the midline of the brain if an artery on one side is occluded. The circle of Willis thereby serves a safety valve function for the brain, allowing collateral circulation (or flow of blood through an alternate route) to take place if the flow is reduced to one area. The state of a person's collateral circulation helps determine the outcome after a vascular insult, such as a stroke, occurs and affects blood flow to the brain.

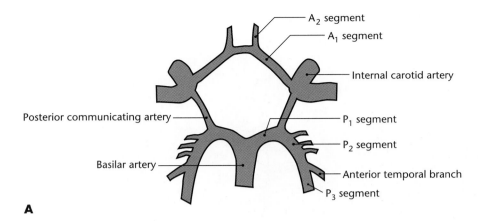

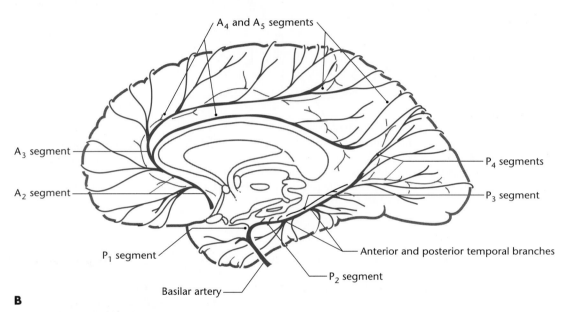

FIGURE 3-21
The cerebral arterial circle (circle of Willis; **A**) and the segments of the anterior (A_1-A_2) and posterior (P_1-P_4) cerebral arteries (**B**). (Reprinted from Haines, D. [2006]. *Fundamental neuroscience* [3rd ed.]. Philadelphia: Churchill Livingstone.)

Development of the Nervous System

The embryologic development of the nervous system is a fascinating sequence of events occurring over a brief period. The spinal cord and brain (with the exception of the cerebellum) reach development of their full number of neurons by the twenty-fifth week of gestation. This includes the almost 10 billion cells of the cerebral cortex. The complete mature cortex contains 50 to 100 billion cells, which are primarily neuroglial cells that continue to develop after birth. Dendrites of the neuronal cells begin to develop a few months before birth but are quite primitive in the newborn.

In the first year of life dendritic processes develop on each cortical neuron to establish the amazing number of connections each nerve cell makes with other neurons. The average number of connections that a single cell will make is within a range of 1000 to 10,000. This pattern of increasing interconnection among neurons continues until young adulthood, at which time the pattern is reversed as neurons begin to die.

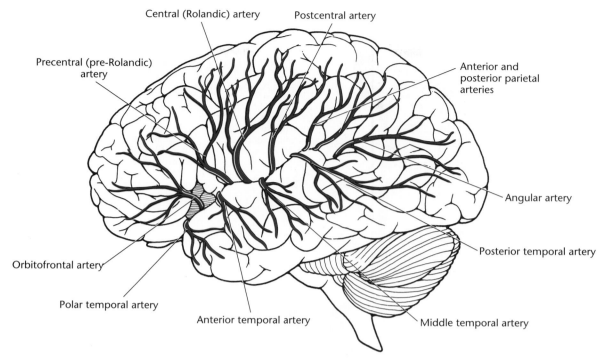

FIGURE **3-22**
Branches of the middle cerebral artery on the lateral surface of the hemisphere. Polar temporal and anterior arteries are branches of M_1; the remaining arteries represent branches of M_4. (Reprinted from Haines, D. [2006]. *Fundamental neuroscience* [3rd ed.]. Philadelphia: Churchill Livingstone.)

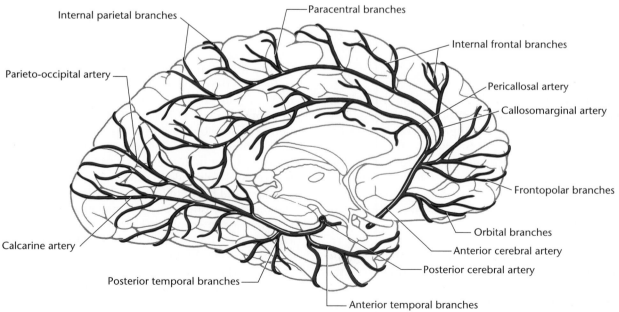

FIGURE **3-23**
Arteries on the medial surface of the cerebral hemisphere and on the inferior surface of the temporal lobe. (Reprinted from Haines, D. [2006]. *Fundamental neuroscience* [3rd ed.]. Philadelphia: Churchill Livingstone.)

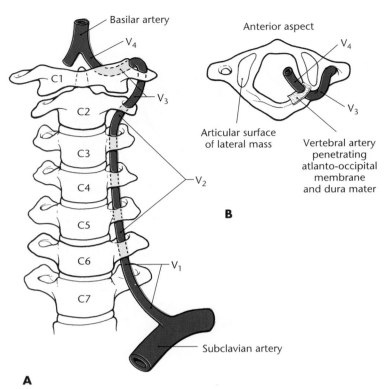

A

FIGURE **3-24**
The origin and course of the vertebral artery and the landmarks used to divide it into segments V₁ to V₄. (Reprinted from Haines, D. [2006]. *Fundamental neuroscience* [3rd ed.]. Philadelphia: Churchill Livingstone.)

EARLY DEVELOPMENT

During the second week after conception, the blastocyst that has been formed from **mitosis** of the zygote is embedded in the uterus. As this process takes place the inner cell mass changes and produces a thick, two-layered plate called the embryonic disk. At the beginning of the third week, this mass is referred to as the **embryo**, and the embryonic period lasts through the eighth week.[3] The ninth week after fertilization until term (or 38 weeks after the last normal menstrual period) is known as the **fetal period**.

Three primary germ layers that give rise to the tissues and organs begin to form at the beginning of the third week. These are the ectoderm, **mesoderm**, and **endoderm**. The embryonic ectoderm gives rise to the epidermis and the nervous system. The mesoderm gives rise to muscle, connective tissues, cartilage, bone, and blood vessels, whereas the endoderm forms the linings of the digestive and respiratory tracts.

Also during the third week a cellular rod called the **notochord** develops. It defines the primitive axis of the embryo and gives it some rigidity. As the notochord develops, the ectoderm over it thickens and forms the neural plate, which eventually gives rise to the CNS. On the eighteenth day of development the neural plate begins folding in along its axis to form a neural groove with neural folds along each side. These folds move together and begin to fuse, with fusion occurring first in the middle and then progressing cranially and caudally. Closure at the cranial end is more rapid than at the caudal end. This fusing of the neural folds forms what is called the **neural tube** (Fig. 3-25), which then separates from the surface ectoderm. The closure of the neural tube is complete by the end of the fourth week.

As the neural tube is rising from the ectoderm, the mesodermal layer of the embryo is forming longitudinal columns that soon divide into paired cubelike structures called somites (see Fig. 3-25). Eventually 42 to 44 pairs of somites develop. They form distinct surface

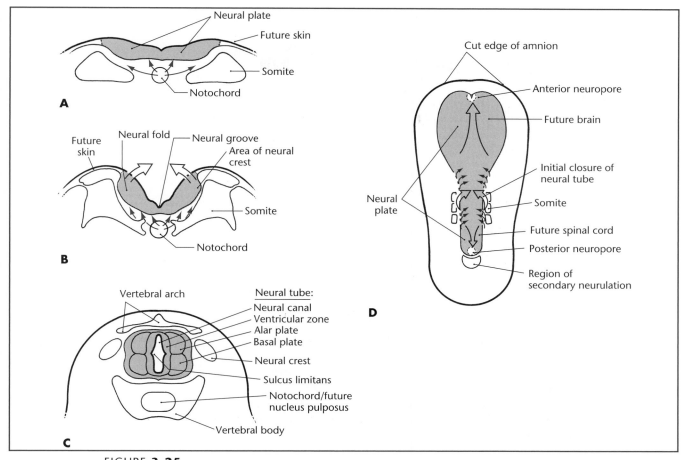

FIGURE **3-25**
Early development of the nervous system. Cross sections (**A** to **C**) show transition from the neural plate (**A**) to neural tube (**C**), and a dorsal view (**D**) of the neural plate shows the point of initial closure and the direction of closure *(small arrows)* toward anterior and posterior neuropores. *Blue arrows* (**A** and **B**) represent induction of neural tube formation. (Reprinted from Haines, D. [2006]. *Fundamental neuroscience* [3rd ed.]. Philadelphia: Churchill Livingstone.)

elevations on the embryo. These somites differentiate into muscle, bone, and connective tissues (i.e., nonneural tissue).

A cross section of the developing embryo (see Fig. 3-25) shows another activity occurring as the neural folds fuse during the fourth week of development. Some of the neuroectodermal cells that lie along the crest of the neural folds break away from the other cells and migrate to the sides of the neural tube. These cells form the neural crest. The neural crest soon separates into two parts that migrate to the right and left dorsolateral aspects of the tube, where they will give rise to various important structures in the PNS and to the ganglia of the autonomic nervous system. The dorsal root ganglia of the spinal nerves are derived from the neural crest, as are parts of the ganglia of cranial nerves V, VII, IX,

and X. In addition to these ganglion cells, the neural crest also is responsible for Schwann cells and cells forming the meninges of the brain and spinal cord.

At the beginning of the fourth week, the embryo is almost straight, and temporary openings called neuropores appear at the cranial and caudal ends of the tube (see Fig. 3-25). These openings close by the end of the fourth week, and a longitudinal folding at the head (midbrain flexure) and the tail (cervical flexure) areas occurs, giving the embryo a characteristic C-shaped curve. Also during this time, four brachial or pharyngeal arches develop in the head area. Primary derivatives of the first arch are the bones of the jaw, as well as the muscles of mastication. The second, third, and fourth arches primarily give rise to the muscles and cartilages of the face, larynx, and pharynx. Figure 3-26

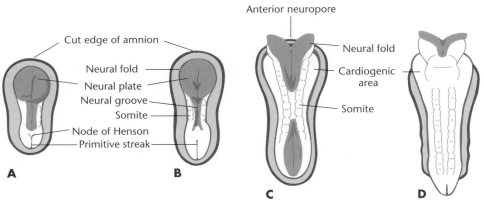

FIGURE **3-26**
Early CNS development. A, 18 days; B, 20 days; C, 22 days; D, 23 days. (Reprinted from Carlson, B. M. [1994]. *Human embryology and developmental biology*. St. Louis: Mosby.)

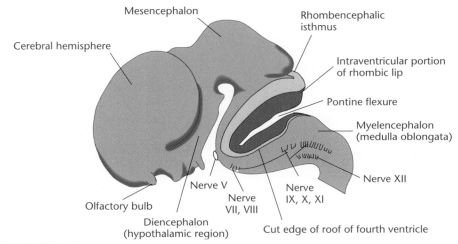

FIGURE **3-27**
Lateral view of the brain vesicles at 8 weeks of development. Note the cranial nerves. (Reprinted from Sadler, T. W. [1985]. *Langman's medical embryology*. Baltimore: Williams & Wilkins.)

shows an 18- to 23-day-old embryo depicting some of these structures.

By the end of the fourth week of development, the neural tube is closed. After closure, an enlarged rostral region develops containing three subdivisions of the brain. The portion of the neural tube cranial to the fourth pair of somites develops into the brain (Fig. 3-27). A narrow region caudal to the fourth pair of somites develops into the primitive spinal cord (Fig. 3-28).

SPINAL CORD

The lateral walls of the developing spinal cord thicken differentially into zones. The marginal zone gradually becomes the white matter of the cord as axons grow

into it. A shallow groove, called the sulcus limitans, develops on the lateral walls of the developing cord. This groove divides the dorsal lamina, or alar plate, from the ventral lamina, or basal plate. The alar plate or dorsal part of the spinal cord is later associated with afferent (sensory) functions and the basal plate or ventral part of the spinal cord with efferent (motor) functions (Fig. 3-29).

Until the third month of development, the spinal cord extends the entire length of the developing vertebral column. At this time the dorsal (sensory) and ventral (motor) roots of the spinal cord extend laterally from the spinal cord and unite in the intervertebral foramina to form the spinal nerves. The vertebral column elongates at a more rapid rate than the spinal cord, thus making the spinal cord shorter than the vertebral column. At birth the end of the cord, called

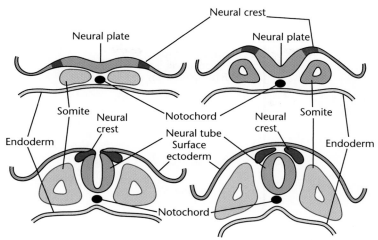

FIGURE **3-28**

Transverse sections showing early stages of spinal cord development. The neural plate, neural groove, and neural tube stages are illustrated. (Reprinted from Brodal, P. [1998]. *The human nervous system* [2nd ed.]. New York: Oxford University Press.)

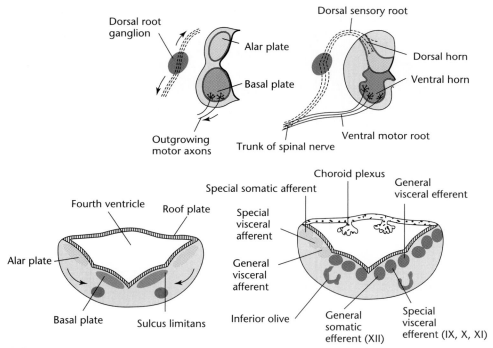

FIGURE **3-29**

Development of the spinal cord (**A**) and brainstem (**B**) showing the relation of the alar and basal plates as they form the sensory and motor nuclei. (Reprinted from Sadler, T. W. [1985]. *Langman's medical embryology*. Baltimore: Williams & Wilkins.)

the conus medullaris, is located at the level of the third lumbar vertebra. In the adult it is located approximately between the first and second lumbar vertebrae. As the differential growth of the two structures takes place, the nerve roots located between the conus medullaris and the intervertebral foramina elongate.

The lumbar, sacral, and coccygeal nerve roots become directed downward at an angle. This elongated bundle of nerve fibers is known as the cauda equinus (horse's tail). A common birth defect in spinal cord embryologic development is known as **spina bifida** (Fig. 3-30).

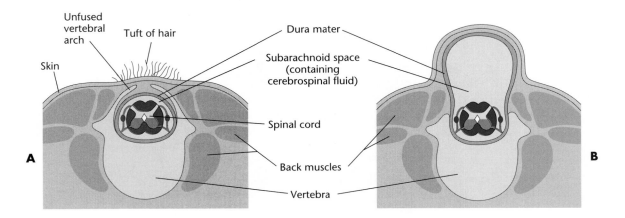

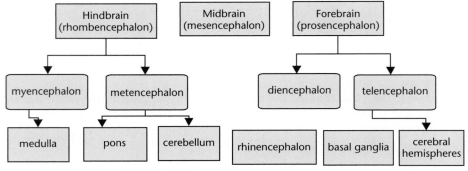

FIGURE **3-30**
Various types of spina bifida. **A**, Spina bifida occulta, with hair growth over the defect.
B, Meningocele. **C**, Myelomeningocele. **D**, Rachischisis. (Reprinted from Carlson, B. M.
[1994]. *Human embryology and developmental biology*. St. Louis: Mosby.)

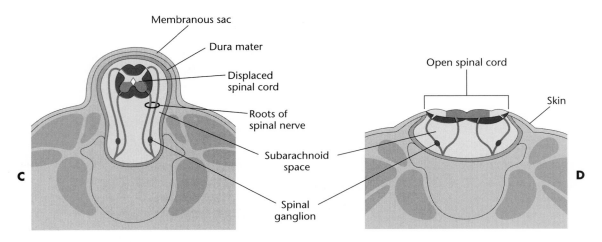

FIGURE **3-31**
Derivates of the three primary brain vesicles.

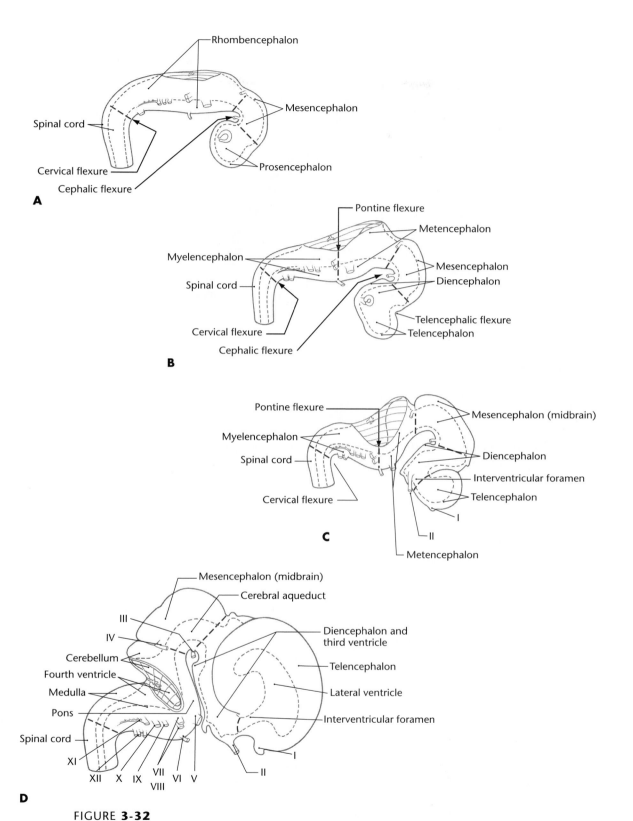

FIGURE **3-32**
Developmental sequence of the brain and head showing cranial nerves. **A**, 4 to 5 weeks of development; **B**, 6 weeks' gestation; **C**, 6½ weeks' gestation; **D**, 8½ weeks' gestation. Ventricles are indicated by *dashed lines* in **A** to **D**; cranial nerves are indicated by Roman numerals. (Reprinted from Haines, D. [2006]. *Fundamental neuroscience* [3rd ed.]. Philadelphia: Churchill Livingstone.)

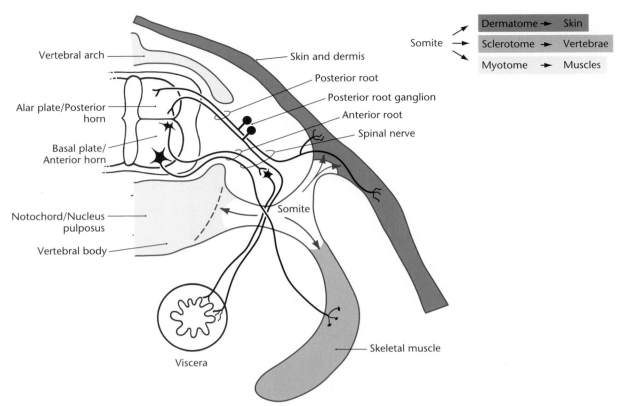

FIGURE 3-33
Derivatives of a somite and the corresponding innervation of structures that originate from the dermatome and myotome. (Reprinted from Haines, D. [2006]. *Fundamental neuroscience* [3rd ed.]. Philadelphia: Churchill Livingstone.)

BRAIN

During the fourth week the neural folds expand and fuse to form three primary brain **vesicles**. These are the **hindbrain**, or **rhombencephalon**; **midbrain**, or **mesencephalon**; and **forebrain**, or **prosencephalon**. The central canal of the neural tube dilates into a rudimentary ventricular system, and in the thin roof of the ventricles the choroid plexus develops to produce CSF. By about the sixth week of development these divisions have further divided, and significant brain development can be noted. The rhombencephalon divides into the myelencephalon, which later becomes the medulla oblongata, and the metencephalon, which is the future pons and cerebellum. The midbrain or mesencephalon does not divide. The prosencephalon divides into the diencephalon and the telencephalon. The diencephalon later becomes the thalamic complex and the third ventricle.

At approximately the third month of development the telencephalon divides into three parts. The rhinencephalon will contain the olfactory lobes. The second division, the striatal area, is the site of the groups of neuronal cell bodies known as the basal ganglia. Only in higher vertebrate and human development does the third division of the telencephalon takes place. This division is the suprastriatal structure called the neopallium. This is what is seen as the cerebral hemispheres and what is called the **cortex**. Figure 3-31 outlines the primary brain vesicles and the ensuing derivational pattern.

The smooth surface of the hemispheres begins to convolute at approximately 20 weeks of gestation, and by week 24 gyri and sulci gradually appear. The first sulcus to appear is the lateral sulcus with its floor, the insula, gradually covered by further development and enfolding. This folding in of the cortical tissue allows this outer layer of neurons to increase greatly, eventually reaching an approximate dimension of 2300 cm^2 without the brain becoming too large for the skull.

The cortex begins to stratify into layers, and at approximately 6 months of gestation the demarcation of the cortex into layers or lamina is present. The allocortex, or archicortex, which is found primarily in the limbic system cortex, is composed for the most part of three layers. The mesocortex is found as transition cortex between the

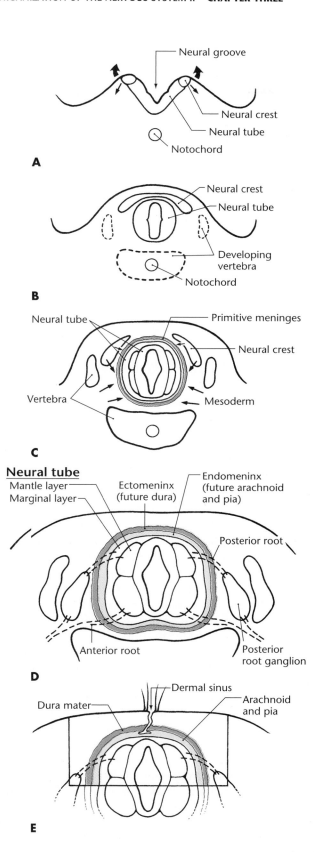

A

B

C

Neural tube

D

E

archicortex and the neocortex. It contains three to six layers and is found in regions such as the insula and the cingulate gyrus. The neocortex, or isocortex, of the cerebral hemispheres is composed of six layers. All six layers can be microscopically differentiated early in development, but the final differentiation of the outer three layers is not complete until middle childhood.

Embryology of the Peripheral Nervous System

The PNS develops mostly from neural cells and is summarized in Box 3-1.

The embryologic development of the neural tube forms the cells that arise from the lateral edge of the neural plate, detach, and move laterally to the neural tube. This neural crest gives rise to most of the PNS, as well as to a number of other structures. This early development of the nervous system is illustrated in Figure 3-25.

The PNS also arises from specialized epidermal cells called placodes that are found in the embryologically developing head region. These cells join neural crest cells, and together placodes and neural crest cells form the ganglia of cranial nerves V, VII, VIII, IX, and X. This embryologic development is shown in Figure 3-32.

The spinal cord develops from caudal portions of the neural tube (see Fig. 3-25). The neural canal of this region becomes the central canal of the spinal cord.

Neuroblasts that give rise to the spinal cord neurons are produced between the fourth and twentieth week of development by a proliferation in the ventricular layer lining the neural canal. These cells migrate peripherally to form four longitudinal plates, which become the gray matter of the spinal cord; a pair of anteriorly located cell masses, which constitute the basal plate; and a pair of posteriorly located masses, which constitute the alar plate. The basal plate develops into the anterior, or ventral, horn of the spinal cord, and the alar plate becomes the posterior, or dorsal, horn of the spinal cord (Fig. 3-33).

FIGURE **3-34**
Development of the meninges. After the neural tube closes (**A** and **B**), cells from the neural crest and mesoderm (**C**, *arrows*) migrate to surround the neural tube and form the primordial of the dura and of the arachnoid and pia (**D**). A dermal sinus (**E**) is a malformation with a channel from the skin into the meninges. (Reprinted from Haines, D. [2006]. *Fundamental neuroscience* [3rd ed.]. Philadelphia: Churchill Livingstone.)

Principal Structures Derived from Neural Crest Cells

Neural Elements

Neurons of:
Posterior root ganglia
Paravertebral (sympathetic chain) ganglia
Prevertebral (preaortic) ganglia
Enteric ganglia
Parasympathetic ganglia of cranial nerves VII, IX, and X
Sensory ganglia of cranial nerves V, VII, VIII, IX, and X*

Nonneural Elements

Schwann cells
Melanocytes
Odontoblasts
Satellite cells of peripheral ganglia
Cartilage of the pharyngeal arches
Ciliary and papillary muscles
Chromaffin cells of the adrenal medulla
Pia and arachnoid of the meninges

Some of the sensory cells in these ganglia arise from placodes.
(From Haines, D. [2006]. *Fundamental neuroscience* [3rd ed.]. Philadelphia: Churchill Livingstone.)

DEVELOPMENT OF THE MENINGES

Embryologically, the meninges develop from the neural crest and the mesoderm, which eventually develop into the CNS. Both the neural crest and the mesoderm form the primitive meninges. Figure 3-34 illustrates the development of the meninges from the neural tube and neural crest.

DEVELOPMENT OF THE VENTRICLES

Embryologically, the ventricle system illustrates brain growth from the neural crest and neural tube. By about the third week of development, the nervous system consists of a tube that is closed at both ends and is somewhat hook shaped. The cavity of this tube, the neural canal, eventually gives rise to the ventricles of the adult brain and the central canal of the spinal cord. Figure 3-35 illustrates the early development of the brain and ventricle system.

CRITICAL PERIODS

The study of abnormal embryonic development is called **teratology**. Teratogens are environmental agents that may induce developmental disruptions after exposure of the mother to these agents during a time when the embryo's organs are forming.[3] Commonly the causes of congenital abnormalities are divided into two categories: (1) genetic factors, such as chromosomal abnormalities, and (2) environmental factors, such as drugs. A fundamental concept of teratology is that certain stages of embryologic development are more vulnerable to teratogens than are other stages. The most critical period for the growth of a particular organ is the period of most rapid cell division for that particular tissue or organ. Thus the critical period varies depending on the organ of concern. For brain development, the most critical period is from 3 to 16 weeks.[3] Major anomalies occur during the third and fourth week as the neural tube and the neural crest form. The fetal period is also quite susceptible to teratogens, such as alcohol, and future cognitive development may be affected, resulting in some degree of mental retardation.

General Principles of Neurologic Organization

Certain fundamental principles of neurologic organization are particularly crucial to the understanding and diagnosis of communication disorders. The following principles will also be built on in later chapters.

CONTRALATERAL MOTOR CONTROL

The first principle to remember is that major movement patterns in human beings have **contralateral** neurologic control in the brain. The arms and legs are represented in the motor strip of the cerebral cortex in a contralateral fashion. In other words, the cerebral hemisphere on one side of the body controls movements of the arm and leg on the other side of the body. This contralateral motor control is brought about by the crossing of the major voluntary motor pathway at the level of the lower brainstem. Auditory and visual sensory systems also have some contralateral organization, a fact that will become clinically important (see Chapters 5 and 6).

If a patient sent to the speech-language pathologist has a severe language disorder and some paralysis of the right arm and leg, these symptoms suggest that the brain lesion causing this motor deficit is probably in the left cerebral hemisphere (Fig. 3-36).

The severe language disturbance accompanying the right limb paralysis serves as a confirming sign of left-sided brain lesion. Why the nervous system provides contralateral motor control of the limbs is not completely known, but the fact illustrates that knowledge of

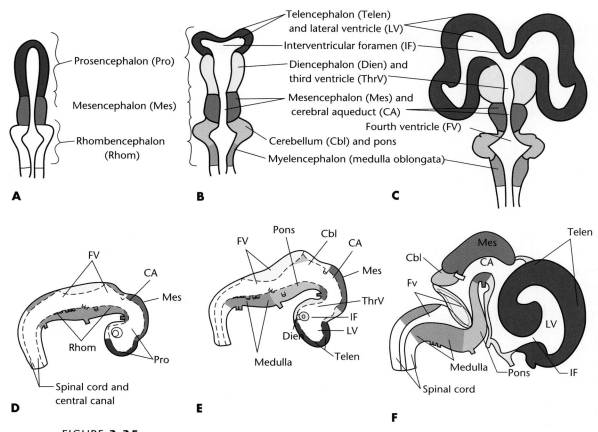

FIGURE 3-35
The early development of the brain and ventricular system, showing how brain growth and the configuration of the ventricles interrelate. Diagrammatic dorsal views (**A** to **C**) correlate in general with lateral views (**D** to **F**) at approximately 5 weeks (**D**), 6 weeks (**E**), and 8½ weeks (**F**) of gestation. The outlines of the ventricles are shown in **D** to **F** as *dashed lines*. (Reprinted from Haines, D. [2006]. *Fundamental neuroscience* [3rd ed.]. Philadelphia: Churchill Livingstone.)

principles of neurologic organization can be used to locate and lateralize causative lesions seen in neurology and speech pathology. Figure 3-37 shows what might happen when a lesion causes either contralateral or, as discussed in the next section, ipsilateral (same side deficit as the lesion) deficits.

IPSILATERAL MOTOR CONTROL

If a lesion occurs in the nervous system below the crossing of the major descending motor pathways, the effect is observed below the level of the lesion on the same side of the body where the lesion occurs. In many spinal cord injuries, paralysis and sensory loss occur below the point of injury. Thus a second important principle is to determine whether effects of lesions are **ipsilateral** or contralateral (see Fig. 3-37). An illustration of how the tongue might deviate ipsilateral to a lesion is shown in

Figure 3-38. In this figure, the tongue is paralyzed on the left side from surgery to remove a lymph node from the left side of the neck, resulting in damage to the hypoglossal nerve fibers on the same side.

BILATERAL SPEECH MOTOR CONTROL

For the most part, the midline muscles of the body in the head, neck, and trunk tend to be represented bilaterally, and the nerve fibers supplying these regions, with certain exceptions, descend from both cerebral hemispheres. This **bilateral** neural control provides smooth, symmetrical movement for those muscles used in speaking: the lips, tongue, soft palate, jaw, abdominal muscles, and diaphragm. The principle of bilateral control of speech muscles suggests that serious involvement of the speech muscles usually results from diseases that affect bilateral neurologic mechanisms. With **unilateral**

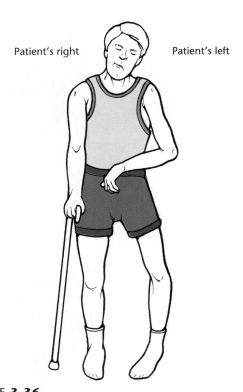

Patient's right   Patient's left

FIGURE 3-36
Patient with a lesion of the internal capsule on the right side. This man exhibits a left hemiparesis, drooping of the lower part of the face on the left, and slight turning of the head to the right (weak right sternocleidomastoid muscle). (Reprinted from Haines, D. [2006]. *Fundamental neuroscience* [3rd ed.]. Philadelphia: Churchill Livingstone.)

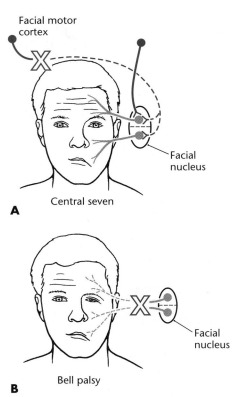

FIGURE 3-37
Illustration of the face after a lesion of the corticobulbar fibers of the facial nerve nucleus (contralateral; **A**) versus a lesion of the root of the facial nerve that causes ipsilateral deviation (**B**). (Reprinted from Haines, D. [2006]. *Fundamental neuroscience* [3rd ed.]. Philadelphia: Churchill Livingstone.)

damage to the nervous system, effects on speech are generally less serious, and compensatory mechanisms are made available from the other side of the midline speech system.

Representation of the body is found in an inverted fashion on the motor areas of the cerebral cortex. Pathways concerned with movements of the lower limbs originate in the upper parts of the motor strip, whereas movements of the head and neck originate at the lower end of the motor strip, just above the sylvian fissure. The area surrounding the left sylvian fissure contains major areas for language processing. The anatomic relations of motor speech areas and language suggest that speech and language disturbances may commonly coexist because of the close proximity of their control areas on the cortex.

An example of bilateral damage effects of motor speech lesions may be seen in spastic dysarthria. When damage to the upper motor neurons occurs, spasticity results. The affected muscles (in this case those

dealing with articulation, respiration, and phonation) indicate an increased resistance to passive movements or movement manipulation. The more rapidly the individual tries to move the articulators (or even an upper or lower extremity, as in cerebral palsy) the greater is the resistance to the movement. In spastic dysarthria, bilateral damage to the upper motor neurons usually is caused by stroke, head trauma, or a degenerative disease (see Chapter 8). The bilateral damage is within both direct activation pathways (corticobulbar and corticospinal tracts) and indirect pathways (extrapyramidal tract). The corticobulbar tract is illustrated in Figure 3-39, and the corticospinal tract is shown in Figure 3-40.

UNILATERAL LANGUAGE MECHANISMS

An impressive facet of cerebral asymmetry is that language mechanisms, for the most part, are unilaterally controlled in the brain, in contrast to the bilateral

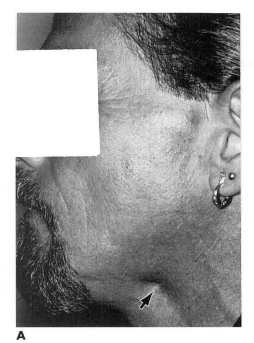

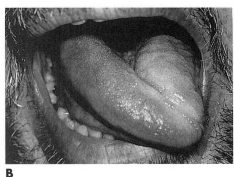

FIGURE 3-38
Paralysis of the tongue on the left side. Removal of a lymph node from the left side of the neck (**A**, *arrow*) inadvertently resulted in damage to peripheral fibers of the hypoglossal nerve on that side. The tongue deviates to the left (side of the lesion) on protrusion (**B**). (Reprinted from Haines, D. [2006]. *Fundamental neuroscience* [3rd ed.]. Philadelphia: Churchill Livingstone.)

speech muscle mechanism. Handedness usually appears between 18 and 48 months of age. Among the adult population, more than 95% of right-handed people have their language mechanisms in the left cerebral hemisphere. Language dominance the world over is primarily in the left brain. Left-handed people are more variable. Some are right brained for language; others have bilateral representation of language. Figure 3-41 illustrates the left hemisphere and its relation to the motor and sensory (receptive) language areas. The obvious clinical principle suggested by these facts

is that major language disturbance is a neurologic sign of left cerebral injury and that the left hemisphere has special anatomic properties for language.

SCHEME OF CORTICAL ORGANIZATION

Students and clinicians should have in mind a general scheme of organization of the cortex because it is the site of most language functions. Although any such scheme is oversimplified and exaggerated, it nevertheless provides a crude but workable framework for conceptualizing functional localization. Later chapters in this text detail the specifics of cortical localization.

The right and left hemispheres may be designated as nonverbal and verbal, and the anterior and posterior portions may be characterized as motor and sensory areas. The central sulcus divides the cerebral hemispheres into anterior and posterior regions. Figure 3-42 provides a lateral view of the cerebral hemisphere, showing lobes and the sensory and motor cortices. In human beings, approximately half of the volume of the cerebral cortex is taken up by the frontal cortex. The frontal lobe contains the primary motor cortex, the premotor cortex, and Broca's area, the primary motor speech association area. In the anterior portion of the frontal lobes are the prefrontal areas, which are generally concerned with behavioral control of both cognitive and emotional functions.

Castro et al[1] described lesions in this area that may produce an "internal agnosia or the inability to communicate with one's limbic system as though suffering from an impairment of the 'sixth sense' that distinguishes appropriate from inappropriate behaviors and right from wrong." Mental shifts become difficult, and perseveration and rigidity are observed, as are a lack of self-awareness and a tendency toward concreteness. In brief, the frontal lobe appears to excel in the control, integration, and regulation of emotional and cognitive behavior. Cortical areas of the left hemisphere that mediate the processing of language are shown in Figure 3-43. Lesions in the inferior frontal lobe may result in **Broca's**, or **expressive, aphasia**, whereas damage to the angular gyrus, the supramarginal gyrus, and the superior temporal gyrus may result in **Wernicke's**, or **receptive, aphasia**.

In contrast, the posterior cortex appears dominated by the control, integration, and regulation of sensory behavior. The defects arising from the posterior cortex are related to the specific sensory association areas implicated by a lesion.

The occipital lobe, as previously noted, contains the primary visual cortex and visual association areas. Deficits in the primary cortex result in blind spots in

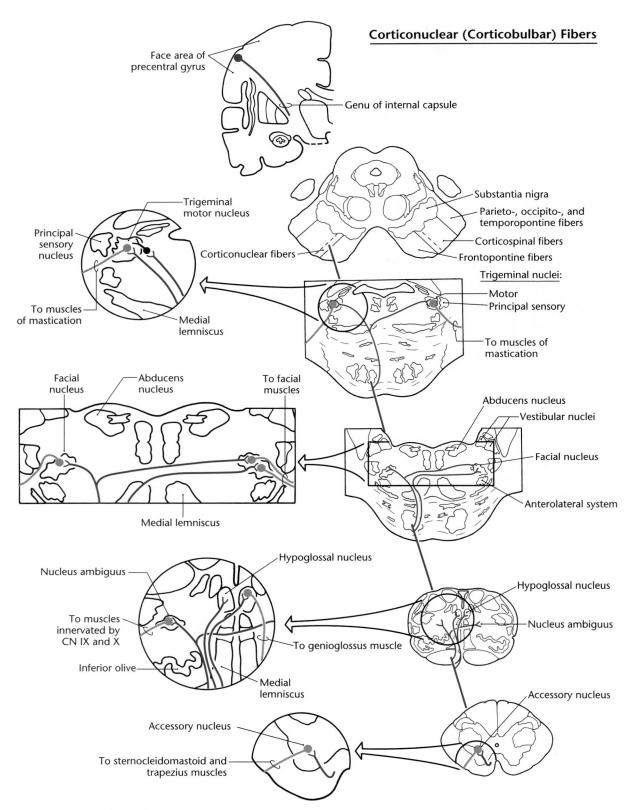

Corticonuclear (Corticobulbar) Fibers

FIGURE **3-39**

The corticonuclear (corticobulbar) system with details shown at the levels of the trigeminal motor, facial motor, hypoglossal and ambiguus, and accessory nuclei. *CN,* Cranial nerve. (Reprinted from Haines, D. [2006]. *Fundamental neuroscience* [3rd ed.]. Philadelphia: Churchill Livingstone.)

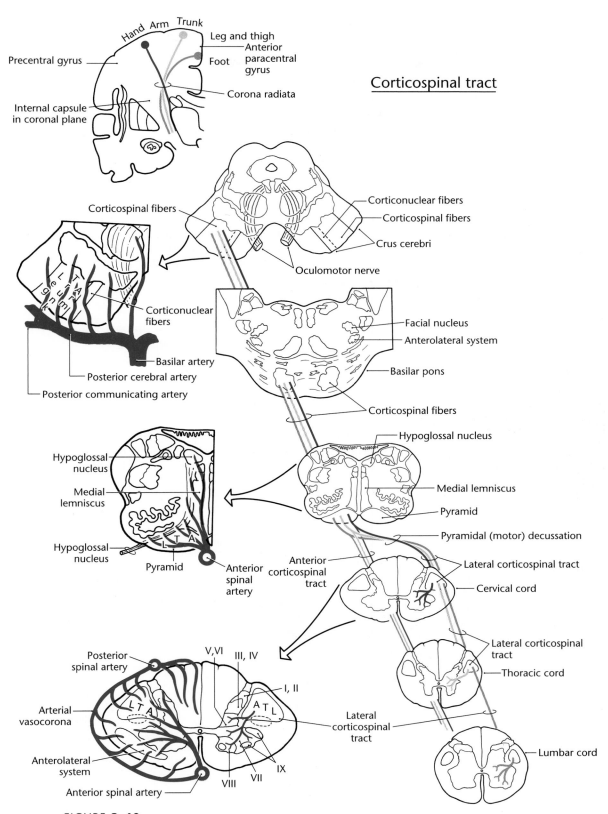

Corticospinal tract

FIGURE **3-40**

The corticospinal system with details showing the blood supply to these fibers in the midbrain, medulla, and spinal cord. (Reprinted from Haines, D. [2006]. *Fundamental neuroscience* [3rd ed.]. Philadelphia: Churchill Livingstone.)

the visual field, and total destruction of the cortex produces complete blindness. Visual imperceptions and agnosias (see Chapter 9) are associated with the visual association areas.

The left parietal lobe is associated with **constructional disturbances** and visuospatial defects. Disorders of recognition, called agnosias, are common. The inferior parietal lobe is concerned with language association tasks, and lesions there cause defects in reading and writing. Contralateral neglect is associated with hemispheric lesions of the nondominant parietal association cortex. Such patients usually neglect stimuli on their left, as illustrated in Figure 3-44. In extreme cases the patient does not recognize the left side of his or her own body, a condition termed asomatognosia. An example is when a patient has a left neglect and ignores the left side when getting dressed or grooming.

The temporal lobe on the left is concerned with hearing and related functions. It contains the primary auditory and auditory association areas. Auditory memory storage and complex auditory perception are among the functions of the temporal lobe. An area known as the speech zone surrounds the sylvian fissure and appears to contain the major components of the language mechanism. Damage in the speech zone produces Wernicke's aphasia (see Fig. 3-43).

With a clinical knowledge of primary sensory and related association areas and behavioral correlates to these areas, the speech-language pathologist is able to infer the approximate location of a lesion from the

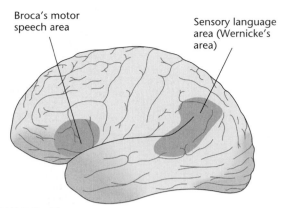

FIGURE **3-41**
Motor and sensory language areas. (Reprinted from Castro, A. Merchut, M.P. Neafsey, E.J., and Wurster, R.D., [2002]. *Neuroscience: An outline approach.* Philadelphia: Mosby.)

patient's behavioral symptoms and to recognize the well-known speech-language syndromes associated with cortical dysfunction. The general clinical principle is that specific cortical deficits can be associated with specific behavioral syndromes.

The organization of the human communication nervous system is fundamental to understand and recall. While studying this text, refer to Appendix 3-1 for a summary figure of the levels and an outline of the most important structures of the CNS.

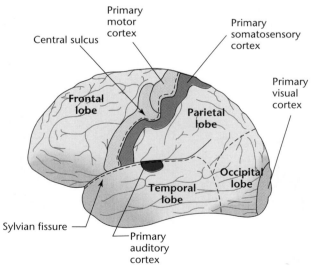

FIGURE **3-42**
Lateral view of the cerebral hemisphere. *Dashed lines* demarcate major lobes. (Reprinted from Castro, A., Merchut, M.P. Neafsey, E.J., Wurster, R.D., [2002]. *Neuroscience: An outline approach.* Philadelphia: Mosby.)

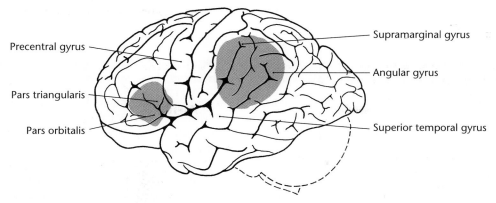

FIGURE **3-43**
Cortical areas that mediate the processing of language. Lesions in the pars orbitalis and pars triangularis of the inferior frontal lobe result in Broca's aphasia, whereas damage in the supramarginal and angular gyri and adjacent superior temporal gyrus results in Wernicke's aphasia. (Reprinted from Haines, D. [2006]. *Fundamental neuroscience* [3rd ed.]. Philadelphia: Churchill Livingstone.)

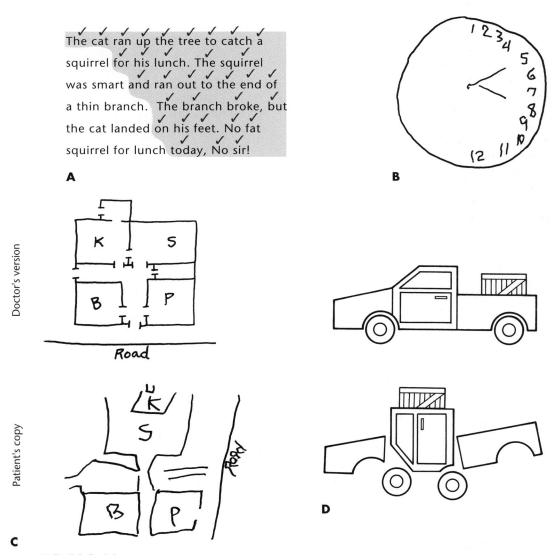

FIGURE **3-44**
Signs (**A** to **D**) of damage to the nondominant parietal association cortex. (Reprinted from Haines, D. [2006]. *Fundamental neuroscience* [3rd ed.]. Philadelphia: Churchill Livingstone.)

Synopsis of Clinical Information or Applications for the Speech-Language Pathologist

- The CNS is the controlling influence for the human communication nervous system.
- The PNS is composed of the cranial nerves, peripheral nerves, and peripheral parts of the autonomic nervous system.
- Mixed nerves carry both sensory and motor fibers.
- Sensory and motor nerves exit at the intervertebral foramina.
- Roots unite to form a spinal nerve, whereas sensory and motor fibers mix.
- A lesion is a damaged area in the brain.
- Injury at the cervical cord (C1-C8) could affect speech production because of respiratory weakness.
- Injury at level C3-C5 could cause cessation of breathing.
- Cord injuries in the caudal portion do not affect speech but would have an effect on language.
- Spinal cord injuries may cause partial or complete loss of function at the level of the lesion.
- Cranial nerves have some relation to the speech, language, and hearing process.
- Seven of the 12 cranial nerves are directly related to speech production.
- Cranial nerves are unprotected and are vulnerable to trauma damage due to their point of exit from the brainstem.
- Some cranial nerves are motor, some are sensory, and some are mixed.
- Cranial nerve I, olfactory: Sensory/afferent; smell
- Cranial nerve II, optic: Sensory/afferent; vision
- Cranial nerve III, oculomotor: Motor/efferent; eye movement
- Cranial nerve IV, trochlear: Motor/efferent; eye
- Cranial nerve V, trigeminal: Mixed; pharynx, mastication, mandible, maxillary, eye, teeth, upper lip, scalp
- Cranial nerve VI, abducens: Motor/efferent; eye
- Cranial nerve VII, facial: Mixed; tongue/taste, oral cavity, facial movement, expression, salivary glands, Bell's palsy
- Cranial nerve VIII, vestibulocochlear: Sensory/afferent; hearing and balance
- Cranial nerve IX, glossopharyngeal: Mixed; gag reflex, swallowing, taste, external ear
- Cranial nerve X, vagus: Mixed; larynx, pharynx, taste buds, heart
- Cranial nerve XI, spinal, accessory: Motor/efferent; sternocleidomastoid muscles, trapezius muscles
- Cranial nerve XII, hypoglossal: Motor/efferent; intrinsic muscles of the tongue, movement, fasciculations, fibrillations of tongue
- The enteric nervous system is part of the autonomic nervous system and controls digestion and deglutition.
- The autonomic nervous system is composed of the sympathetic (flight or fight reaction) and parasympathetic (calming effect of bodily functions) systems.
- The autonomic nervous system involves neural control of smooth and cardiac muscles and gland secretions.
- The autonomic nervous system allows homeostasis to be maintained.
- The brain and spinal cord are protected and covered by meninges and a cushioning layer of tissue from CSF.
- Dura mater is the outermost layer of protection for the brain from rotary displacement.
- Arachnoid mater and subarachnoid space are the middle layer in the meninges; all cranial nerves and cerebral arteries and veins pass through this space.
- Pia mater is the most internal layer of meninges; it adheres to the surface of the brain and contains blood supply.
- The brain has a three-part ventricle system: the lateral (two), third, and fourth ventricles.
- The ventricles are connected by small ducts and canals.
- Each ventricle contains a choroid plexus, which is responsible for the production of CSF.
- CSF is a clear, colorless fluid that cushions the CNS from the surrounding bones and protects against direct trauma.
- CSF helps regulate intracranial pressure, remove waste products, and nourish the nervous tissues.
- Hydrocephalus is a blockage of CSF or failure to absorb CSF.
- Elevated intracranial pressure may also be indicative of a tumor, hemorrhage, meningitis, or encephalitis.
- The brain requires approximately 25% of the body's oxygen.
- Two large internal carotid arteries and two vertebral arteries are the main suppliers of blood to the brain.
- The internal carotid divides into the anterior and middle cerebral arteries.
- The internal carotid also divides into the ophthalmic artery, and the posterior communicating artery, posterior cerebral artery, which are part of the circle of Willis.
- The anterior communicating artery joins anterior cerebral arteries at the circle of Willis.
- The internal carotid supplies much of the cerebral hemisphere.
- The middle cerebral artery is the largest branch of the internal carotid.

Synopsis of Clinical Information or Applications for the Speech-Language Pathologist

- The vertebral artery divides into the meningeal branch, posterior spinal branch, anterior spinal branch, posterior inferior cerebellar artery, and medullary branches.
- The basilar artery divides in the pontine arteries, labyrinthine artery, anterior inferior cerebellar artery, and superior cerebellar artery.
- The circle of Willis is formed by the anastomosis of the two internal carotids with the two vertebral arteries and its branches.
- During embryologic development of the brain, the ectoderm becomes the epidermis and nervous system.
- During embryologic development of the brain, the mesoderm becomes the muscles, connective tissues, cartilage, bone, and blood vessels.
- During embryologic development of the brain, the endoderm becomes the linings of digestive and respiratory tracts.
- The ectoderm thickens and forms a neural plate that gives rise to the CNS.
- Neural folds fuse to form the neural tube, which separates from the ectoderm.
- The neural tube closes by the fourth week.
- The neural crest is formed from the sides of the neural tube to eventually form parts of the PNS and autonomic nervous system, including spinal nerves, cranial nerves, Schwann cells, and cells that form the meninges of the brain and spinal cord.
- At 20 weeks' gestation, the brain begins to convolute from a smooth surface.
- At 24 weeks' gestation, the gyri and sulci are formed.
- The neural crest and mesoderm are primitive meninges.
- Teratology is the study of abnormal embryonic development.
- Teratogens are environmental agents that may induce developmental interruptions after exposure to the mother.
- Genetic factors affecting development include chromosomal abnormalities.
- Environmental teratogens include drugs and chemicals.
- The most critical period for growth of a particular organ is the period of most rapid cell division; critical periods vary depending on the organ.
- The critical period for brain development is from 3 to 16 weeks' gestation.
- Major problems may occur during the third or fourth week as the neural tube and neural crest form.
- Contralateral refers to a lesion affecting the opposite side of the body.
- Ipsilateral refers to a lesion affecting the same side of the body.
- Major movements in human beings have contralateral neurologic control because of fiber decussation (crossing) at the medullary location.
- Left cerebrovascular accident (stroke) results in contralateral (right side) paralysis or paresis (weakness).
- Right cerebrovascular accident (stroke) results in contralateral (left side) paralysis or paresis (weakness).
- If a lesion occurs after decussation, the affected side is ipsilateral.
- Bilateral damage to cortical areas (upper motor neurons) controlling speech musculature results in spastic dysarthria.
- In general, the right hemisphere of the brain governs nonverbal activity and the left hemisphere of the brain governs verbal activity.
- In general, the anterior portions of the brain govern motor activity and posterior portions of the brain govern sensory activity.

REFERENCES

1. Castro, A. J., Merchut, M. P., Neafsey, E. J., & Wurster, R. D. (2002). *Neuroscience: an outline approach.* St. Louis: Mosby.
2. Heimer, L. (1994). *The human brain and spinal cord. Functional neuroanatomy and dissection* (2nd ed.). New York: Springer-Verlag.
3. Moore, K. L., & Persaud, T. V. N. (1993). *Before we are born: Essentials of embryology and birth defects* (4th ed.). Philadelphia: W. B. Saunders.

Appendix 3-1

A vast amount of information is provided in Chapters 2 and 3. Figure 3-45 is a summary drawing of the levels of the CNS to organize the information in Chapter 2. Referring to this figure while reading subsequent chapters will be helpful. An outline of the most important structures discussed in these chapters is also provided for review and organization. For each item, ask the following questions:

- What is it?
- Where is it?
- What does it do?

When appropriate, attempt to label drawings of some of the various structures for which illustrations were used. The effort put into doing this will be rewarded in understanding subsequent chapters.

I. The human nervous system
  A. CNS
    1. Brain
      a. Cerebral hemispheres
        (1) Four lobes
        (2) Fissures
        (3) Sulci
        (4) Gyri
        (5) Association cortex
        (6) Connecting fibers
      b. Basal ganglia
        (1) Corpus striatum
          (a) Caudate nucleus
          (b) Lentiform nucleus: putamen, globus pallidus
        (2) Claustrum
      c. Limbic system
      d. Cerebellum
      e. Brainstem
        (1) Medulla oblongata
          (a) Pyramids
          (b) Olives
          (c) Peduncles
        (2) Pons
        (3) Mesencephalon
          (a) Tectum
          (b) Colliculi
    2. Spinal cord
      a. Spinal nerves
      b. Peripheral nerves
      c. Five regions
    3. Meninges
      a. Dura mater
      b. Arachnoid mater
      c. Pia mater
    4. Ventricles
      a. Choroid plexus
      b. CSF
    5. Blood supply
      a. Internal carotid artery and its branch
      b. Vertebral artery and its branches
      c. Circle of Willis
  B. PNS
    1. Spinal peripheral nerves
      a. Anterior horn cell
      b. Efferent fibers
      c. Afferent fibers

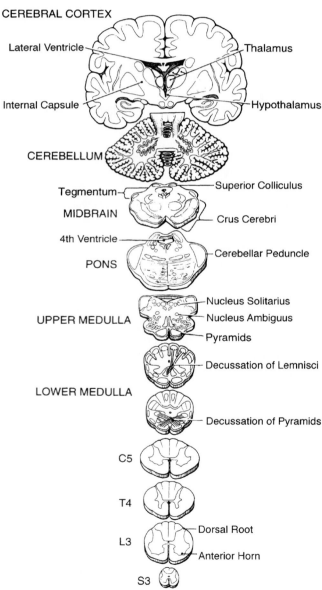

CEREBRAL CORTEX

Lateral Ventricle — Thalamus

Internal Capsule — Hypothalamus

CEREBELLUM

Tegmentum — Superior Colliculus
MIDBRAIN — Crus Cerebri

4th Ventricle
PONS — Cerebellar Peduncle

UPPER MEDULLA — Nucleus Solitarius
— Nucleus Ambiguus
— Pyramids

— Decussation of Lemnisci
LOWER MEDULLA

— Decussation of Pyramids

C5

T4

— Dorsal Root
L3
— Anterior Horn

S3

FIGURE 3-45
The levels of the CNS.

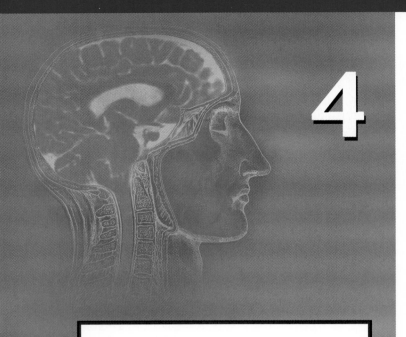

4

Neuronal Function in the Nervous System

But strange that I was not told
That the brain can hold
In a tiny ivory cage
God's heaven and hell.
　　　　Oscar Wilde, *Poems and Fairy Tales of Oscar Wilde*, 1932

KEY**TERMS**

absolute refractory period	motor endplate
action potential (AP)	multipolar cell
adequate stimulus	myasthenia gravis
anastomosis	myelin
anion	necrose
anterograde	neurofilaments
axon	neuron
axonal regeneration	neurotransmitter
axoplasm	orthograde transneuronal atrophy
bipolar cell	osmotic force
bouton	perikaryon
cation	postsynaptic terminal potential
cerebrovascular accident (CVA)	presynaptic terminal
concentration gradient	proximal
convergence	pseudounipolar cell
dendrite	relative refractory period
depolarization	resting potential
distal	retrograde
divergence	retrograde transneuronal degeneration
excitatory postsynaptic potential (EPSP)	saltatory transmission
graded potential	sodium-potassium pump
hyperpolarization	soma
interstitial fluid	synapse
irritability	synaptic cleft
ligand-sensitive channel protein	
microtubules	

CHAPTER**OUTLINE**

Neuronal Physiology
　Neuron
　Chemical and Electrical Properties of Cells
　Ionic Concentration Gradients
　Electrical Forces
Cellular Potential
　Neural Messaging
　Action Potential
　Graded Potentials
　Hyperpolarization
Myelin
　Development of Myelin
　Myelin Disorders
The Synapse
　Neurotransmitters
　Chemical Transmission in the Motor System
Principles of Neuronal Operation
　Degeneration and Regeneration
　　Central nervous system regeneration

Neuronal Physiology

NEURON

The **neuron**, or nerve cell, is the basic anatomic and functional unit of the nervous system, underlying all neural behavior, including speech, language, and hearing. Each neuron consists of a cell body known as a **soma**, or **perikaryon**. These cell bodies actively synthesize proteins, illustrated by the large size of the cell nucleus of diffuse chromatin and at least one nucleolus where RNA is synthesized. In the cell's cytoplasm, ribosomes are abundant and endoplasmic reticulum and Golgi complex are extensive. (Review Figure 2-1 for a refresher of the basic structure of the neuron.)

Neurons vary greatly in size, but most of the billions of neurons of the central nervous system (CNS) are small. Three types of neurons generally are based on cell shape: **multipolar**, **pseudounipolar**, and **bipolar cells**. Figure 4-1 outlines diagrammatically the various types of neurons. Each neuron contains a cell nucleus and one to a dozen projections of varying length. These projections receive stimuli and conduct neural impulses. Those receiving neural stimuli, called **dendrites**, are the shorter and more numerous projections of the nerve cell. The dendrites of a neuron generally are no more than a few millimeters in length.

Dendrites usually branch extensively, giving an appearance similar to a tree branch configuration. The dendrites receive signals from other neurons through the synapse (contacts with other neurons) by specialized receptors. Information travels from **distal** to **proximal** along dendrites to the cell body.

Dendrites sometimes display a variety of extensions called dendritic spines (see Fig. 4-1), usually on the most distal branches of the dendrite "tree." These are usually the sites of the synaptic contacts, forming an **anastomosis**, or connection.

The other process of a neuron is the **axon**, a longer single fiber that conducts nerve impulses away from the neuron to other parts of the nervous system, glands, or muscle (see Fig. 4-1). Axons arise from the cell body at an area called the axon hillock. Axons do not contain ribosomes, which is how scientists distinguish them from dendrites at the ultrastructural level. Axons range in length from several micrometers to more than 2 m. The diameter of individual axons varies greatly, and their conduction velocity ranges from 2 to 100 m/s depending on the fiber size. The larger the diameter, the greater the conduction velocity. In a physiologic sense, the term axon refers to a nerve fiber that conducts impulses away from a nerve cell body. Any long nerve fiber, however, may be referred to as an axon regardless of the direction of the flow of nervous impulses.

The cytoplasm of the axon, called **axoplasm**, contains dense bundles of **microtubules** and **neurofilaments**. Each axon ends at a terminal button, or **bouton**, that corresponds to the points of contact or synapse.

The site at which one axon terminal communicates with another neuron is called the **synapse**. The synapse is usually the point of contact between one neuron (typically the axon of that neuron) with another neuron's cell body, dendrites, or axon. Axonal transport occurs either slowly or fast. If the transport occurs from the cell body toward the axon terminal, it is known as **anterograde**. Transport up the axon from the terminal toward the cell is also possible and is called **retrograde**. Characteristics of axonal transport are outlined in Table 4-1. Figure 4-2 shows anterograde and retrograde axonal transport.

Neurons do the work of the nervous system by transmitting electrical signals or neural impulses to glands, muscles, and other neurons. In the peripheral nervous system (PNS) many neuromuscular (i.e., neuron to muscle fiber) transmissions take place. In the brain itself, most of the neurons conduct neural impulses to other neurons, which are clustered quite close together, providing a high neuronal density in the cerebrum. This high density creates an almost unlimited capacity for complex neuronal activity. This neuronal activity, or brain activation, produces perceptions and thoughts as well as nerve signals for voluntary muscle movement. Activation is the result of rapid biochemical and biophysical changes at the cellular level and in the neurons and glial cells of the brain.[3]

CHEMICAL AND ELECTRICAL PROPERTIES OF CELLS

As discussed in Chapter 2, the neuron is enclosed by a membrane composed of protein channels and a bilipid layer. Water makes up a large percentage of our body (an estimated 55% to 65% of an adult's body weight), and the brain contains more water than many other parts. A well-functioning nervous system depends on an appropriate volume of water content in the cells of the CNS and PNS. Too much water cannot be allowed in the cell, however, or it will swell and its integrity may be compromised. The chemical composition

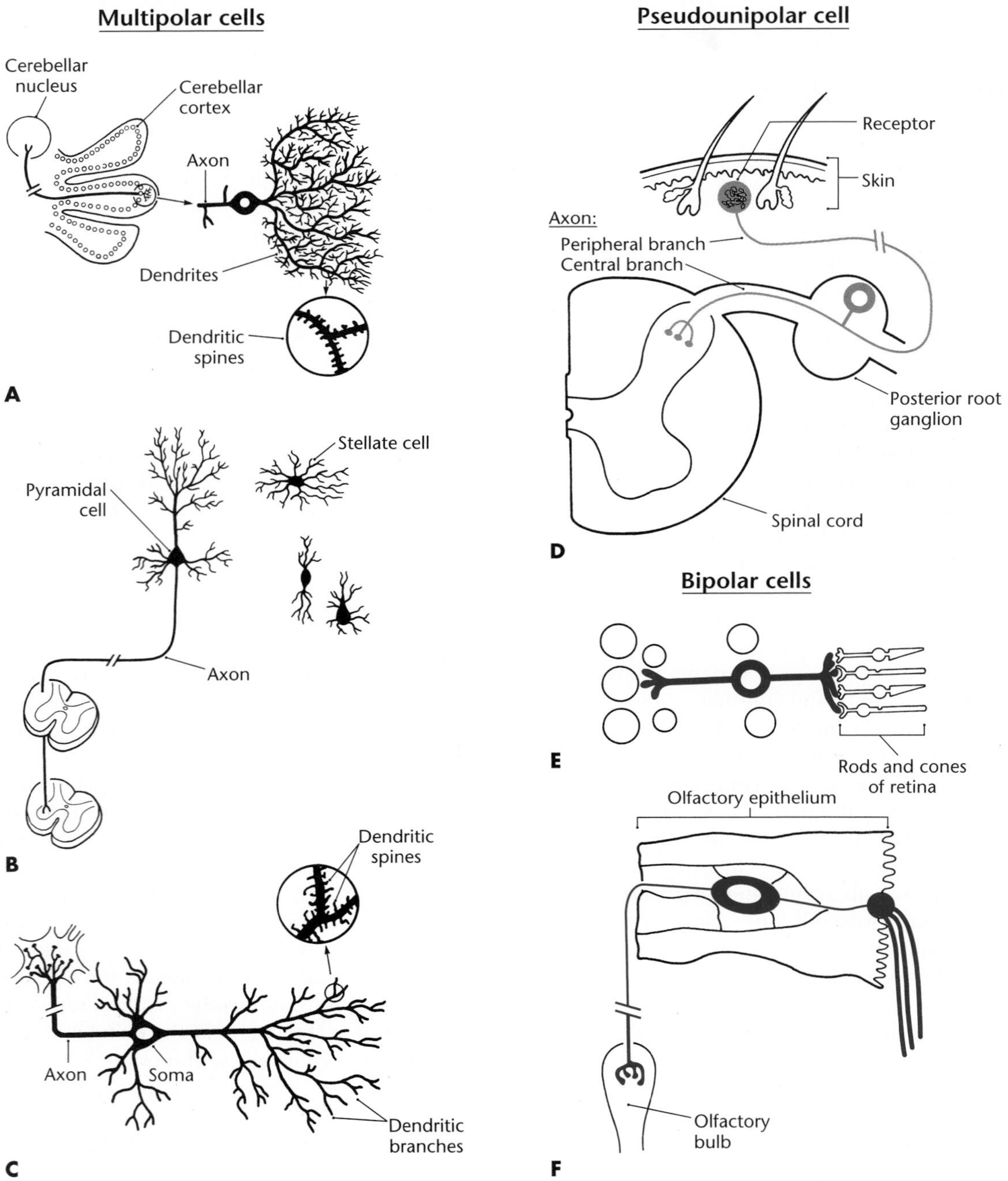

Multipolar cells

A

B

C

Pseudounipolar cell

D

Bipolar cells

E

F

FIGURE **4-1**
Various types of neurons showing the dendrites, somata, and axons of multipolar cells from the cerebellar cortex (**A**) and the cerebral cortex (**B** and **C**). Compare these with a pseudounipolar cell of the posterior root ganglion (**D**) and bipolar cells from the retina (**E**) and olfactory epithelium (**F**). (Reprinted from Haines, D. [2006]. *Fundamental neuroscience* [3rd ed.]. Philadelphia: Churchill Livingstone.)

of the fluid inside and outside the cell membrane of the neuron ensures that this balance will be maintained. This chemical make-up of the intracellular and extracellular fluid also adapts the nervous system for both the chemical (primarily) and electrical signaling that must take place for neural transfer of information to occur. What is this chemical composition?

The membrane of the neuron is permeable to the diffusion of the small molecules that compose water. It is not permeable to large protein ions that make up

TABLE 4-1
Characteristics of Axonal Transport

DIRECTION OF TRANSPORT	SPEED OF TRANSPORT	PROPOSED MECHANISM	SUBSTANCES CARRIED
Anterograde	Fast (100-400 mm/day)	Kinesin/microtubules Neurotransmitters in vesicles, mitochondria	Proteins in vesicles
	Slow (~1 mm/day)	Unknown	Cytoskeletal protein components (actin, myosin, tubulin) Neurotransmitter-related cytosolic enzymes
Retrograde	Fast (50-250 mm/day)	Dynein/microtubules	Macromolecules in vesicles, "old" mitochondria Pinocytotic vesicles from axon terminal

(Reprinted from Haines, D. [2006]. *Fundamental neuroscience* [3rd ed.]. Philadelphia: Churchill Livingstone.)

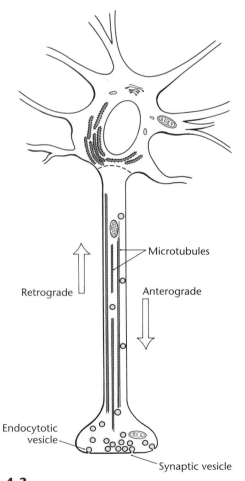

FIGURE **4-2**
Anterograde and retrograde axonal transport. (Reprinted from Haines, D. [2006]. *Fundamental neuroscience* [3rd ed.]. Philadelphia: Churchill Livingstone.)

part of the intracellular fluid of a neuron. These large proteins, carrying a negative electrical charge, displace space that would be taken up by water if they were not there. The fluid in and outside the nerve cell also contains solutions of sodium, potassium, calcium, and chloride. The extracellular fluid (or **interstitial fluid**) bathing the cells of the brain and spinal cord is cerebrospinal fluid, which contains the same chemical ions and a much higher concentration of water than the intracellular fluid. Therefore the fluid inside the cell is said to be less dilute (a lower concentration of water molecules) because of the presence of the large protein molecules, which are not present in the extracellular space. Because the laws governing the movement of fluids along a concentration gradient dictate that fluids normally move from a region of higher concentration to region of lower concentration (movement by **osmotic force**), a mechanism must change the concentration gradient across this permeable membrane to balance the fluid content of a cell by counteracting these osmotic forces. The presence of a high concentration of sodium in the extracellular fluid provides this balance. The membrane of the neuron ordinarily is impermeable to sodium ions; they cannot diffuse across the membrane, although they can be transported through selective channel proteins on the membrane. Because the sodium ions do not easily move across the membrane and they are in very high concentration in the extracellular space, the dilution of the extracellular fluid becomes more like that inside the cell and the concentration gradient is more balanced so that water volume is not excessive.

IONIC CONCENTRATION GRADIENTS

The **concentration gradient** required for the appropriate ion ratio across the membrane is also primarily maintained by channels and pumps in the cell membrane (Fig. 4-3). Channel proteins in the cell membrane consist of water-filled proteins that allow small molecules of a certain ion to pass back and forth depending on the need. The channels are selective to one ion only. Important to neuronal function are sodium, potassium, and chloride channels in the membrane of a neuron. The channels are classified according to the way that they open. Some are nongated; that is, they are always open. Gated channels, on the other hand, open under certain conditions and can close and open quickly. Some channel proteins are voltage gated, meaning that they open and close at specific membrane potentials operated by a voltage sensor mechanism in the protein. Others are chemical or **ligand-sensitive channel proteins** that open or close in the presence of certain chemicals or neurotransmitters. Sometimes opening of these chemical-gated channels depends on depolarization caused by the voltage gating before the chemical can affect an opening.

The pumps in the membrane are also water-filled proteins but open only on one side of the membrane at a time. The **sodium-potassium pump** is the most important

---

BOX 4-1

Key Protein Membrane Channels and Pumps

Channel Proteins

- Allow small molecules to pass back and forth through a membrane; selective to one ion only
- Sodium, potassium, and chloride channels in membrane of neuron important to neuronal function
- Nongated: channels that are always open
- Gated: channels that open and close conditionally and quickly
- Voltage-gated: channels that open and close by voltage-sensitive mechanisms
- Ligand-sensitive: channels that open and close in the presence of chemicals or neurotransmitters

Protein Pumps

- Pumps open one side of a membrane at a time
- Sodium-potassium pump: most important neuronal pump; provides energy to a cell along an electrical gradient powered by positively charged ions (cations) and negatively charged ions (anions)

---

to the neuron, helping maintain the steep gradient of sodium to potassium and providing energy to a cell by increasing sodium transport into the cell. For every two potassium ions that enter through the pump, three sodium ions leave the cell. The concentration of sodium to potassium also plays an important part in the generation of chemical and electrical signals in the nervous system. A summary of membrane channels and pumps is outlined in Box 4-1 and illustrated in Figure 4-3.

ELECTRICAL FORCES

Neurons, like other cells, must exist at a steady state; that is, they must at times be at rest, without communication or action. As previously mentioned, osmotic forces are balanced so that the steady state is partially reached in healthy cells. Electrical forces across a cell membrane also must be balanced so that this steady or resting state can be maintained in all cells at some time. Positively charged ions are called **cations**, and any negatively charged ion is called an **anion**. The sodium, potassium, and chloride ions that make up the solute inside and outside the cell all carry a particular electrical charge. Chloride ions carry a negative charge and sodium and potassium carry a positive charge. Calcium ions are also present and carry two positive charges. Their particular role is discussed later in this chapter.

The intracellular portion of the neuron contains a high concentration of potassium and a low concentration of sodium and chloride in relation to the extracellular fluid. Also remember that large, negatively charged protein anions are found in the intracellular fluid. In the extracellular fluid, no protein anions are present and the concentration of the other ions is reversed. Sodium and chloride are found in high concentrations, approximately 10 times greater than inside the cell, and potassium is found in low concentration. The difference in chemical concentration produces ionic differences across the membrane of the cell. These ionic differences create small electrical potentials across the surface membrane of the neuron and may produce a flow of electrical current.

Cellular Potential

Potential is defined as the relative amount of voltage in an electrical field. Think of the neuron as having two electrical fields, one outside and one inside the cell. The electrical charge within the nerve cell is negative

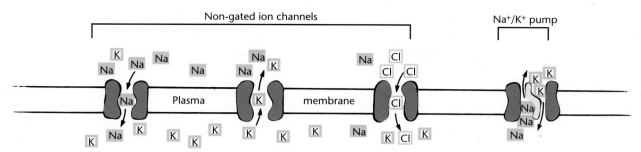

FIGURE **4-3**

All membranes have pumps and channels. Channel proteins have water-filled pores that selectively allow small molecules to pass through the membrane. Illustrated are three variations of these channels that are continuously open: one selective for sodium, one for potassium, and one for chloride. According to the diagrammed concentration gradients, sodium tends to enter the cell and potassium tends to leave the cell, as does chloride. Pumps differ from channels because their water-filled cavity is open to only one side of the membrane at a time. Here the sodium pump is shown first accepting three intracellular sodium ions. After being phosphorylated by adenosine triphosphate, the pump becomes closed to the interior and opens to the exterior, losing its affinity for the sodium ions, which consequently diffuse away. Next, two potassium ions enter the pump, and when the high-energy phosphate group is lost the pump closes to the outside and opens to the inside, losing its affinity for the potassium ions. Consequently, they diffuse away and the cycle is set to begin again. (Reprinted from Haines, D. [2006]. *Fundamental neuroscience* [3rd ed.]. Philadelphia: Churchill Livingstone.)

(dominated by the presence of the protein anions) relative to the outside of the cell (dominated by sodium ions).

The importance of ions to nervous system functioning may be understood through a discussion of their electrical properties and movements. The major functions of neurons, including integration (i.e., cognition or thinking), always depend on their electrical properties and how the ions move. Most of the energy consumed by the nervous system is used for ionic movement. Ion currents are responsible for the creation of electrical events in biologic systems. This occurs through the movements of both positive and negative ions in the opposite direction of each other. The direction of the currents is arbitrarily assigned to the positive and negative ions as they move in opposite directions. During stimulation of some part of the body (e.g., oral mechanism for speaking, brain cells for thinking), negative ions attract positive ions and repel other negative ions; the opposite occurs for a positive ion. Ions move because of voltage gradients (opposite ions attract and same ions repel), chemical gradients, and metabolic activity (sodium and potassium ions expending high-energy phosphates, thus producing what is known as metabolic energy). The sodium-potassium pump allows sodium and potassium to move against their gradient when needed to provide extra energy to a cell.

The ionic difference across the membrane at steady state is called the cell's **resting potential**. At resting potential, the difference in potential, or the separation of electrical charge, across the cell membrane is calculated to be approximately −70 mV. This means that a probe inserted into the cytoplasm inside the cell would find its charge to be 70 mV more negative than the charge measured in the fluid outside the cell. The resting potential is one aspect of the cell's characteristic **irritability**, or ability to respond to outside influences. At the resting potential the cell is not responding to any outside influences and it is not firing an impulse. An **adequate stimulus** is required, one that is capable of changing the cell's potential, to change the resting state. An adequate stimulus may be mechanical, thermal, electrical, or chemical in nature.

NEURAL MESSAGING

What an adequate stimulus may do to the membrane of a neuron is perturb it enough to (1) cause ion channels to open and (2) allow movement of the ions across the cell membrane, effecting a change in the relative charge across the membrane. An influx of the positively charged sodium ions causes a depolarization of the cell. **Depolarization** means that the inside of the cell has become less negative (or more positive) than at rest relative to the outside of the cell. If the change in potential reaches a certain threshold (approximately −55 mV), the stimulus will be adequate enough to cause depolarization at the axon hillock and begin the generation of an **action potential (AP)** down the axon of the cell. The AP is the neural impulse that travels to another cell body, another dendrite, or another cell's axon.

ACTION POTENTIAL

APs are brief electrical transients visible when recorded as intracellular voltages or extracellular currents (Fig. 4-4).[2]

APs occur throughout the body's tissues, regulating secretions of hormones and even signaling fertilization of the egg by the sperm. In a nervous system, APs serve to integrate neural messages sent to cell bodies from sense organs and from other parts of the nervous system. If the neural signal is strong enough to depolarize the receiving cell at the point called the axon hillock, the result will be an electrical impulse, or action current, sent down the axon of that cell.

The action current is propagated along an axon for long distances without a change in the waveform and at a constant velocity. Once an AP is initiated at the axon hillock, a series of these depolarizations along the cell membrane of the axon is begun. This means that all the

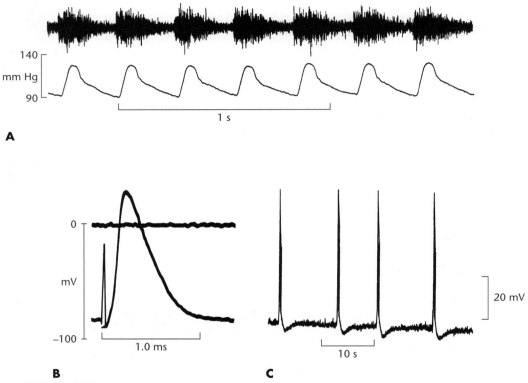

FIGURE **4-4**
APs take many forms. An extracellular recording of a small bundle of baroreceptor afferents (**A**) measures the electrical currents of APs that fire in response to changes in blood pressure, plotted in the lower trace. An intracellular recording from a myelinated nerve axon measures the voltages associated with an AP: a 50-μs electrical stimulus at time zero, the rapid upstroke to a peak voltage greater than 0 mV, and a complete recovery by 1 ms (**B**). Intracellular recordings of APs in most other neurons have complex waveforms, such as hippocampal pyramidal cells that fire a burst of a half-dozen spikes that are terminated with a 1- or 2-second long after hyperpolarization (**C**). (Reprinted from Haines, D. [2006]. *Fundamental neuroscience* [3rd ed.]. Philadelphia: Churchill Livingstone.)

neuronal signals of coded information transmitted along axons in the nervous system are conveyed by a series of uniformly sized impulses. The information transmitted is therefore signaled by the frequency of APs generated rather than by their amplitude. The AP functions in an all-or-nothing manner. A stimulus sets up either a full-sized impulse or nothing.

During the passage of an AP across a nerve cell membrane, that part of the membrane becomes incapable of responding to another stimulus. This period of unresponsiveness is called an **absolute refractory period**. The absolute refractory period is relatively short, lasting approximately 0.8 ms. After the absolute refractory period, an AP initially may be produced by an intense stimulus and then by stimuli of less intensity. The period after the absolute refractory period is called the **relative refractory period**. The absolute refractory period prevents an AP from traveling back up the axon, thus forcing the impulse down the fiber toward the terminal bouton of the axon (Fig. 4-5).

GRADED POTENTIALS

Graded potentials are primarily generated by sensory input, causing a change in the conductance of the membrane of the sensory receptor cell. They also are generated at a localized place on the cell membrane where an excitatory or inhibitory synapse has taken place. Graded potentials (also called local, or generator, potentials), which are excitatory in nature, are generated in the same way an AP is generated at the axon hillock, that is, by the influx of positively charged sodium ions into the intracellular fluid, decreasing the negativity of the charge inside relative to the outside of the cell. If this change in difference across the membrane reaches a certain threshold, a graded potential is generated at a segment of the cell membrane of the neuron or dendrite at which the stimulation occurred; that is, the change in the positive to negative ratio causes a local flow of current.

Unlike an AP, which is an all-or-nothing phenomenon, a graded potential may or may not initiate a series of depolarizations along the membrane; the current may remain more localized with the flow of sodium ions decreasing. A graded potential may decrease in strength the further along the membrane it spreads. If the graded, or generator, potential initially is not strong enough to reach the threshold required for generation of an AP, it likely will decrease by the time it travels along the membrane to the axon hillock and an AP will not be generated at that time. Because of this decrement, graded potentials usually must summate either in time (a number of graded potentials occurring on the cell membrane at once) or in space (a number of graded potentials occurring at the same point on the membrane) to generate a signal strong enough to generate an AP.

HYPERPOLARIZATION

The ionic exchange that takes place as the cell's resting potential is changed may also result in state called

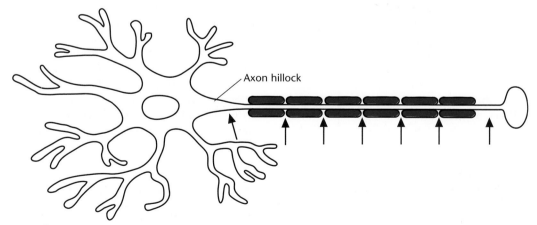

FIGURE **4-5**
A neuron with myelin sheathing of its axon. The interruptions in the myelin sheath are the nodes of Ranvier. The *arrows* indicate regions of high-density, voltage-sensitive sodium channels; current flow; and AP generation. (Reprinted from Nadeau, S., Ferguson, T. S., Valenstein, E., Vierck, C. J., Petruska, J. C., Streit, W. J., & Ritz, L. A. [2004]. *Medical neuroscience*. Philadelphia: Saunders.)

hyperpolarization, in which the likelihood is decreased that an AP will be generated without a much greater stimulus being provided. In this case, the inside of the cell has become more negative relative to the outside of the cell. This occurs because of the influx of chloride anions.

Myelin

Nerve fibers, or axons, may be classified as myelinated or unmyelinated. Large peripheral nerves and the large axons of the CNS acquire a white fatty sheath of wrapping as the brain develops. Layers of **myelin** are incorporated in the cells that produce myelin—oligodendrocytes in the CNS and Schwann cells in the PNS. Myelin is white, contrasting these nerves sharply with the gray unmyelinated nerves, and the myelin sheet is thick. It can be revealed by a special myelin stain. The thick insulation of myelin is interrupted at intervals by structures called the nodes of Ranvier. Because of how the myelin sheaths are designed, they enhance rapid propagation of the electrical impulse along the nerve fiber. The impulse moves along the myelinated fiber by hopping from node to node without any active contribution from the long internodal spaces.

APs develop only at the nodes (see Fig. 4-5). This mode of transmission is extremely efficient compared with the slow gliding along of the nerve impulses on unmyelinated fibers. The type of transmission in myelinated fibers is called **saltatory transmission**. The efficiency of saltatory transmission is achieved because of the insulation that prevents current flow between nodes; in addition, little leakage of current from the fibers occurs. The conduction velocity of a myelinated fiber is directly proportional to the diameter of the fiber, whereas in an unmyelinated fiber the velocity is approximately proportional to the square root of the diameter. On average, transmission along a myelinated fiber is roughly 50 times as fast as one along an unmyelinated fiber.

Unmyelinated fibers are more common in the smaller nerve fibers of the PNS, although the cranial nerves, which are part of the PNS, are relatively large in diameter and are myelinated. Six of the cranial nerves innervate the speech muscles and provide neuromotor control for talking. The rapidity of transmission in these nerves helps supply neural innervation for the rapid muscular movements underlying speech.

DEVELOPMENT OF MYELIN

Myelin is laid down in the nervous system as the brain develops. At birth, the human brain is relatively low in myelin. Most of the pathways that have been formed in prenatal life are unmyelinated, so the gray matter of the cortex is hard to distinguish from the white matter of the subcortical tissue at birth. The major increase in the formation of the myelin lipid sheaths occurs during the first 2 years of life. The development of myelin parallels the development of glia in the brain.

Because the infant brain shows a distinct lack of myelin at birth, its development has frequently been considered a significant index, among several others, of the maturation of the nervous system. Specific attempts have been made to relate major speech and language milestones, such as the appearance of babbling, first words, and word combinations, to the development of myelin in the nervous system. Although a case can be made for a positive relation between communicative milestones and development of myelin, insufficient evidence exists to suggest that delays in the development of myelin are necessarily related to syndromes of speech and language delay. The area of neurologic developmental delays of myelin awaits further research.

MYELIN DISORDERS

In demyelinating disease such as multiple sclerosis, groups of oligodendrocytes and their myelin segments degenerate and are replaced by astrocytic plaques. This loss of myelin results in an interruption of the propagation of the AP. The axons that become demyelinized survive temporarily, and some may even regenerate. But the particular variety of motor, visual, or general sensory losses in multiple sclerosis reflects the location of the demyelization processes. Multiple sclerosis is caused by an autoimmune inflammatory response that damages the myelin sheath. If this inflammatory reaction is intense, the axons, too, may be damaged, producing irreversible neurologic deficits that show irregular fluctuating periods of exacerbation and remission.

Approximately half of the population with multiple sclerosis have speech defects. A speech disorder resulting from involvement of the neuromuscular aspect of the nervous system is called dysarthria. Clinical symptoms of dysarthria are detailed in Chapter 8.

The Synapse

As the electrical nerve impulse, in the form of an AP, moves along an axon, it comes to a point where it must be transmitted to another neuron, a gland, or a muscle. This point is known as a synapse. Until the discovery that small junctures occur at the synapse, researchers assumed that neurons were connected in one continuous network.

Science now knows that between the end of the axon (called the **presynaptic terminal**) and the membrane of the receiving cell (called the **postsynaptic terminal**) is a small space called the **synaptic cleft**.

The transmission of a neural impulse across this synaptic juncture or gap is primarily a chemical process, sometimes an electrical process, and occasionally a combination of both. Electrical synapses are thought to occur infrequently in mammals. When they do occur, it is primarily at gap junctions between dendrites or between two closely adjacent neuron cell bodies. No neurotransmitter is involved, and no delay at the synapse occurs. Thus no modulation of the transmission would be possible. According to Fitzgerald and Folan-Curran,[1] electrical synapses occur to ensure that neurons that must participate in a common activity fire in synchrony. An example of this occurs in the medulla for synchronous discharge during inspiration.

Most neural transmission is carried out through chemical messaging accomplished at the synapse. The transmission of nerve impulses to muscle in the PNS was the first well-established example of chemical synaptic transmission and remains the best understood. Approximately 50 years ago, many neurophysiologists believed that the impulse transmission of one thousandth of a second was too fast for any type of chemical mediation. An electrical nerve impulse was believed to excite the muscle fiber directly. The large electrical mismatch, however, between the tiny nerve fiber and the large muscle fiber indicated that an electrical explanation would be faulty by at least two orders of magnitude. In the 1930s researchers established that synaptic transmission in nerve-to-muscle synapses was entirely attributable to chemical mediation by a substance called acetylcholine.

Neurons primarily communicate with each other by this special type of junction called the synapse. The synapse includes a presynaptic nerve terminal, a postsynaptic nerve, and usually a space between called the synaptic cleft. When a nerve impulse is generated down the axon through the AP, it travels to a point called the terminal bouton. At this point the AP causes opening of special voltage-gated calcium channels, allowing calcium to rush into the nerve terminal. This causes vesicles, called the synaptic vesicles, which contain neurotransmitters, to fuse with the presynaptic membrane and release their neurotransmitter. The chemical released diffuses across the synaptic cleft and binds to specific protein receptors on the postsynaptic membrane. What happens after the binding to the receptor depends on the particular neurotransmitter. Once the neurotransmitter is released, it must be rapidly inactivated so that too much is not released at one time. This inactivation

may occur through action of an enzyme within the synaptic cleft, a mix of reuptake and enzyme action, or a mix of diffusion out of the cleft and reuptake. The steps in neurotransmitter processing are shown in Figure 4-6.

The most frequently used example of neurotransmitter action is that of a neurotransmitter such as glutamate, which is excitatory to the postsynaptic cell. In this kind of transmission (and in many others), the transmitter release changes the potential of the receptor membrane to a receptor potential by opening ionic channels. In an **excitatory postsynaptic potential (EPSP)** the neurotransmitter binds to chemical-gated sodium channel receptors. The conductance of these channels is briefly increased and sodium is allowed to flow into the cell. This partially depolarizes the membrane. If a sufficient number of EPSPs arrive at the membrane in a synchronous fashion, the depolarization is larger in strength. If strong enough, the threshold to open the voltage-gated sodium channels at the axon hillock is reached and an AP is generated. If the EPSP is not strong enough and does not summate, it decreases and an AP is not generated at that time. Figure 4-7 illustrates this sequence.

NEUROTRANSMITTERS

Neurotransmitters are the fundamental basis for chemical action in the nervous system. Table 4-2 illustrates the criteria necessary to define a substance as a neurotransmitter.

Neurotransmitters may have excitatory or inhibitory effects on the postsynaptic membrane, but most serve to modulate the excitability of the neuron. For classification purposes, neurotransmitter specificity also can be used to describe neurons and their axons. For example, cells that contain the neurotransmitter dopamine are called dopaminergic neurons. If they contain glutamate, they are called glutamatergic. Many of these chemical messengers are present in the CNS (Box 4-2).

The majority of chemical signaling within the nervous system is carried on by amino acid neurotransmitters. γ-aminobutyric acid (GABA) and glutamate are the two most prevalent of the neurotransmitters. Glutamate is the major excitatory neurotransmitter in the nervous system, whereas GABA is the major inhibitory neurotransmitter. Neurotransmitters involved in within-system neural modulation modify the actions of other transmitters of neural signals and usually exert their effect within single neural systems. Neuropeptides are the most important of these modulatory neurotransmitters.

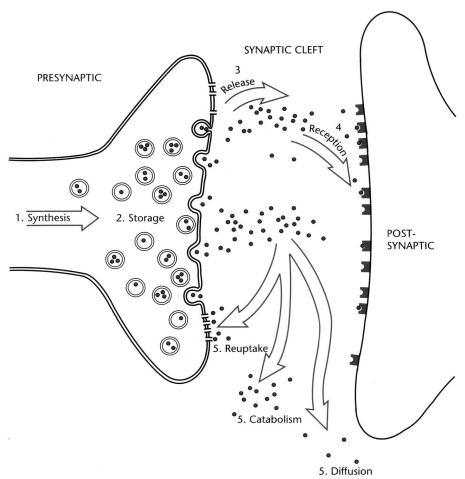

FIGURE **4-6**
The major steps in neurotransmitter processing. (Reprinted from Nadeau, S., Ferguson, T. S., Valenstein, E., Vierck, C. J., Petruska, J. C., Streit, W. J., & Ritz, L. A. [2004]. *Medical neuroscience*. Philadelphia: Saunders/Elsevier.)

Speech-language pathologists and audiologists often are confronted with patients who are diagnosed with disorders of neurotransmitter metabolism. Parkinson's disease results from a decrease in dopamine production in the substantia nigra. The decreased dopamine production accounts for the characteristic tremor and the inability to control movements. Research in Parkinson's disease is striving to determine what triggers the rapid death of the dopaminergic cells.

The original treatment for Parkinson's disease included administration of a form of L-dopa, a precursor of dopamine. This helped the nervous system increase dopamine synthesis, but it did not last long. More current Parkinson's therapy includes a combination of L-dopa with carbidopa because carbidopa cannot cross the blood-brain barrier (see Chapter 2).

Carbidopa decreases L-dopa metabolism in the peripheral tissues, thus making it more readily available for the CNS to increase dopamine synthesis in the healthy neurons that are left.

Patients with seizures experience the effects of abnormal activity of glutamatergic neurons. Because it is an excitatory neurotransmitter, rapid and sustained firing of even a small group of these neurons in one area of the brain may lead to successive excitation of other similar neurons until a region, or in the case of a grand mal seizure, the entire brain, experiences a paroxysmal discharge, which is the seizure activity. Pharmacologic treatment is targeted toward utilization of GABA transmitters to inhibit neural firing. Drugs such as phenobarbital are used for long-term management of seizures.

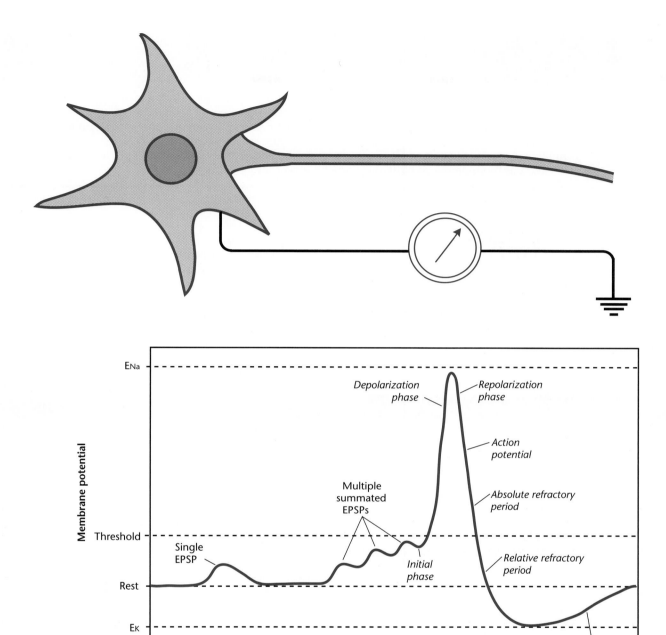

FIGURE **4-7**

Response of the neuron to the release of excitatory neurotransmitter by presynaptic neurons. The membrane potential (ordinate) becomes more positive as the binding of neurotransmitter released by firing of the presynaptic neuron increases sodium permeability through chemical-gated sodium channels, producing an EPSP. One EPSP of exaggerated amplitude is shown, after which sufficient EPSPs occur in quick succession to summate and elicit enough membrane depolarization to open up voltage-sensitive sodium channels. This reaches the threshold of depolarization necessary to generate an AP. The AP is terminated as the various sodium channels are inactivated, and voltage-sensitive potassium channels open and repolarize the membrane and, in this example, actually hyperpolarize it through efflux of potassium through opened potassium channels. (Reprinted from Nadeau, S., Ferguson, T. S., Valenstein, E., Vierck, C. J., Petruska, J. C., Streit, W. J., & Ritz, L. A. [2004]. *Medical neuroscience*. Philadelphia: Saunders/Elsevier.)

TABLE 4-2

What Makes a Chemical Substance a Neurotransmitter?

Localization	A putative neurotransmitter must be localized to the presynaptic elements of an identified synapse and must also be present within the neuron from which the presynaptic terminal arises.
Release	The substance must be shown to be released from the presynaptic element upon activation of that terminal and simultaneously with depolarization of the parent neuron.
Identity	Application of the putative neurotransmitter to the target cells must be shown to produce the same effects as those produced by stimulation of the neurons in question.

(Reprinted from Haines, D. [2006]. *Fundamental neuroscience* [3rd ed.]. Philadelphia: Churchill Livingstone.)

CHEMICAL TRANSMISSION IN THE MOTOR SYSTEM

In peripheral nerve-to-muscle transmission, or neuromuscular transmission, the nerve is known to be a structure on the muscle surface, making contact with the muscle fiber but not fusing with it. A special structural enlargement of the muscle fiber is at the synaptic junction called the **motor endplate**. In the PNS, electrical currents generated by the action of the transmitter substance acetylcholine flow across the synapse to the postsynaptic membrane. In nerve-to-muscle impulses, this is the membrane of the motor endplate. An impulse is then generated along the muscle fiber, which sets off a complex series of events for muscle contraction.

BOX 4-2

Chemical Messengers in the Central Nervous System

Small Molecules

Amino Acids
GABA
Glycine
Glutamate
Aspartate
Homocysteine
Taurine
Biogenic Amines
Acetylcholine
Monoamines
    Catecholamines
        Dopamine
        Norepinephrine
        Epinephrine
    Serotonin
Nucleotides and Nucleosides
Adenosine
Adenosine triphosphate
Other
Nitric oxide

Neuropeptides

Opioid Peptides
Methionine enkephalin
Leucine enkephalin
β-Endorphin
Dynorphin
Neoendorphin
Posterior Pituitary Peptides
Arginine vasopressin
Oxytocin
Tachykinins
Substance P
Kassinin
Neurokinin A
Neurokinin B
Eledoisin
Glucagon-Related Peptides
Vasoactive intestinal peptide
Glucagon
Secretin
Growth hormone–releasing hormone
Pancreatic Polypeptide–Related Peptides
Neuropeptide Y
Other
Somatostatin
Corticotropin-releasing factor
Calcitonin gene-related peptide
Cholecystokinin
Angiotensin II

(Reprinted from Haines, D. [2006]. *Fundamental neuroscience* [3rd ed.]. Philadelphia: Churchill Livingstone.)

Myasthenia gravis is an unusual disorder of neuro-transmitter transmission in the motor system. With this neuromuscular disease, the patient shows muscle weakness on sustained effort. Neuromuscular transmission appears to fail after continuous muscle contraction as a result of reduced availability of acetylcholine at the synapse between nerve and muscle. Antibodies interfere with the transmission of the acetylcholine. These antibodies are an autoimmune disease reaction to postsynaptic receptor protein, with an involvement of the postsynaptic membranes. In the earlier stages, if the muscle is allowed to rest, normal function is restored until further use again depletes the acetylcholine.

The primary symptom of weakness often affects the speech muscles. The nerves innervating the larynx and palate are sometimes the first to be affected by the disease. The weakened vocal folds do not close appropriately, and the voice becomes breathy and weak in intensity. A hypernasal voice quality may develop after sustained speaking because of weakness of the soft palate. As the speech deteriorates, the tongue, lips, and respiratory muscles may be involved. Speech symptoms are discussed further in Chapter 8.

Certain drugs (e.g., neostigmine [Prostigmin] and edrophonium [Tensilon]) temporarily and promptly relieve the symptoms and help the neurologist diagnose the disease. Treatment to reduce the antibodies blocking the acetylcholine transmission is effective in reversing the neuromuscular problem in the muscles of the body, as well as the speech muscles.

Principles of Neuronal Operation

The CNS is constantly bombarded by volleys of sensory nerve impulses. The excitatory and inhibitory influences of the nervous system provide a process of selectivity of impulses for transmission at the level of the synapse. This selectivity of transmission of nerve impulse may be the basic function of the synapse. The synapse also allows transmission in an all-or-nothing manner. In other words, all that can be transmitted is either a full-sized response for the condition of the axon or nothing.

Furthermore, the CNS is characterized by the principle of **divergence**. Charles Sherrington observed that within the human nervous system are numerous branchings of all axons with a great opportunity for wide dispersal of impulses because the impulses discharged by a neuron travel along its branches to activate all its synapses. Thus the CNS is composed of an almost infinite series of sources and routes for widespread or accessory neuronal activity. This accessory neuronal activity forms what may be considered neuronal pools of activity.

A complementary principle of **convergence** exists in the nervous system. This principle, also enumerated by Sherrington, implies that all neurons receive synaptic information from many other neurons, some of an excitatory nature and some of an inhibitory nature. The number of synapses on individual neurons is generally large, measured in hundreds or thousands, with the largest being approximately 80,000. Therefore both excitation and inhibition play a large role in the nervous system.

Principles of divergence and convergence also suggest that, although individual neurons are neither excitatory nor inhibitory, certain neuronal systems primarily act as either excitatory or inhibitory mechanisms for effective overall neuronal functioning. An example is the large excitatory and inhibitory neuronal system in the reticular formation deep within the brain, which both activates and suppresses levels of consciousness during wakefulness and sleep, respectively. Box 4-3 summarizes the principles of divergence and convergence.

The complexity of the neuronal firings and synaptic connections, particularly on the surface of the brain called the cerebral cortex, provides an intricate weaving of impulses into complex spatial and temporal patterns. Sherrington has compared this neuronal activity with the weaving of an enchanted loom. No doubt these ever-changing neuronal designs are the basis for the integrative activity of the nervous system and are the foundations of emotion, thought, language, and action, as well as that most human of behaviors—speaking.

BOX 4-3

Principles of Divergence and Convergence

Divergence
- Branching of all axons within the human nervous system allows activation of all proximate synapses
- Creates limitless pathways for potential neuronal activity
- Allows grouping of neuronal activity: excitation or inhibition

Convergence
- Individual neurons receive multiple signals simultaneously from many other neurons
- Signals from multiple neurons can be conflicting (some that excite and some that inhibit)
- Activation or suppression of an individual neuron is based on these incoming signals

The range of behavior that is assumed to specifically be human, including our rich and complex language system, is sometimes difficult to grasp. Even harder to believe is that this range ultimately can be reduced to and equated with the mere ebb and flow of minute chemical and electrical changes in tiny, but intricate, synaptic mechanisms. This contemporary interpretation of neuronal function, reductionist as it appears, highlights the vast and mysterious frontier between mind and brain that faces the neuroscientist. Despite this great gulf between mind and matter, the speech-language pathologist should remember that this view of neuronal functioning provides the neurophysiologist with a basis for seeing the workings of the brain as a vast abstract complex of neuronal design on the enchanted loom of Sherrington. Despite the sophistication of studying neuronal function, the specifics of the neuronal patterns for understanding and producing language and speech in the brain are unknown.

DEGENERATION AND REGENERATION

Primary neuronal loss refers to the immediate necrotic degeneration of neurons directly affected by, for instance, anoxia, physical trauma, or vascular insult such as a **cerebrovascular accident (CVA)**. Secondary neuronal loss, on the other hand, refers to the degeneration of neurons that occurs hours, days, or weeks after the primary insult. The secondary insult neuronal loss is variable and can have an effect on prognosis. In the case of CVA (stroke), it occurs in the region adjacent to the primary area of infarction. Several variables have an effect on the mechanisms of degeneration. These could include blood flow levels, the integrity of the blood-brain barrier, edema, and inflammation.

In the adult nervous system, neurons that are lost through disease or brain trauma are not replaced, although current research is indicating that the adult brain is capable of much greater cortical reorganization (neuroplasticity) than once thought (see Chapter 10). The adult CNS still contains some stem cells, but neuronal proliferation is a rare event outside the olfactory epithelium and hippocampus. In diseases of the CNS such as Parkinson's or Alzheimer's disease, the neurons die in great numbers, leaving areas of the brain relatively nonfunctional for efficient motor or cognitive functioning. However, if the axons are simply damaged but the cell bodies remain intact, regeneration and return of function are possible in certain circumstances.

Two types of damage may occur in axons. Anterograde degeneration usually accompanies the disintegration of the myelin sheath and depends on the Schwann cells or oligodendrocytes. Retrograde response is characterized by swollen cell bodies, an enlarged nucleus, and the dissolution of endoplasm.

Axonal regeneration most likely occurs in the PNS when a peripheral nerve is either compressed or crushed but not severed and permanently damaged. The injured axon degenerates distal to the lesion and the myelin sheath begins to break up. Monocytes from the blood enter and become macrophages to clean up the debris. The macrophages also signal the Schwann cells to secrete trophic substances to feed and guide the growth of new axonal sprouts. The axonal sprouting begins at the site of injury days to weeks after the injury. If regeneration is to be successful, the sprouting axons must make contact with the Schwann cells of the distal stump. The sprouting axons exhibit swellings on their tips. These swellings are called growth cones. The Schwann cells on the distal stump send out processes toward these growth cones. Regeneration usually proceeds at approximately 5 mm/day in the larger nerve trunks, with growth in the finer branches at approximately 2 mm/day.

If the nerve trunk of a peripheral nerve has been completely severed, spontaneous regeneration is not as successful because the axonal sprouts are not as likely to reach the appropriate distal stump targets. If the proximal axon sprouts fail to make contact, a neuroma may form, with whorls of these regenerating axons trapped in scar tissue at the injury site. Surgical repair of a severed nerve trunk is not usually attempted for a few weeks; delay is desired so that connective sheaths can thicken somewhat to be able to hold sutures better.

Central Nervous System Regeneration

If injury occurs to white matter in the CNS, degeneration distal to the point of injury occurs as it does in the PNS. However, clearance of the debris by the microglial cells and monocytes proceeds quite slowly, with debris found months later. Rather than the chromatolysis, or loss of color, noted in parent cell bodies of peripheral nerves, the neurons in the CNS that are injured tend to **necrose**, or die. Surviving neurons in the area may appear wasted and usually do not make many synaptic contacts. This large-scale death of neurons is caused by a process known as **orthograde transneuronal atrophy**. Neurons of the CNS normally have a trophic effect on each other; that is, they sustain each other. When the main input to a group of neurons is damaged and no longer effective, the whole group is likely to waste away. Sometimes a phenomenon called **retrograde transneuronal degeneration** occurs in neurons upstream to those initially affected by the lesion. Astrocytes may initiate the formation of a glial scar, which replaces the neuronal debris in the case of a small lesion. With a large lesion, cystic cavities containing cerebrospinal fluid and blood may be left.

Animal studies in the laboratory have provided hope that CNS neurons have regenerative capacity because they have shown sprouting of axons and invasion of planted peripheral nerves. Deterrents to spontaneous regeneration, as seen in the PNS, are the glial scar tissue that develops and the growth inhibition caused by breakdown of oligodendrocyte products (unlike the active signaling for growth to the Schwann cells in the PNS). In general the CNS in mammals seems to lack trophic factors required to initiate the significant sprouting of axons. Injured motor and sensory pathways will regenerate only for a few millimeters, and if synapses develop, they are usually on nearby neurons.

At this writing, the most active area of research for provision of trophic factors for regeneration in the CNS is the use of embryonic nervous tissue. Embryonic central neurons have an abundant supply of trophic factors and have been shown to grow well when transplanted into the adult brain. The most successful attempt in human beings at this point has been the transplantation of fetal dopaminergic neurons into the caudate nucleus of patients with Parkinson's disease. In many cases this treatment allowed the patient's drug regimen to be reduced. Current controversy regarding the procurement of stem cell lines for use in research or treatment has slowed the forward progress in this type of neurobiologic research.

Synopsis of Clinical Information or Applications for the Speech-Language Pathologist

- A neuron is a nerve cell that is the basic anatomic and functional unit of the nervous system.
- Neurons have a cell body that synthesizes proteins.
- The three types of neuronal cells are classified by shape: multipolar, pseudounipolar, and bipolar.
- Each cell contains a nucleus and 1 to 12 projections of varying length that receive stimuli and conduct neural impulses.
- Dendrites receive neural stimuli; shorter ones receive signals from other neurons.
- Axons are longer single fibers that conduct nerve impulses away from the neuron to other parts of the nervous system, glands, and muscles.
- A synapse is the point of contact between the axon of one neuron and another neuron's cell body.
- This action produces neuronal activity or brain activation, thus producing perceptions, thoughts, and voluntary muscle movements.
- Cellular potential is the relative amount of voltage in an electrical field.
- Neurons have two electrical fields—one inside and one outside the cell body.
- Functions of neuron integration (thinking or cognition) depends on electrical properties and how the ions move.
- Resting potential is the ionic difference across the membrane at a steady state in the cell.
- AP is the neural impulse that travels to another cell body, dendrite, or axon.
- APs are brief electrical transients visible when recorded.
- APs occur throughout the body's tissues and regulate secretions of hormones and signal fertilization of the egg by the sperm. In a nervous system, APs integrate neural messages from cell bodies from sense organs.
- Nerve fibers, or axons, are either myelinated or unmyelinated.
- Myelin is a white, fatty, lipid substance that surrounds the axon for protection and transmission.
- Myelin in the CNS are oligodendrocytes.
- Myelin in the PNS are Schwann cells.
- Myelin is white, as opposed to the nonmyelinated cells that appear gray.
- Myelin develops as the brain develops from the embryonic state.
- Multiple sclerosis is an autoimmune inflammatory response that damages the myelin sheath; it may cause irreversible damage.
- Dysarthria is a speech disorder found in multiple sclerosis.
- The synapse is the point at which an electrical nerve impulse in the form of an AP must be transmitted to another neuron, gland, or muscle.
- The presynaptic terminal is at the axon sending the impulse.
- The postsynaptic terminal is the receiving area of the receiving axon.
- The synapse between the presynaptic and postsynaptic space, called the synaptic cleft, is transmitted by chemical reaction.
- Chemical substances known as neurotransmitters are released by the presynaptic terminal; they diffuse across the synaptic cleft and bind with receptors in the postsynaptic terminal.

Synopsis of Clinical Information or Applications for the Speech-Language Pathologist—cont'd

- Neurotransmitters provide excitatory action from the presynaptic terminal; to ensure completion of the synapse across the cleft, neurotransmitters also provide an inhibitory action from the postsynaptic terminal.
- Neurotransmitters are the fundamental basis for chemical action in the nervous system.
- Neurotransmitter types are named specifically to describe the neurons and axons that are part of the synapse process.
- The neurotransmitter dopamine has cells called dopaminergic neurons; if the cells contain glutamate, they are called glutamatergic cells.
- GABA and glutamate are the most prevalent neurotransmitters.
- Glutamate is a major excitatory neurotransmitter.
- GABA is a major inhibitory neurotransmitter.
- Disorders of neurotransmitter metabolism include Parkinson's disease, which is caused by a decrease in dopamine in the substantia nigra.
- Myasthenia gravis is a condition caused by reduced acetylcholine at the synapse between nerve and muscle.

- Primary neuronal loss is necrotic degeneration of neurons affected by anoxia or CVA.
- Secondary neuronal loss is degeneration of neurons that occurs within hours, days, or weeks after a primary insult; it may include effects on blood flow, integrity of the blood-brain barrier, edema, and inflammation.
- Neurons in the adult brain that are lost to trauma or disease are not replaced.
- In Parkinson's and Alzheimer's disease, neurons die in large numbers and leave those areas of the brain nonfunctional for motor function or cognition.
- If axons are simply damaged, then regeneration may be possible.
- Axonal damage is categorized as anterograde or retrograde.
- Anterograde damage is disintegration of the myelin sheath that depends on the Schwann cells or oligodendrocytes.
- Retrograde damage is characterized by swollen cell bodies, an enlarged nucleus, and dissolution of endoplasm.
- Large-scale death of neurons is called orthograde transneuronal atrophy.

REFERENCES

1. Fitzgerald, M. J. T., & Folan-Curran, J. (2002). *Clinical neuroanatomy and related neuroscience* (4th ed.). Edinburgh: W. B. Saunders.

2. Haines, D. E. (2006). *Fundamentals of neuroscience* (3rd ed.). St. Louis: Elsevier.

3. Roland, P. E. (1993). *Brain activation.* New York: John Wiley & Sons.

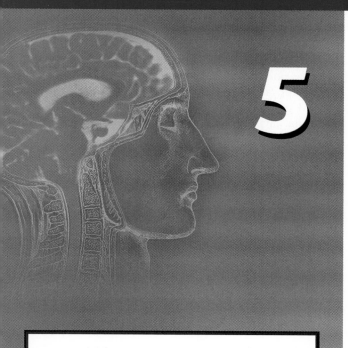

5

Neurosensory Organization of Speech and Hearing

Speech is normally controlled by the ear.
Raymond Carhart, *Hearing and Deafness*, 1947

KEY**TERMS**

analgesia
anterior spinothalamic
  tract
astereognosis
atopognosis
audition
auditory agnosia
auditory brainstem
  responses (ABRs)
cochlear duct
dermatome
dorsal column pathway
endolymph
equilibrium
esthesiometer
exteroceptors
fasciculi
Gerstmann syndrome
helicotrema
hemianopsia
Heschl's gyrus
hyperalgesia
hyperesthesia
hypoalgesia
hypoesthesia
interoceptors
lateral spinothalamic
  tract
masking

mechanicoreceptors
nociceptor
olfaction
optic chiasm
optic disk
organ of Corti
perilymph
peristriate cortex
photoreceptors
proprioception
proprioceptors
Reissner's membrane
Romberg test
scalae
simple receptive field
spinocerebellar
  pathway
splenium
stereocilia
stereognosis
striate cortex
tectal (collicular)
  pathway
tectorial membrane
temporal visual cortex
tonotopic
trigeminal (gasserian)
  ganglion
visual agnosia

Classification

During the nineteenth century, neurophysiologists primarily conceived the execution of skilled motor acts as the result of programming in the motor areas of the cerebral cortex, with some additional influences on the descending motor impulses from cerebellar and extrapyramidal mechanisms. This view of the nervous system was modified during the twentieth century to include the concept of sensory feedback control in motor acts. Audition, of course, plays a special and primary feedback role in the control of speech. More recently, specific efforts have been directed at determining the nature of other neurosensory controls exercised in speaking. Before discussion of sensory control in speech, an understanding of the general types of sensation mediated by the nervous system is necessary.

SHERRINGTON'S SCHEME

Charles Sherrington[10] proposed a classification of sensation that has application for the sensory control of speech. He divided the sensory receptors into three broad classes: exteroceptors, proprioceptors, and interoceptors. **Exteroceptors** mediate sight, sound, smell, and cutaneous sensation. Cutaneous superficial skin sensation includes light touch or pressure, fine touch (also known as two-point or discriminative touch), superficial pain, temperature, itching, and tickling. **Proprioceptors** mediate deep somatic sensation from receptors beneath the skin, in muscles and joints, and in the inner ear. Proprioception includes the senses of

movement, vibration, position, deep pain, and **equilibrium**. **Interoceptors** mediate sensation from the viscera as well as visceral pain and pressure or distention. Pain receptors, either from cellular or tissue injury, are known as **nociceptors**.

Neurophysiologists have classified the senses as special and general. The term special senses reflects the traditional layperson's concept that certain senses are primary. For the neurophysiologist, hearing, vision, taste, smell, and balance are the special senses. The general senses, in this classification scheme, include the remainder of the senses. Further breakdown into visceral and somatic sensations has also been added to the classification schemes. General visceral afferent interoceptors monitor events within the body, including bladder distention and pH changes in the blood. Special visceral afferent receptors are those of taste and smell (**olfaction**). Special somatic afferent receptors are concerned with vision, audition, and balance or equilibrium.

SENSORY ASSOCIATION CORTICES

In Chapter 2 the functional typology of association cortex was discussed, with unimodal and polymodal association cortices found in the sensory processing areas of the brain. Afferent projections of sensory information initially are processed in unimodal cortex found in the primary sensory cortices, including the visual cortex (area 17 along the calcarine fissure), the auditory cortex (areas 41 and 42 in Heschl's gyrus), and the somatosensory cortex (areas 1, 2, and 3 in the postcentral gyrus). Areas around the primary sensory cortices usually are polymodal association cortex. The visual association cortex includes the entire medial surface of the occipital lobe beyond the primary area, the lateral surface of the occipital lobe (areas 18 and 19), the inferior and middle temporal gyri, and the entire inferior surface of the temporal lobe (areas 20, 21, and 37). The auditory association cortices include the areas around Heschl's gyrus and area 22, a portion of the superior temporal gyrus. In the left temporal lobe, area 22, however, is considered more of a supramodal association area than simply a polymodal processor because of the language processing capability.

Recognition and identification or classification of a sensory stimulus is a critical function and can preclude or complicate evaluation of communication skills. Perception of a word requires adequate hearing acuity, but the stimulus must also be recognized to be a word. The features must be visually, audibly, or tactilly perceived before an object can be recognized. Sensory disorders resulting in an inability to interpret a sensory stimulus and recognize it are called agnosias.

The term agnosia was introduced to neurology by Sigmund Freud (1856-1939) in 1891. Agnosia is a disorder of recognition caused by cerebral injury. Classic theory places the lesion responsible for the disorder in the sensory association areas of the cerebral cortex, leaving the primary sensory receptor areas intact. To diagnose the classic disorder correctly, certain precautions must be observed. First, the lesion must be determined to be at the level of the cortical association area rather than at the level of sensory receptor, the sensory pathway, or the primary sensory receptor area in the cortex. Second, unfamiliarity with the test item must be ruled out as a reason for failure to recognize the sensory stimuli. To establish basic knowledge of an item, the patient should match items. If an item can be matched or recognized in other modalities, unfamiliarity can be ruled out as a possible cause for the lack of recognition. The concept of agnosia has been highly criticized in contemporary neurology (see Chapter 9). Although true agnosias are not common, some patients in clinical practice appear to demonstrate a tactile, visual, or auditory agnosia. Table 5-1 defines the various types of agnosias that may be seen in a clinical practice specializing in neurobehavioral disorders.

TABLE 5-1
Agnosias

TYPE OF AGNOSIA	CHARACTERISTICS
Agnosia	A disorder of recognition caused by damage to cortical sensory association areas or pathways
Visual agnosia	Inability to recognize objects, colors, and pictures
Auditory agnosia	Inability to comprehend speech or nonspeech sounds (pure forms: auditory nonverbal agnosia, and pure word deafness)
Tactile syndrome	Inability to recognize objects by touch; characterized by bilateral parietal lobe lesions
Gerstmann syndrome	Includes finger agnosia, right-left disorientation, acalculia, and agraphia; usually characterized by left parietal lobe lesions

Anatomy of Sensation

SOMATIC SENSATION

The neuroanatomy of the senses is complex. The general somatic sensory pathways—those dealing with bodily sensation—use the spinal cord and spinal nerves. Sensation to the head and vocal mechanism—larynx, pharynx, soft palate, and tongue—use the cranial nerve pathways.

The pathways of somatic sensation generally are composed of a three-neuron pathway from the periphery to the cerebral cortex. Some variation exists within this three-neuron organization for the sensations of light touch, pain, temperature, and proprioception. For most bodily sensations carried to the brain through spinal nerves, the first-order, or prime, neuron is found on the dorsal or posterior spinal root in a mass known as a spinal ganglion. For instance, the superficial sensations of light touch, pain, and temperature begin in special receptors in the skin and are transmitted by spinal nerves to the spinal cord through the spinal ganglion. From the first-order neuron, an axon ascends or descends one or two spinal segments, traveling in a tract called Lissauer's tract, or the dorsolateral fasciculus. It then synapses on the second-order neuron in the dorsal gray column of the spinal cord. Fibers of the second-order neuron then cross the midline, and an axon ascends to the third-order neuron in the ventral posterolateral nucleus of the thalamus. A general name for the tract formed by the axon of the second-order neuron is lemniscus.

Lateral Spinothalamic Tract

The crossed ascending sensory pathway in the spinal cord, known as the **lateral spinothalamic tract**, transmits the sensations of pain and temperature and perhaps itch (Fig. 5-1). The fibers enter the cord through the spinal root ganglion, travel up or down a few segments in Lissauer's tract, and end in the dorsal root of the gray matter. At this point the first-order neuron synapses with the second-order neuron and promptly crosses to the other side of the spinal cord. There the fibers enter the lateral white column or the lateral spinothalamic tract and ascend to the ventral posterior lateral nucleus in the thalamus. The axons of the lateral spinothalamic tract synapse with a third-order neuron that leaves the thalamus, ascends in the internal capsule, and reaches the postcentral cortical gyri in the parietal lobe (areas 3, 1, and 2). This is the primary somatic sensory area of the brain, and pain and temperature sensations as well as pressure and touch are interpreted here.

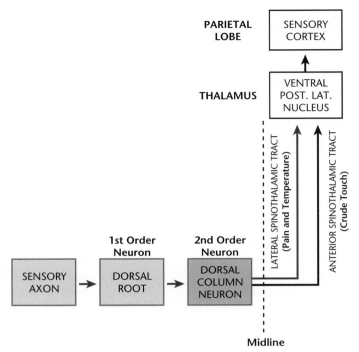

FIGURE 5-1
Flowchart depicting the lateral spinothalamic tract, which mediates pain and temperature, and the anterior spinothalamic tract, which mediates light or crude touch. *POST.,* Posterior; *LAT.,* lateral.

Anterior Spinothalamic Tract

Approximately 10% of the spinothalamic fibers are sometimes separated in anatomical texts and presented to be fibers of the **anterior spinothalamic tract**. Mentions of the spinothalamic tract, spinal lemniscus, or the anterolateral system all refer to the combined lateral and anterior tracts. The anterior (or ventral) spinothalamic tract carries sensory information of light touch, including light pressure and touch and tactile location (see Fig. 5-1). The light touch fibers synapse within the dorsal gray horn cells in the spinal cord and ascend in the anterior spinothalamic tract to the brainstem and the posterior ventral nucleus of the midbrain. The tract also ends in the postcentral gyrus of the parietal lobe.

Other fibers are given off as the spinothalamic tract ascends. These terminate on the reticular nuclei in the brainstem; fibers from the nuclei then project to the thalamus, hypothalamus, and hippocampus. Somatic and visceral responses to pain, such as changes in respiration and heartbeat as well as nausea and fainting, are mediated through descending fibers from these structures.

Damage to the spinothalamic tracts of pain and temperature usually result in loss to the opposite side of the body. The fibers of light touch take two routes, one ipsilateral and one contralateral. The ipsilateral fibers ascend with the proprioceptive fibers in the dorsal columns, and the crossed fibers ascend in the spinothalamic tract. The fibers of light touch branch extensively; because of this branching, touch is unlikely to be abolished by injury to a specific pathway in the spinal cord.

Proprioception Pathways

Proprioception, two-point discrimination, vibration, and form perception follow different pathways than do those of the spinothalamic tracts. Proprioception is the sense of knowing exactly where body parts are in space and in relation to one another. Two-point discrimination allows two adjacent points on the skin to be distinguished. Two-point sensitivity varies over the brain surface. The lips and fingertips are the most sensitive and the back the least sensitive. Vibratory sensation allows the recognition of vibration from touch. Form perception allows recognition of objects by touch alone. Table 5-2 summarizes the human proprioceptive pathways.

Spinocerebellar Tract

Proprioception is conveyed by fibers from muscle tendons and joints and takes two major routes after entering the spinal cord. One of these major pathways is the

TABLE 5-2 **Human Proprioceptive Pathways**	
PATHWAY	DESCRIPTION
Proprioception	Allows temporal and spatial comprehension among body parts
Two-point discrimination	Cognition of adjacent points on dermis
Vibratory sensation	Sensory pathway to detect vibrations by touch
Form perception	Recognition of objects by touch

spinocerebellar pathway and the other is the **dorsal column pathway**.

The spinocerebellar pathways are of lesser importance in human neurology because of the poor localizing information available about these tracts. The spinocerebellar pathway has two tracts, dorsal and ventral. These tracts arise from the posterior and medial gray matter of the cord. The dorsal tract ascends ipsilaterally, but the ventral tract crosses in the cord. Both tracts terminate in the cerebellum and allow proprioceptive impulses from all parts of the body to be integrated in the cerebellum. The spinocerebellar pathway has been proposed to function in unconscious perception of already-learned motor patterns.

Dorsal Columns

Conscious proprioception, two-point discrimination, and form perception have been called the sensory modalities of the dorsal, or posterior, columns of the spinal cord. The first-order neuron of the posterior column pathway can be found in the dorsal root ganglion (Fig. 5-2). The axon of the first-order neuron enters the spinal cord and ascends to the medulla aggregately as the dorsal white columns. However, two fiber bundles, or **fasciculi**, comprise these columns. Axons entering the cord at the sacral and lumbar regions, which mediate proprioception from the leg and lower body, travel in the fasciculus gracilis, which comprises the medial dorsal column. Axons from the thoracic and cervical regions, generally related to the arm and upper body, travel in the fasciculus cuneatus, comprising the lateral dorsal columns. These first-order neuron axons terminate in the nucleus gracilis and nucleus cuneatus in the medulla. The second-order neuron axons then cross over to the other side of the medulla, where they form a bundle called the medial lemniscus. Fibers of the medial lemniscus ascend to the third-order neuron in the ventral posterior nucleus of the thalamus and then proceed to the somatosensory cortex in the parietal lobe.

PROPRIOCEPTIVE DEFICITS

Damage to the postcentral gyrus of the parietal lobe, the dorsal columns, or the dorsal root ganglion may produce a loss of proprioception, astereognosis, loss of vibratory sense, and loss of two-point discrimination in the trunk or extremities. If damage to these dorsal column fibers occurs below the level of the medulla, the loss in proprioception is on the same side of the injury. Damage above the level of the medulla produces a loss in proprioception on the opposite side of the body.

Sensory Examination

The neurologist uses several traditional and standard procedures for determining sensory loss. These are incorporated into the standard neurologic examination (see Appendix C).

The senses of light touch, pain, and temperature are mediated by the fibers of the dorsal root of the spinal cord, which come from a circumscribed area of the skin known as a **dermatome**. In peripheral nerve injuries, impairment of touch corresponds to dermatomal zones; however, at the boundary of each segmental dermatome is an overlap area supplied by the adjacent segmental nerves. For instance, if the fifth thoracic nerve (T5) is severed, T3 and T6 will carry many of the pain and temperature sensations supplied by T5. This segmental overlap also is present in the spinal cord. Thus overlap is greater for pain and temperature than for touch.

LIGHT TOUCH

The sense of light touch is tested by determining the patient's ability to perceive light stroking of the skin with a wisp of cotton. Disorders of the sensory pathways from skin to cortex show abnormal sensory reactions. Decreased tactile sensation is called **hypoesthesia**, and complete loss of sensation is called anesthesia. Abnormally increased tactile sensation is known as **hyperesthesia**.

Inability to localize touch is called **atopognosis**. Topagnosia is tested by touching the patient's body. With the eyes closed, the patient is asked to point to the spot where touch occurred. The neurologist compares similar areas on both sides of the body. Atopognosia usually is associated with a lesion of the parietal lobe.

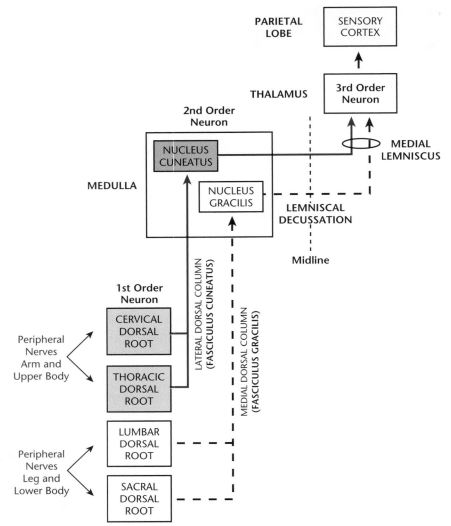

FIGURE **5-2**
Flowchart of pathways mediating proprioception. The pathways are known as the dorsal column modalities.

TWO-POINT DISCRIMINATION

Two-point discrimination, or the ability to discriminate the shortest distance between two tactile points on the skin, is sometimes tested with points of a caliper. Right and left sides of the body are compared. Loss of discrimination suggests a parietal lobe lesion.

Double stimulation may also be used to determine a cortical sensory disorder. Two simultaneous tactile stimulations are presented to both sides of the body in similar areas or to different areas. Lateralized sensory loss can then be determined. Sensory pathway or cortical sensory losses frequently accompany lesions that produce cerebral language disorders.

PAIN AND TEMPERATURE

Pain and temperature disturbance are more likely to be sensory pathway disorders, and lesions of the ventral and lateral spinothalamic tracts may be present. Pain perception is lost on the side contralateral to the lesion. Pain is tested by the ability to perceive a pinprick or deep pressure. Increased pain, or tenderness, is called **hyperalgesia**. A diminished sense of pain is **hypoalgesia**, and a complete lack of pain sensibility is **analgesia**.

Temperature disturbances are tested by the ability to distinguish between warm and cold. For this test, the neurologist usually asks the patient to identify a test tube of warm water and one of cold water.

RECOGNITION OF LIMB POSITION

The patient with proprioceptive deficits may not be able to determine, without looking, whether a joint of an arm, hand or leg is in flexion or extension, and may have difficulty identifying the direction of displacement of limbs or digits during movement.

STEREOGNOSIS

Stereognosis is the ability to perceive the weight, form, and other details of a body by touch. **Astereognosis** is the inability to recognize common objects, such as coins, keys, and small blocks, by touch. The examiner has the patient close his or her eyes and then places various objects in the person's hand, first one and then another, to be identified.

If this recognition disorder is caused by a cortical sensory lesion rather than a dorsal column proprioceptive lesion, it is called tactile agnosia. A lesion in the right somesthetic association area or in the corpus callosum may produce a true tactile agnosia in the right hand. Beauvois et al[1] have reported a syndrome, which they named bilateral tactile aphasia, in a bilaterally damaged patient. This aphasia is analogous to the auditory and visual agnosia disorders. The patient was unable to name objects by touching them but could give the name when hearing the sound an object made. In this disorder, the lesion is presumed to be in both parietal lobes.

VIBRATORY SENSIBILITY TEST

The sensation evoked when a vibrating tuning fork is applied to the base of a bony prominence is lost with dorsal column problems. The patient cannot differentiate a vibrating tuning fork from a silent one on bony surfaces.

BODY SWAY TEST

This test, called the **Romberg test**, requires the patient to stand with the feet together. The neurologist notes the amount of sway with the patient's eyes open and compares it with the amount of sway with the eyes closed. An abnormal accentuation of swaying with the eyes closed or actual loss of balance is called a positive Romberg sign. The visual sense can compensate for this loss of proprioception of muscle and joint position if it is caused by a dorsal column disorder, so the patient may correct balance problems by opening his or her eyes. If the lesion is in the cerebellum rather than the dorsal columns, the cerebellar ataxia of balance will not be corrected by visual compensation, as is the case in the sensory ataxia of the dorsal column.

Neuroanatomy of Oral Sensation

The neuroanatomy of oral sensation is different from that of the trunk and extremities in that the cranial and oral sensations are mediated by the cranial nerves, as opposed to mediation by the spinal nerves, as in bodily sensations. The sensory innervation of the speech mechanism is summarized in Table 5-3. Of particular importance to oral sensation is the trigeminal nerve (cranial nerve V). This cranial nerve is the primary somatic sensory nerve for the skin of the face, the anterior portion of the scalp, the anterior two thirds of the tongue, the teeth, and the outer surface of the eardrum. It mediates the sensations of pain, temperature, touch, pressure, and proprioception for the oral and cranial regions.

The glossopharyngeal nerve (cranial nerve IX), which is primarily sensory, also plays a role in mediating general somatic sensation in the cranial and oral regions. It mediates sensation from the posterior third

TABLE 5-3

Sensory Innervation of the Speech Mechanism

STRUCTURE	CRANIAL NERVE	FUNCTION
Face	V	Pain, temperature, touch to face
	VII	Proprioception to face
Tongue	V	Touch to anterior two thirds
	IX	Touch to posterior third
Palate	IX	Sensory to soft palate
Pharynx	IX	Sensory to lateral and posterior pharyngeal walls
	X	Sensory to lower two thirds of pharynx (forms pharyngeal plexus with cranial nerve IX)
Larynx	X	Sensory to most of the laryngeal muscles

of the tongue, the palatopharyngeal mucosa, and the external ear.

SENSORY PATHWAY OF CRANIAL NERVE V

In studying the spinal pathways for sensation, it is logical to separate the pathways for pain and temperature and the pathways for touch and pressure. This general model of the pathways for sensation is similar, with minor variations, for both the oral-cranial regions as well as the body and extremities. As Table 5-3 shows, cranial nerve V mediates pain and temperature for the face and touch from the face and the anterior tongue.

Pain and temperature receptors in the skin and mucous membranes in the face project to the neural cell bodies of the **trigeminal** or **gasserian ganglion**. This ganglion in the face is analogous to the dorsal root ganglion of the spinal nerves. The gasserian or trigeminal ganglia are called first-order neurons. Axons from the ganglion enter the pons and become a fiber bundle called the descending tract of cranial nerve V. The descending tract may sometimes reach the upper cervical region of the spinal cord. Fibers enter the adjacent spinal nucleus of cranial nerve V and synapse with second-order neurons. These axons cross over to the contralateral side on leaving the nucleus. Those contralateral fibers, called the secondary trigeminothalamic tract, then ascend to the level of the thalamus. From the thalamus, third-order neuron axons pass into the internal capsule and finally terminate in the primary somatosensory cortex in the postcentral gyrus of the parietal lobe.

The pressure and touch pathways of cranial nerve V have the same general organizational plan as the pain and temperature pathways. First-order neurons are the cell bodies of the gasserian or trigeminal ganglion. The axons of the cell bodies terminate in the main sensory nucleus of the trigeminal nucleus complex in the pons. The trigeminal nucleus complex is a large collection of cells in the brainstem extending from the midbrain to the medulla. The complex also includes the mesencephalic nucleus and the spinal nucleus of cranial nerve V. Second-order neurons of the pressure and touch pathway of cranial nerve V reach the thalamus via the secondary ascending tract of cranial nerve V found within the medial lemniscus. Fibers travel both ipsilaterally and contralaterally, unlike the pain and temperature pathways of nerve V. The third-order neurons are the relay fibers from the thalamus to the postcentral gyrus of the cerebrum.

The contralateral pathway organization of pain and temperature and the bilateral organization of pressure and touch can be observed clinically if a unilateral sensory cortex lesion is present. The patient incurs no major loss of touch or pressure from the face but loses pain and temperature sensations on the side of the face contralateral to the lesion.

Proprioceptive pathways of cranial nerve V are composed largely of fibers from the muscles of mastication and the temporomandibular joint. The primary afferents enter at the pons and synapse on the first-order neurons, the cell bodies of the mesencephalic nucleus, which are located in the midbrain. These primary sensory neurons are unique in the central nervous system because they are the only ones whose cell bodies are inside the central nervous system. Because they are first-order neurons, they do not synapse in the nucleus. Most of the processes from these first-order neurons descend through the tegmentum of the pons and synapse onto the motor nucleus of cranial nerve V. This enables initiation of stretch reflexes for the muscles of mastication.

SENSORY PATHWAY OF CRANIAL NERVE IX

The glossopharyngeal nerve primarily is a sensory nerve mediating sensation from the oropharynx, tonsils, faucial pillars, posterior third of the tongue, and the mucosa of the soft palate and the upper third of the pharynx. The glossopharyngeal nerve has its first-order neuron in the ganglion of cranial nerve IX (petrosal ganglion). Fibers pass from the ganglion to the nucleus tractus solitarius in the medulla. The route of the second-order neuron, the ascending central pathway to the thalamus, is not precisely known but probably involves many fibers projecting to the reticular formation, with additional fibers terminating in the thalamus. The path of the third-order neuron to the cortex is likewise unknown.

In summary, the sensory pathway plan in the orofacial region, like the rest of the body, involves a sensory ganglion close to the primary sensory receptors. This is a first-order neuron. A second-order neuron is the pathway to the thalamus, and a third-order neuron projects from the thalamus to the primary sensory cortex in the parietal lobe.

Oral Sensory Receptors

Sensory receptors in the oral region and respiratory system generally are excited by chemical or mechanical stimulation. Taste, of course, is based on chemical stimulation. **Mechanicoreceptors** respond when stimuli distort them. For instance, the tongue touching the teeth, alveolar ridge, or palate compresses mechanicoreceptors, and the receptors in turn generate electrical impulses to the fibers.

The tongue mucosa and the tongue surface in particular are served by many different types of mechanicoreceptors. The endings in these receptors have been divided into diffuse, or free, endings and compact, or organized, endings. Some speech experts believe that free endings provide a general sense of touch in sensory control of speech articulation and that organized endings provide sensitive acuity in speech articulation.

ORAL PROPRIOCEPTORS

In addition to receptors in the mucosa of the oral region, receptors are present in the oral muscles themselves, in the joints of the jaw, and in the membranes of the teeth. The receptors in the temporomandibular muscles, the pterygoids, the masseter, and the temporalis, place stretch on the joint.

The periodontal receptors are fine filaments in the teeth that are responsive to extremely slight touch on the teeth. The pressure sense of these receptors is quite sensitive and no doubt plays a role in sensory control of articulation.

STUDYING ORAL SENSATION

The role of the tactile receptors in the oral region has been widely studied in the speech science laboratory since the 1980s. Two-point discrimination for tactile sensation is assessed by speech scientists with an instrument called an **esthesiometer**. Subjects are asked to discriminate whether there are one or two points on the surface of the tongue. Healthy individuals can separate two points on the tongue tip when the points are only 1 to 2 mm apart. The sensitivity of the tongue tip is extremely delicate, but the back of the tongue and the lateral margins are less sensitive. Differences of less than 1 cm cannot be clearly distinguished at these points.

To determine the significance of tactile sensation in the sensory control of speech, the technique of nerve block has been used. An anesthetic, usually lidocaine, is injected into the branches of the trigeminal nerve. Tactile sensation of the tongue is mediated by the lingual branch of cranial nerve V (Fig. 5-3). Nerve block techniques have resulted in some distortion of the articulation of speech, but for the most part speech remains intelligible. The consonants /s/ and /z/ are frequently distorted with tongue anesthetization.

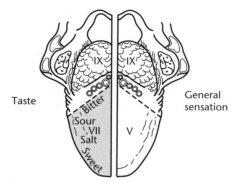

FIGURE **5-3**
Cranial nerve sensory innervation for mediation of taste and general sensation for the tongue.

SENSORY CONTROL MODALITIES

The sensory recognition abilities of the tongue raise the question of the relative significance of the various sensory control mechanisms in speech production. Intuitively, audition appears to be the most powerful sensory mechanism controlling speech. If a person misspeaks, as in uttering a "slip of the tongue," the person often hears the error and corrects it. Additionally, congenitally deaf individuals, who do not hear their speech, show deviations in articulation and voice. Under certain conditions, hearing one's own speech provides a strong sensory control. But individuals who have developed normal speech and then lose their hearing do not immediately show articulation and vocal deviations. Persons with acquired deafness rely on sensory mechanisms other than audition to control most of their speech performance. For many speech sounds, the average auditory processes that provide feedback occur too late to be of help in ongoing speech. Where the tactile sensory receptors of the tongue have been interfered with by nerve block of the trigeminal nerve, the addition of auditory **masking** does not increase the articulation error scores significantly.

Tremblay et al[11] tested the adaptation of subjects to a mechanical load that altered jaw movement, and thus somatosensory feedback, but had no perceptible or measurable effect on the acoustic output. Over time, the subjects corrected for the effect of the mechanical load, showing a dissociation of somatosensory and auditory feedback. This study supports the hypothesis that targeted somatosensory inputs associated with articulatory positions may be a speech movement goal in the nervous system independent of the auditory signal. The possible importance of somatosensory feedback calls into question whether strategies in treatment to enhance this feedback in training of speech production, especially for individuals who are deaf, should be given more attention in addition to the usual emphasis on auditory training. Orosensory testing has not been widely used by neurologists or speech-language pathologists. More refined methods are needed. Issues surrounding these aspects of speech physiology and their disorders are still primarily relegated to laboratory studies.

SPEECH PROPRIOCEPTION

According to Sherrington's classification,[10] proprioception refers to sensory receptors within the body itself. Most critical for speech are the muscle spindles, which are encapsulated structures within striated muscle, including muscles of the speech mechanism. Muscle spindles serve as the primary afferent proprioceptor within striated muscle. The distribution of muscle spindles varies considerably within the speech musculature. Muscle spindles are found in all intercostal muscles. Kent[6] summarized research of muscle fiber types and spindle receptors in craniofacial muscles. Interarytenoids of the larynx have been found to have spindles, and spindles are abundant in one quadrant of the thyroarytenoid, the primary adductor, but sparse in other parts of it. The muscles that elevate the jaw have abundant spindles, whereas the depressors have many fewer. The facial muscles, including the lips, have very few. Spindles have been shown to be present in the palatal muscles, the tensor veli palatine, the levator veli palatine, and the palatoglossus. The tongue, the primary articulator for speech, appears to have muscle spindles present in both extrinsic and intrinsic muscles. Key musculature found with muscle spindles for oromotor functions can be found in Box 5-1.

BOX 5-1

Muscle Spindle Location in Oromotor Function

Arytenoids: Abundant spindles found in interarytenoids but only in one quadrant of the thyroarytenoid

Jaw muscles: Jaw elevators include large quantities of muscle spindles, whereas depressors have far fewer

Facial muscles: Very few muscle spindles

Palatal muscles: Spindles found in tensor veli palatine, levator veli palatine, and palatoglossus

Tongue: Both extrinsic and intrinsic tongue muscles include spindles

---

In summary, the oromotor mechanism is richly endowed with exteroceptors and proprioceptors for control of the neuromuscular activity of speech, but no single type of sensory input is superior to another in the control of speech muscles. Different types of articulation probably demand different types of sensory feedback. Alveolar stops, for instance, may use primarily tactile sensation, whereas articulations with no contact, such as back vowels, may use auditory and proprioceptive feedback.

Visual System

RETINA

The visual system processes and decodes a wealth of information, more than any other afferent system in the body. To begin this processing, the eye absorbs the light from an image and passes it through the pupil. The image is then passed into the lens, where it is reversed and inverted. The lens focuses and projects the light onto the retina, which is a light-sensitive 10-layer formation of nerve cells lining the inside of the eyeball. The retina is composed of two types of **photoreceptors** (rods and cones) and four types of neurons (bipolar cells, ganglion cells, horizontal cells, and amacrine cells). Rods play a special role in peripheral vision and in vision under low light. Cones, on the other hand, function under bright light and are responsible for discriminative vision and color detection. The rods and cones synapse with the first-order neurons, the bipolar cells. These cells in turn synapse with the ganglion cells, which are second-order neurons. The axons of these cells converge to leave the eye within the optic nerve. After leaving the eye the axons acquire myelin sheaths.

This series of transmissions from first- to third-order sensory neurons is modified by horizontal cells and amacrine cells. They essentially sharpen the response of the ganglion cells to certain formations of light.

PATH OF THE OPTIC NERVE

The point of exit for the optic nerve is called the **optic disk**, which can be seen through an ophthalmoscope. Because rods and cones do not overlay the optic disk, it is essentially a small blind spot in each eye. The area on the retina for central fixated vision during good light is the macula. A small central pit in the macula called the fovea centralis is composed of closely packed cones, and vision here is sharpest and color vision most acute.

The optic nerve conveys visual impulses. It consists of approximately 1 million nerve fibers, which course through the optic canal of the skull to form the

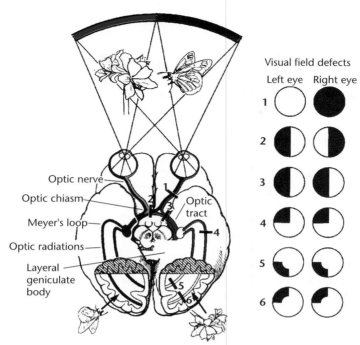

FIGURE **5-4**
Visual pathways with lesion sites and resulting visual field defects. The occipital lobe has been cut away to show the medial aspect and the calcarine sulci.

optic chiasm (Fig. 5-4). The fibers from the retina of each eye originate from two different areas on each retina. The retinal fibers can be thought of as exiting either as temporal fibers, which come from the lateral half of the retina nearest the temple, or as nasal fibers, which originate from the lateral half nearest the nose. As Figure 5-4 shows, at the optic chiasm the nasal fibers from each eye decussate while the temporal fibers continue ipsilaterally. This shift makes stereoscopic three-dimensional vision possible.

Figure 5-4 shows that the optics of the eye are such that the temporal half of one retina and the nasal half of the other retina receive information from the same half of the visual field. In other words, the temporal fibers of the left retina and the nasal fibers of the right retina carry information from the right half of the visual field, and the temporal fibers of the right retina and the nasal fibers of the left retina receive information from the left side of the visual field. Because of the decussation of the nasal fibers at the optic chiasm, all the information from the contralateral side of the visual field travels in one pathway down the optic tract to the visual cortex. The visual cortex in the left hemisphere receives information about the contralateral right side of the visual field, whereas the right hemisphere processes information from the left visual field. This information is critical to understanding how a visual field deficit occurs after brain injury.

After passing the point of the optic chiasm, most of the axons forming the optic tract course to the lateral geniculate body, which is a small swelling located under the pulvinar of the thalamus. They then pass through the internal capsule and around the lateral ventricle, curving posteriorly. Some fibers travel far over the temporal horn of the lateral ventricle and form what is called the temporal loop, or Meyer's loop (see Fig. 5-4). These fibers terminate in the visual cortex below the calcarine sulcus. Meyer's loop carries fibers representing the upper part of the central visual field. Other optic fibers travel from the lateral geniculate body to the visual cortex above the calcarine sulcus. These fibers represent the lower part of the central visual field.

Some retinal ganglion cells terminate in the superior colliculus of the midbrain. The superior colliculus also receives synapses from the visual cortex. Fibers from the superior colliculus project to the spinal cord through the tectospinal tracts. These tracts control reflex movements of the head, neck, and eyes in response to visual stimuli.

PRIMARY VISUAL CORTEX

The characteristics of neurons in the visual cortex and the responses of individual cells have been studied in a wide variety of experimental animals. Scientists are interested in how patterns are perceived and recognized by the eye. Hubel and Wiesel,[5] among others, have found many different types of receptive fields in the neurons of the visual cortex. These receptive fields are termed simple, complex, hypercomplex, and higher order hypercomplex. **Simple receptive field** cells respond to a slit of light of particular width, slant or orientation and place on the retina. Complex receptive fields respond to slit-shaped stimuli over a large area of the retina rather than a specific place. For hypercomplex fields, the line stimulus must be of a certain length. Cells with higher order hypercomplex fields require more elaborate visual stimuli to respond.

The visual cortex is organized in columns of cells with similar properties. Some columns respond only to one eye and are monocular. Others respond to both eyes and are binocular. Because the eyes are located in different positions on the head, a difference of position exists on the retinas for a stimulus, giving binocular disparity to the columnar cells. This provides information about the depth of objects.

In addition to the primary visual pathways, two other major visual pathways can be distinguished: the **tectal**, or **collicular, pathway** and the pretectal nuclei pathway. Thus fibers from the optic tracts do not all go to the lateral geniculate body. Some of them project to the subcortical pretectal nuclei and ascend to the thalamus and out from there to various regions of the cortex. This system seems to be important in the control of certain visual reflexes, such as the pupillary reflex, and certain eye movements.

The tectal, or collicular, pathway projects to the superior colliculi in the brainstem and to the thalamus and out to many regions of the cortex. The superior colliculi also receive input from somatosensory and auditory systems. The tectal pathway seems to be involved in a major way in the ability to orient toward and follow a visual stimulus.

The visual pathways do not operate independently. They are interconnected at every level from retina to cortex, and each receives descending input from the cerebral cortex, providing for the richness of visual perception.

VISUAL ASSOCIATION CORTEX

The area surrounding the **striate cortex**, the **peristriate cortex** (Brodmann's areas 18 and 19), is composed of neurons that have firing properties much like those of the primary visual cortex; however, these neurons also tend to show regional specialization for analyzing more complex aspects of visual stimuli such as motion, color, and form. Anatomists have been able to identify at least

five different regions of this peristriate area, each with a different processing role.

The second major part of the visual association cortex is the **temporal visual cortex** located within the middle and inferior temporal areas. This association area receives input from the peristriate cortex and has four major cortical output pathways: (1) to the contralateral temporal visual area, (2) to the prefrontal cortical area, (3) to the ipsilateral posterior association cortex of the superior temporal area, and (4) to the paralimbic and limbic areas of the medial temporal lobe. As with other neurons in primary and secondary visual cortex, neurons in the temporal visual association areas are sensitive to properties of the visual stimulus such as wavelength, size, length, and movement. These neurons, however, also seem to trigger in response to specific objects, including faces. Thus this part of the visual system may extract complex features from visual stimuli so that neurons become responsive to individual patterns rather than to isolated stimulus features. This may provide the mechanism for object discrimination. Box 5-2 outlines the two different cortices associated with vision.

VISUAL INTEGRATION

As Mesulam[7] points out, object recognition or identification requires interaction between the visual representation in the association areas and other components of

---

BOX 5-2

Cortical Output Regions and Pathways for Vision Association

Peristriate Cortex

- Consists of five different regions, each having a different role in processing visual stimuli.
- Includes neurons that function as those of the primary visual cortex *and* show regional specialization for analyzing complex stimuli.

Temporal Visual Cortex

Consists of cortical output pathways to the following four areas:

1. Contralateral temporal visual area
2. Prefrontal cortical area
3. Ipsilateral posterior association cortex of the superior temporal area
4. Paralimbic and limbic areas of the medial temporal lobe

- Neurons trigger in response to specific objects and individual patterns
- May play key role in object discrimination

mental operation, including integration with past experience. This process requires relay of information from these temporal visual association areas to paralimbic and limbic areas of the brain.

Damage to the association areas in the peristriate cortex or temporal lobes or to their connections to other parts of the brain may have a number of different effects on visual processing. Mesulam lists the following four consequences as possibilities:

1. Impaired specialized visual processing and impaired formation of visual templates
2. Loss of visual templates previously formed
3. Disconnection of visual-auditory, visual-motor, visual-somatosensory, and visual-verbal pathways caused by interruption of input from the visual association areas to the frontal and parietal association areas
4. Interruption of pathways providing input to paralimbic and limbic structures from the visual association area

Lesions in the peristriate areas have been noted to cause specific disorders such as difficulty with color vision or movement perception, yet they cause no disturbance to other visual functions. In 1982, Mishkin and Ungerleider,[8] scientists at the National Institutes of Health, published a study discussing two cortical pathways separating the function of object perception and recognition from location and movement perception. Nadeau et al[9] refer to these as the "what" and "where" systems in vision. This differentiation of visual processing capabilities begins at the retina, with rod and cone receptors projecting to both pathways. The "where" system allows visually guided hand and eye movements, permitting individuals to direct the eyes at what they want to look at and coordinate the touching or capture of a desired object with a part of the body. The "where" pathway is described as beginning in the occipital cortex and extending dorsally and medially into the parietal cortex (Fig. 5-5).

The "what" system is critical because it allows perception and recognition of objects located anywhere in the visual field; that is, independent of location, the abstract features of an object can be perceived and recognized. The pathway for this system begins in the occipital cortex and extends ventrally along the inferior temporal cortex, progressing into anterior areas of that cortex (see Fig. 5-5). With anterior progression, neurologic responsiveness of the visual receptive fields increases both in the number of neurons responding and the complexity of the stimulus features that generate a response. As Mesulam implies, a point exists at which what is seen is paired with what is already known, and the stimulus can be recognized in many different

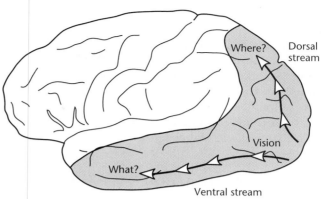

FIGURE 5-5
Dorsal and ventral parallel processing streams shown emerging from the primary visual cortex in the occipital lobe. The dorsal stream, directed toward the parietal lobe, processes where the stimulus is, its direction of movement, and its speed of movement. The ventral stream, directed toward the temporal lobe, processes stimulus shape, what the stimulus is, and what it is called. (From Castro, A. et al. [2002]. *Neuroscience: An outline approach.* Philadelphia: Mosby/Elsevier.)

orientations and backgrounds. Lesions in this pathway may result in impairment of object recognition or a visual agnosia.

VISUAL AGNOSIA

Analyzed in disconnection terms, classical **visual agnosia** is produced when visual associations are lost because of a disconnection of the visual areas from the language area. Also known as associative visual agnosia, the condition results in difficulty in recognizing pictures and objects along with a surprisingly good ability to describe, copy, and match visual stimuli. Patients correctly name the stimulus after tactile or auditory presentation. Bilateral occipital lobe lesions with extension on one side or the other into the medial temporal lobe involving the hippocampus have been found on autopsy. With such lesions both the naming and the memory of objects presented visually are affected.

Visual agnosia may also result from unilateral lesions. With destruction of the left visual cortex in addition to a lesion of the **splenium** of the corpus callosum, or extensive involvement of the white matter of the association cortex of the left occipital and parietal lobes, a unilateral left visual agnosia may result.

Benson[2] observed that in the few cases of visual agnosia reported, associated findings are common. These may include **hemianopsia** and prosopagnosia, a visual agnosia for faces. In addition, other associated disorders include constructional impairment, alexia without agraphia, amnesia, and some degree of anomia. A color-naming deficit may also be present; this inability to match seen colors to their spoken names is called color agnosia by Benson[2] and color anomia by Geschwind.[4] Lesions in the calcarine fissure and splenium are usually present. These lesions, according to Geschwind, disconnect the right visual cortex from the left language areas.

Central Auditory Nervous System

A major aspect of speech and language function depends on audition. **Audition** generally is classified as one of the special senses and as an exteroceptive sense. Knowledge of the neurologic functions of the central auditory pathways is crucial for an understanding of the mechanisms of the communication nervous system.

Before discussing the specific levels of the central auditory pathway, a review of how sound is transmitted to the inner ear and the auditory nerve, cranial nerve VIII, is warranted. The physical signal known as sound undergoes a series of complex transformations for it to be heard. These transformations begin when a mechanical disturbance causes molecules in the air to alternately expand and compress (vibrate) and sets up a displacement that is passed along among the molecules. The resulting sound waves are channeled by the external ear structures into the external auditory meatus, or ear canal, the resonating canal that ends at a taut membrane called the eardrum, or tympanic membrane (Fig. 5-6). The eardrum is at the entrance to the middle ear, an air-filled cavity containing the three tiniest bones of the body, the malleus, incus, and stapes, collectively known as the ossicles. This ossicular chain has one end attached to the eardrum and the other to a small opening at the inferior part of the cavity called the oval window. Mechanical transmission of vibration through the ossicular chain helps increase the force that reaches the oval window. The force causes the oval window to move and transmit the movement into the fluid-filled cavity of the inner ear. The inner ear contains the coiled cochlea. On the membranes of the cochlea are the sensory hair cells that contain neurotransmitters to be released to stimulate the auditory nerve, cranial nerve VIII. This auditory nerve then carries this signal to the cochlear nucleus in the brainstem and on to its final destination, the auditory cortex.

RECEPTOR LEVEL

The cochlea of the inner ear serves as an acoustic transducer, changing fluid vibrations to nerve impulses. The design and function of the cochlea are incredibly complex and intricate. A summary of this fascinating structure for study by the speech-language pathologist is, of necessity, brief. More in-depth information can be found in other texts.[3,12]

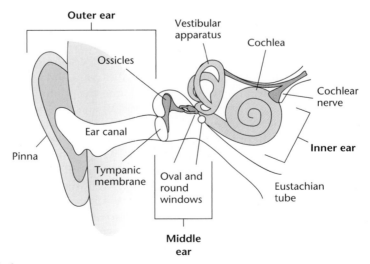

FIGURE **5-6**
Three divisions of the ear. In the outer ear sound waves are directed to the middle ear, where they are converted to oscillations of the ossicles. In the inner ear the oscillations are converted to pressure waves, which in turn are converted to neuronal activity. (From Castro, A. et al. [2002]. *Neuroscience: An outline approach.* Philadelphia: Mosby/Elsevier.)

The cochlea has a central bony, hollow core called the modiolus, which is in the axis of the internal auditory meatus. Running through the modiolus is the cochlear division of cranial nerve VIII. The cell bodies of its neurons form the spiral ganglion. These are the primary neurons of the auditory system. Forming a coil of two and a half turns around the modiolus are three separate fluid-filled columns called **scalae**. The upper compartment is the scala vestibuli and the lower chamber is the scala tympani. These two chambers communicate at the apex of the modiolus at a site called the **helicotrema**. Between these two compartments is a third chamber called the scala media, also known as the **cochlear duct**. The scala vestibuli and the scala tympani are filled with a fluid called **perilymph**. The cochlear duct is filled with a different fluid, **endolymph**. These two fluids do not mix because of a tight barrier of epithelium lining the cochlear duct. The vestibular membrane, or **Reissner's membrane**, separates the cochlear duct and the scala vestibuli and the basilar membrane separates the cochlear duct from the scala tympani.

Membranes of fibrous connective tissue also run between the epithelium and the bones of the cochlea. The spiral lamina projects from the modiolus. Attached to the tip of the spiral lamina is the basilar membrane.

This membrane reaches across the cavity of the cochlea, forming the floor of the cochlear duct, and attaches to the spiral ligament on the outer wall of the cochlea. Figure 5-7 shows a cross section of the cochlea, looking at it in an upright position rather than its usual position on its side.

The basilar membrane is an important structure because it contains the **organ of Corti**, the sensory epithelium of hearing. When sound occurs, causing vibration of the tympanic membrane and movement of the ossicles of the middle ear, movement of the oval window leading into the scala vestibule occurs. This creates a pressure wave in the perilymph in the scala vestibuli. The pressure waves are transmitted through the vestibular membrane to the basilar membrane. This movement then sets up a neural chain of events in the organ of Corti.

In the organ of Corti are several types of cells, with the two most important being the inner hair cells and the outer hair cells. These cell types are separated by a central tunnel, with the outer hair cells located on the outer side of the tunnel. The hair cells rest on supporting cells; other ancillary cells also are in the structure. On the top of the hair cells are **stereocilia**, extremely long microvilli extending from the surface. Overlying the hair cells and their stereocilia is a gelatinous structure called

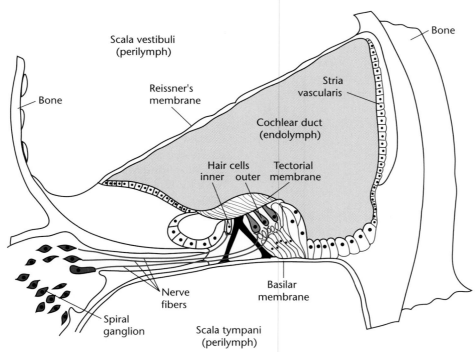

FIGURE 5-7
Cross section of the cochlear duct. (From Nadeau, S. et al [2005]. *Medical neuroscience.* Philadelphia: Saunders/Elsevier.)

the **tectorial membrane**. The stereocilia of the inner hair cells lie just below the tectorial membrane, whereas those of the outer hair cells are embedded in the tectorial membrane (see Fig. 5-7). The outer hair cells outnumber the inner cells by approximately 3:1, but most of the neurons of the spiral ganglion innervate inner hair cells, with up to 20 large afferent neurons synapsing on each inner hair cell. These myelinated neurons innervating the inner hair cells are called type I cells, and each one responds best to a certain frequency.

The organ of Corti also receives efferent innervation coming from the olivocochlear bundle of the superior olivary complex in the brainstem. Thus some information comes from the brain to the cochlea rather than its all being unidirectional, from cochlea to brain. Some neurons go to the outer hair cells. These well-myelinated neurons (medial olivocochlear bundle) typically cross the midline and exit the brain with the vestibular portion of cranial nerve VIII. They eventually join the cochlear division and travel in the spiral ganglion. They then enter the organ of Corti and synapse on the outer hair cells. Although none of the efferent fiber functions of the auditory system are well understood, these cells are believed to inhibit or reduce the movement of the outer hair cells, effectively reducing the sensitivity of the cochlea at that particular region.

Some neurons also go to the inner hair cells (lateral olivocochlear bundle); these are unmyelinated, usually do not decussate, and follow the same pathway to synapse just under the inner hair cells. These fibers appear to influence the type I spiral ganglion cells by making them more difficult to excite. These efferent pathways of innervation to the cochlea are believed to combine to assist the auditory system in selective listening so that certain auditory input can be attuned to and background noise or other input can be ignored.

CRANIAL NERVE LEVEL

The nerve of hearing, cranial nerve VIII, has two divisions: the cochlear branch, associated with hearing, and the vestibular branch, associated with balance. Central processes of the cochlear nerve (the first-order neurons) proceed from the spiral ganglion through the internal auditory canal. The cochlear nerve is accompanied by cranial nerve VII, the facial nerve, in the auditory canal. The two nerves enter the brainstem at the sulcus between the pons and the medulla, an area known as the cerebellopontine angle. The cochlear nuclear complex spans the border between the pons and the medulla.

BRAINSTEM LEVEL

The fibers of the cochlear division of cranial nerve VIII end in the dorsal and ventral cochlear nuclei, which are draped around the inferior cerebellar peduncle. The cochlear nuclei contain the second-order neurons of the auditory pathway. From the cochlear nuclei, most fibers of the auditory pathway proceed to the upper medulla and pons and cross the midline. Other fibers ascend in the brainstem ipsilaterally. Fibers course upward in the ascending central auditory pathway of the brainstem called the lateral lemniscus. The fibers take one of several routes, and synapses in the auditory system may occur at one or more of the following structures: the superior olives, the trapezoid body, the inferior colliculus, and the nucleus of the lateral lemniscus. All ascending auditory fibers terminate in the medial geniculate body, a thalamic nucleus.

AUDITORY RADIATIONS AND CORTEX

The fibers arising from the medial geniculate body, coursing to the temporal cortex, are called auditory radiations. They pass through the internal capsule in their route to the bilateral primary auditory areas of the brain in the superior and transverse temporal gyri. These areas are numbered 41 and 42 and are known as **Heschl's gyrus**.

The nuclei of the auditory pathway—the trapezoid body, the superior olivary complex, the nucleus of the lateral lemniscus, and the inferior colliculi—serve as relay nuclei as well as reflex centers. The reflex centers make connections with the eyes, head, and trunk, where automatic reflex actions occur in response to sound.

Descending efferent fibers, in addition to the ascending afferent fibers, are present in all parts of the central auditory pathway. They probably serve as feedback loops within the pathways. Figure 5-8 shows a simplified schema of connections along the auditory pathway.

AUDITORY PHYSIOLOGY

Sound is transmitted to the central auditory pathways by a traveling wave set up on the basilar membrane of the cochlea. The basilar membrane is narrower at the base of the cochlea than at its apex. The mechanics of the membrane on which the organ of Corti is located vary slightly from base to apex. Traveling pressure waves of a specific frequency cause the basilar membrane to

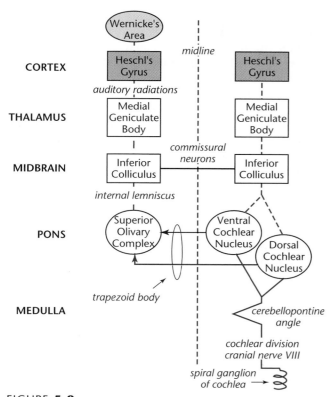

FIGURE **5-8**

The afferent pathways of the central auditory system and the major auditory way stations. The *bold lines* indicate that the majority of fibers in the auditory pathways decussate, though some do travel ipsilaterally *(dotted lines)*. For most of the population, perceptual analysis and comprehension of language occur in Wernicke's area of the left hemisphere, and information coming in to the left ear has to cross to Wernicke's area on the left after reaching Heschl's gyrus in the right hemisphere.

vibrate maximally at a specific point along the length of the membrane. Higher pitched sounds (high-pitched frequency waves) cause the shorter fibers at the basal turn of the cochlea to absorb their energy, whereas lower pitched sounds are absorbed by the longer fibers at the apical turn of the cochlea. Thus the basilar membrane is said to be **tonotopic** in its organization of fibers. This tonotopic organization extends to the inner hair cells as well. These hair cells receive afferent input from the peripheral processes of the spiral ganglion cells. When a local response to a certain frequency occurs in the hair cells, the vibration produces shearing forces causing depolarization. Electrical charges in the dendrites of the spiral ganglion are set up and, in turn, cause the nerve cells to fire, releasing excitatory neurotransmitters.

Auditory nerve impulses ascend in the pathways of the central auditory nervous system. The organ of Corti

serves as an analyzer of sound frequencies. Because of its tonotopic organization, the highest frequencies stimulate hair cells in the most basilar portion of the cochlea, where the basilar membrane is narrowest. The lowest frequencies stimulate the portions of the membrane at the apex. Frequency discrimination is therefore dependent on the frequency of the tone and the spatial response of the basilar membrane. Intensity discrimination depends on the length of the basilar membrane set in motion and the amplitude of the vibration. Displacement of a longer area of the membrane activates more nerve fibers, and a greater amplitude of vibration increases the frequency of the neural discharge.

Localizing the source of a sound depends on a comparison between the arrival time and the intensity of the sound at the two ears. Localization of sound occurs at higher levels in the auditory pathways. Central auditory structures, generally above the level of the inferior colliculus, are capable of making appropriate comparisons for sound localization. Thus in mammals and human beings the temporal auditory cortex is not needed for simple sound recognition, but it is essential for sound localization and recognition of changes in the temporal sequencing of sounds.

Temporal sequencing is a crucial higher auditory function because it is a significant aspect of speech. Sound localization probably requires the inferior colliculus and auditory cortex, whereas temporal sequencing may require the cochlear nuclei, the medial geniculate nuclei, and the auditory cortex. A tonotopic organization is present in all the central auditory nuclei, but the nuclei are used for analysis of several auditory properties of sound other than the recognition of tones or different frequencies.

LESIONS OF THE AUDITORY SYSTEM

The integrity of part of the central auditory system, the auditory brainstem, may be assessed by recording **auditory brainstem responses** (**ABRs**). Surface electrodes are placed on the mastoid bone and on the top of the head. Repetitive clicks are presented, evoking responses in a large number of central fibers of cranial nerve VIII. These responses stimulate activity at the cochlear nuclear level, the superior olivary complex, the lateral lemniscus tracts, and the inferior colliculi. The combined potential is enough to be picked up by the skin electrodes. This method may be used to assess hearing objectively in infants and persons who cannot cooperate in subjective testing. A normal ABR is a strong indication that the middle ear, cochlea, and auditory brainstem are functioning normally. Abnormal ABRs may be caused by a middle ear or cochlear problem or may indicate a pathologic condition at sites in the brainstem such as at the level of the geniculate bodies, the medial colliculus, and the lateral lemniscus. If abnormal ABRs are found, further testing is necessary.

If a lesion occurs unilaterally and involves the auditory nerve in its path from the ear and includes the cochlear nuclei, the person will be deaf in one ear. The results of unilateral cortical damage do not produce complete deafness. Lesions in Heschl's gyrus bilaterally may produce cortical deafness, nonverbal agnosia, or auditory agnosia.

The term **auditory agnosia** usually refers to the inability to identify auditory nonlinguistic stimuli, although many use the term when referring to the inability to recognize nonlinguistic as well as verbal stimuli. Most appropriate is the label "auditory nonverbal agnosia" for a pure deficit in which identification of nonlinguistic stimuli is impaired and the term "pure word deafness" if referring to the disorder in which nonverbal stimuli can be identified but speech cannot be understood. All auditory agnosias occur in the face of normal hearing acuity. The site of lesion for auditory nonverbal agnosia is in dispute but is assumed to be in the auditory association areas of both hemispheres.

Pure word deafness is an uncommon syndrome in which the patient cannot comprehend verbal language but usually reads, speaks, and writes functionally. Errors in speech are often noted and a mild measurable language disorder (aphasia) may be present. Both unilateral and bilateral temporal lobe lesions have been described. Unilateral lesions are deep in the temporal lobe in the fibers projecting to Heschl's gyrus. Bilateral lesions usually have been described as occurring in the mid-portion of the superior temporal gyri of both hemispheres. Geschwind[4] notes that in pure word deafness with a unilateral lesion, the lesion must be located subcortically in the left temporal lobe so that the auditory radiations as well as the callosal fibers from the opposite auditory region are interrupted, preventing Wernicke's area from receiving auditory stimulation.

In bilateral pure word deafness, the lesions in the temporal lobe spare Heschl's gyrus. The lesions on the left are assumed to cut off connections between the primary auditory receptor cortex and Wernicke's area. A lesion on the right would cut off the origin of the callosal fibers from the right auditory cortex. Auditory nonverbal agnosia, in addition to pure word deafness, may be the basis of the syndrome known as cortical deafness, which is probably associated with bilateral temporal lobe lesions.

Synopsis of Clinical Information and Applications for the Speech-Language Pathologist

- The lateral and anterior spinothalamic tracts carry sensory impulses of pain and temperature, light touch and pressure, and tactile discrimination from the periphery to the sensory cortex.
- The two tracts of the dorsal column pathways convey proprioceptive sensations of movement, posture, vibration, and stereognosis from the upper and lower extremities.
- Cerebral lesions marked by language loss may have accompanying sensory loss involving the parietal lobe or subcortical pathways.
- An agnosia is a disorder of recognition of a sensory stimulus. Agnosias result from bilateral damage to the primary cortical receptor areas associated with the particular sensory input affected.
- The oral cavity is rich in sensory receptors and the tactile receptors of the mouth, tongue, pharynx, and teeth; however, the role of sensory feedback in speech production currently is not clear and no standard clinical method of assessment is widely accepted.
- Interruptions of the visual pathway from the retina to the occipital cortex cause visual field deficits, with the extent and type of deficit depending on the point of interruption in this double-crossed pathway.

- Patients with language disorders caused by posterior lesions are most at risk for visual field deficits that particularly affect reading and writing.
- The speech-language pathologist should be quite familiar with the auditory pathways and vigilant in identification of possible hearing loss.
- The central auditory pathway is complex, with the primary auditory receptor in the spiral ganglion of the organ of Corti of the cochlea of the inner ear. The auditory nerve (cranial nerve VIII) enters at the pontomedullary juncture, and damage in this area or to the auditory nerve often results in accompanying damage to cranial nerve VII (the facial nerve) because it also runs through the auditory canal.
- Bilateral damage to Heschl's gyrus or the temporal lobe auditory processing areas produces a spectrum of deficits, including cortical deafness, nonverbal agnosia, and auditory agnosia. Unilateral cortical damage to Heschl's gyrus does not produce total deafness.
- A unilateral lesion along the auditory nerve pathway from the ear and including the cochlear nuclei causes deafness in one ear.

CASE**STUDY**

A 26-year-old male soldier was on duty in Iraq, driving a supply truck. An improvised explosive device detonated on the road near the left side of the truck, causing some damage to the truck and breaking the left window. The soldier had some cuts to his face and arm from the glass and also experienced severe difficulty hearing from both ears after the incident. Fortunately, rupture of the tympanic membranes was ruled out on examination. In approximately 2 weeks, he found that he could hear out of the right ear much better than from the left. He was sent for audiometric testing and consequent radiographs. The radiographs showed a fracture of the left temporal bone.

QUESTIONS FOR CONSIDERATION:

1. What type of hearing loss would the audiogram show as resulting from a fracture of the temporal bone?
2. What part of the ear would most likely be affected?
3. What cranial nerve would be involved?
4. Why did the hearing on his right side eventually improve?

REFERENCES

1. Beauvois, M. F., Sailliant, B., Meininger, V., & Lhermitte, F. (1978). Bilateral tactile aphasia: A tacto-verbal dysfunction. *Brain, 101*, 381-402.
2. Benson, D. F. (1979). *Aphasia, alexia and agraphia.* New York: Churchill Livingstone.
3. Cohen, H. (1999). *Neuroscience for rehabilitation.* Philadelphia: Lippincott Williams & Wilkins.
4. Geschwind, N. (1965). Disconnection syndromes in animals and man. *Brain, 88,* 237-294; 585-644.
5. Hubel, D. H., & Wiesel, T. N. (1968). Receptive fields and functional architecture of the monkey striate cortex. *Journal of Physiology, 206,* 419-436.
6. Kent, R. D. (2004). The uniqueness of speech among motor systems. *Clinical Linguistics and Phonetics, 18,* 6-8, 495-505.
7. Mesulam, M. M. (1985). *Principles of behavioral neurology.* Philadelphia: F. A. Davis.
8. Mishkin, M., & Ungerleider, L.G. (1982). Contribution of striate inputs to the visuospatial functions of the parieto-preoccipital cortex in monkeys. *Behavioral Brain Research, 6,* 57-77.
9. Nadeau, S. E., Ferguson, T. S., Valenstein, E., Vierck, C. J., Petruska, J. C., Streit, W. J., & Ritz, L. A. (2004). *Medical neuroscience.* St. Louis: Elsevier.
10. Sherrington, S. C. (1926). *The integrative action of the nervous system.* New Haven: Yale University Press.
11. Tremblay, S., Shiller, D. S., & Ostrey, D. J. (2003). Somatosensory basis of speech production. *Nature, 423,* 866-869.
12. Webster, D. B. (1999). *Neuroscience of communication.* San Diego: Singular Publishing Group, Inc.

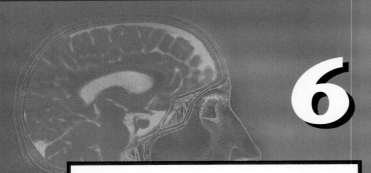

6

Neuromotor Control of Speech

We cannot state exactly the number of muscles that are necessary for speech and that are active during speech. But if we consider that ordinarily the muscles of the thoracic and abdominal walls, the neck and the face, the larynx and pharynx, and the oral cavity are all properly coordinated during the act of speaking, it becomes obvious that over 100 muscles must be controlled centrally.

Eric H. Lenneberg, *Biological Foundations of Language*, 1967

KEY**TERMS**

action tremor
adiadochokinesia
  (dysdiadochokinesia)
akinesia
alpha motor neuron
areflexia
asynergia
ataxia
ataxic dysarthria
athetosis
atrophy
Babinski sign
bilateral innervation
bilateral symmetry
chorea
clonus
contralateral
  innervation
corticonuclear fibers
corticospinal tract
decussation
denervation
dyskinesia
dysmetria
dystonia
extensor
extrapyramidal system
facilitation
feedback
feedforward
flocculi
gamma-aminobutyric
  acid (GABA)
gamma motor neurons
genu
globus pallidus (GPi)
Golgi tendon organs
hemiparalysis
  (hemiplegia)
hyperkinesia
hyperreflexia

hypertonia
hypokinesia
hyporeflexia
hypotonia
ideational apraxia
ideomotor apraxia
intention tremor
limb apraxia
lower motor neurons
motor unit
muscle spindle
muscle tone
myoclonus
neocerebellum
nystagmus
paralysis
paraplegia
paresis
peduncles
phasic tone
plantar
postural tone
premotor area
pyramidal system
quadriplegia
rest tremor
reticulospinal tract
rubrospinal tracts
servomechanism
  control system
spasticity
supplementary motor
  area (SMA)
synergy
tardive dyskinesia
tremor
unilateral innervation
upper motor neurons
vestibulospinal
  tracts
volitional

CHAPTER**OUTLINE**

Motor Control for Speech Production
  Motor Planning
  Premotor and Supplementary Motor Areas
  Limb Apraxia
  Ideomotor Apraxia
  Motor Speech Programmer
The Pyramidal System
  Corticospinal Tract
    Decussation
    Brainstem centers for tone and posture
  Corticonuclear Fibers
  Upper and Lower Motor Neurons
    Upper motor neurons
    Lower motor neurons
  Bilateral Symmetry
    Contralateral and unilateral innervation
  Indicators of Upper versus Lower Motor Neuron
    Damage
    Paralysis, paresis, and plegia
    *Upper motor neuron signs and symptoms
       other confirmatory signs*
    Lower motor neuron signs and symptoms
  Neuromuscular Control
    Alpha motor neurons
    Muscle spindles
    Gamma motor neurons
    Golgi tendon organs
The Extrapyramidal System
  Indirect Activation Pathway

Speech is one of the most complex behaviors performed by human beings. On average, a person utters approximately 14 recognizable speech sounds per second when asked to produce nonsense syllables as rapidly as possible. This unusually brisk rate is maintained even when speaking conversationally or reading aloud. The number of separate neural events supporting this complex coordination of the articulatory muscles is, of course, quite large, and the degree of neural integration in the motor system for routine, everyday talk is truly amazing. The statement that normal speech production requires the finest motor control in the body is no exaggeration.

Motor Control for Speech Production

The motor system for all voluntary and reflexive movement is considered a hierarchical system that becomes progressively less sophisticated as it is descended or more sophisticated as it is ascended. The great neurologist Hughlings Jackson asserted that each level of this hierarchy has a certain autonomy, but the autonomy at the lower levels is partially constrained by the higher levels of the motor system. Speech production, as does other major motor activity, requires the action of major mechanisms at every significant motor integration level of the nervous system. The Jacksonian principle that higher centers bring more refinement to neuronal processing but also tonically inhibit lower centers is often demonstrated when disease or injury to the motor system occurs. This will become clear when signs and symptoms of the different motor speech disorders are discussed in subsequent chapters. An attempt must first be made to understand the functioning of the motor system as a whole for any type of movement.

MOTOR PLANNING

At the highest level of the motor system hierarchy is the cortical input of areas involved in motor planning to the primary motor area of the cortex. For body movements, this is primarily the premotor and supplementary motor areas (Brodmann's area 6). When considering motor planning for speech production, Broca's area, and perhaps the insula, must also be discussed.

PREMOTOR AND SUPPLEMENTARY MOTOR AREAS

The **premotor** area is usually active bilaterally, if at all. It has a major projection to the brainstem nuclei that gives origin primarily to the reticulospinal tracts and has minor projections to the pyramidal tract. Its primary function appears to be bilateral postural fixation as needed to fixate the shoulders and stabilize the hips. It receives cognitive input from the prefrontal cortex in terms of motor intention and from the parietal lobe in regard to tactile and visual signals. It does get quite active when motor routines are run in response to visual or somatosensory cues (e.g., reaching for an object). The premotor area responds mostly to external cues, whereas the **supplementary motor area (SMA)** responds to internal cues. The SMA is involved in motor planning, activated by the frontal lobe the moment a movement is intended. It seems to primarily be for preprogramming movement sequences already in motor memory. Projections are to the primary motor cortex and the pyramidal tract. Unilateral lesions are associated with poor initiation of movement of the contralateral arm and leg. Bilateral lesions cause severe difficulty in initiating movements, including speech initiation.

LIMB APRAXIA

Limb apraxia refers to a wide spectrum of higher order motor disorders that affect the performance of skilled motor acts with the upper limbs. The lower limbs and trunk may also be affected in some cases. Speech-language pathologists are most concerned with limb apraxia when it impairs the ability to gesture for communication (Table 6-1).

TABLE 6-1 **Apraxias**	
TYPE	DESCRIPTION
Apraxia	A disorder in performing voluntary learned motor acts caused by a lesion in motor association areas and association pathways, in which similar automatic gestures are intact.
Ideomotor apraxia	A disorder in which motor plans are intact but individual motor gestures are disturbed.
Ideational apraxia	A disorder in performing the steps of complex motor plans.
Apraxia of speech (AOS)	A disorder of motor programming of speech.
Oral apraxia (buccofacial apraxia)	A disorder of nonspeech movements of the oral muscles.
Childhood apraxia of speech (CAS)	A disorder in which motor speech programming is disturbed in childhood.

IDEOMOTOR APRAXIA

Ideomotor apraxia is the most common type of apraxia. In this condition the patient fails to carry out a motor act on the examiner's verbal command. In general, simple motor gestures are disturbed when attempts are made to elicit them by verbal command, but the level of ideation for the plan of the motor gesture is retained.

Ideomotor apraxia can be demonstrated on examination. For example, a patient may be unable to lick his lips with his tongue on command but may show appropriate licking movements during eating. This deficit in tongue movements involves an apraxia of oral muscles. Difficulties, for instance, in saluting or waving the hand or in kicking a ball on command are limb apraxias. Difficulties in bending at the waist as in a bow or swinging an imaginary baseball bat are trunk apraxias.

The ability to perform learned movements on verbal command is associated with the integrity of the language areas in the dominant left hemisphere. Because adequate verbal comprehension is a prerequisite for testing praxis, Wernicke's area in the left hemisphere must be intact. After the verbal command is recognized and comprehended through the linguistic processing of Wernicke's area, neural impulses are most likely transmitted to the left supramarginal gyrus for matching to kinesthetic memories of required motor acts. This information is then transmitted forward by neural impulse along the arcuate fasciculus to the premotor area, where a motor plan for the required gesture is evoked. This motor plan is relayed to the motor area of the precentral gyrus. At the precentral gyrus the pyramidal tract is activated to carry out the motor gesture. Presumably, according to disconnection theory, a lesion at any point in this complex pathway produces an apraxic disturbance on the right side because motor activities on the right are controlled by motor areas and pathways in the left hemisphere.

A verbal command to the right motor cortex for a learned movement on the left side of the body must be transferred from the left premotor cortex to the right premotor cortex by the anterior fibers of the corpus callosum. Any interruption of the anterior callosal fibers produces an apraxia of the left side, particularly left-handed apraxia. This has been called a sympathetic apraxia in individuals who have Broca's aphasia and right hemiplegia. It has also been called a callosal apraxia. This disorder was described by Liepmann in 1900 and elaborated on by Geschwind in 1975. Figure 6-1 illustrates the pathways proposed by Geschwind that may be interrupted when a limb apraxia is present. Some researchers[13] in apraxia have proposed that the movement patterns or engrams are stored in the left inferior

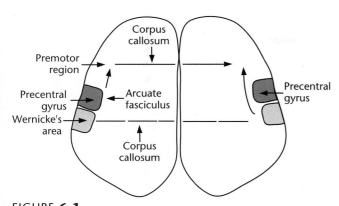

FIGURE **6-1**
A superior view of the model of the central language mechanism showing the corpus callosum and the interhemispheric motor pathways that may be involved in apraxia. (Reprinted from Geschwind. N. [1975]. The apraxias: Neural mechanisms of disorders of learned movements, *American Scientist, 63*, 188-195.)

parietal lobule and translated into an innervation pattern in the SMA rather than in the premotor area, as proposed by Geschwind.

The posterior callosal fibers could theoretically transmit motor information to the right premotor area, but as Geschwind[11] points out, lesions in the posterior callosal area rarely result in a left apraxic hand. Apparently, the posterior callosal pathway is rarely used to transmit interhemispheric motor impulses that are affected in such a way that apraxia results.

MOTOR SPEECH PROGRAMMER

The subconscious planning and programming for the sequencing of the muscle movements that achieve the cognitive and linguistic goals of what is to be said rely heavily on the prefrontal and premotor areas, especially Broca's area and the SMA of the left, or dominant, hemisphere. (Review the discussion of Broca's area and Fig. 2-7 in Chapter 2.) Broca's area contributes to both simultaneous and sequential movements. The organization of the resulting movement commands is based on input from sensory modalities and areas involved in linguistic formulation. Guenther et al[12] propose a neural model for syllable production that includes the ventral premotor cortex, which is located in the area around the ventral precentral sulcus as well as Broca's area. They note, however, differentiating this sulcus from the posterior part of Broca's area (pars opercularis) in neuroimaging studies is challenging; thus, the finite neuroanatomic correlations are still located around the traditional Broca's area.

The SMA connects with Broca's area as well as the primary motor cortex, basal ganglia, and structures of the limbic system. It seems to be tied to cognitive and emotional processes that drive or motivate action and thus is important in initiation of propositional speech as well as its control. A study of the computed tomography (CT) scans of patients with acquired apraxia of speech by Dronkers[6] strongly implicated the left superior precentral gyrus of the insula in motor programming for speech production, with follow-up studies continuing to show the involvement of this area in all studied patients who had apraxia of speech.[15]

The Pyramidal System

Voluntary movement of the muscles of speech is primarily controlled by the **pyramidal system**. In fact, the pyramidal tract itself is the major voluntary pathway for all movement. It is composed of the corticospinal tract, the corticonuclear tract (previously referred to as the corticobulbar tract), and the corticopontine tract. The corticospinal tract controls the skilled movements in the distal muscles of the limbs and digits and is particularly responsible for the precise movements made by the hands and fingers. The corticonuclear tract controls the cranial nerves, many of which directly innervate the muscles of speech. The corticopontine tract goes to the pontine nuclei, which in turn project to the cerebellum. The corticospinal, corticonuclear, and corticopontine tracts are called corticifugal pathways, meaning that they originate in or pass away from the cortex. Figure 6-2 shows the corticospinal and corticonuclear fiber pathways of the pyramidal system.

CORTICOSPINAL TRACT

The **corticospinal tract** descends from the cerebral cortex to different levels of the spinal cord; it begins in the motor cortex of the two cerebral hemispheres. A majority of the corticospinal fibers originate from pyramidal neurons in area 4 of the primary motor cortex, though some originate from the premotor and supplementary motor cortices. Descending corticospinal fibers also originate from the parietal lobe in the postcentral gyrus and the superior parietal lobule. These fibers of sensory area origin terminate on sensory relay nuclei in the brainstem and in the dorsal horn of the spinal cord; they modulate sensory transmission. Besides the efferent output of the cortical motor areas, afferent input into these areas also is present. There are primarily ipsilateral, but also bilateral, afferent projections to the primary motor cortex from both the premotor areas and SMAs. These inputs serve to direct the motor cortex, which primarily is initiating simple muscle contractions to combine simple movements into more complex motor movements. The primary motor cortex also receives afferent input from the primary sensory cortex and the dorsal column sensory nuclei in the spinal cord. The basal ganglia and the cerebellum also serve as "consultants" to the cortical motor system, influencing timing and coordination of movement.

The corticospinal system is actually composed of several tracts that innervate spinal neurons and, eventually, muscles controlled by spinal nerves. The corticospinal tract itself descends from the motor cortex in each hemisphere to subcortical white matter in a fan-shaped distribution of fibers called the corona radiata, or radiating crown. The fibers converge to enter into an L-shaped subcortical structure called the internal capsule. The corticospinal fibers pass through the posterior limb of the internal capsule. As they pass through the internal capsule they join axons from other areas, such as those projecting to and from other cortical areas, to the thalamus and the brainstem. Damage to the pathway through the internal capsule can result in devastating motor deficits because of the number of fibers going through this narrow point.

From that point of the internal capsule, fibers enter the midbrain and form the middle third of the crus cerebri. These fibers then enter the basis of the pons, giving off collaterals that synapse on pontine nuclei, providing circuits from the motor cortex that reverberate through the cerebellum and return impulses to the cerebral cortex after cerebellar modulation. After the fibers cross the basis pontis, they aggregate on the anterior surface of the medulla, coursing through the pyramids of the medulla situated at the medullary-cervical juncture. Again, collaterals are given off by the axons, the innervating nuclei of the inferior olivary complex, the posterior column nuclei, and some reticular nuclei of the medulla.

At the level of the pyramids, approximately 85% to 90% of the corticospinal fibers cross over (decussate) to the other side of the neuraxis, providing contralateral motor control of the extremities.

Decussation
The crossing of the right and left corticospinal tract is known as **decussation**. The few fibers, variable in number, that do not cross are collectively known as the anterior corticospinal tract. The primary crossed corticospinal tract is the lateral corticospinal tract. The decussation means that a lesion interrupting the fibers above the crossing has an effect on the side of the body opposite the site of the lesion. If the corticospinal tract

is interrupted in the cerebrum or at any level above the pyramids of the medulla, voluntary movement of the innervated structure is limited on the contralateral side of the body. By contrast, a lesion below the decussation impairs voluntary movement on the same, or ipsilateral, side.

Brainstem Centers for Tone and Posture
When a cross section of the spinal cord is examined, other descending motor tracts besides the lateral and anterior corticospinal tracts can be seen. These additional descending motor tracts found terminating in the spinal cord are the reticulospinal tracts, vestibulospinal tracts, tectospinal tracts, and rubrospinal tracts. These tracts can be considered a part of the extrapyramidal system because they are outside the pyramidal tracts. Duffy[8] refers to these tracts as the indirect activation pathway. These fiber pathways provide primary input to motor neurons for maintenance of normal tone, body posturing, and reflex responses to sensory stimuli.

Muscle tone is the resistance of the muscle to stretch. The two types of tone are phasic and postural. **Phasic tone** is a rapid contraction to a high-intensity stretch (or change in muscle length) and is assessed by testing tendon reflexes. **Postural tone** is a prolonged contraction in response to a low-intensity stretch. Gravity provides a low-intensity stretch on antigravity muscles, which respond with prolonged contraction and the normal posturing of the head, neck, and extremities that persons without neurologic damage usually maintain.

The **reticulospinal tracts** can be divided into pontine reticulospinal and medullary reticulospinal, with the name referring to the origin of the tract in the brainstem. They are important in the maintenance of flexor and **extensor** muscle tone to sustain posture and gait. They also are involved in the stabilization of proximal body parts that form a platform, allowing movement of the distal portion of the body part and thus enhancing movement capability. The pontine fibers receive input from the vestibular system, and they both receive input from the cerebral cortex, cerebellum, and the spinal cord, with the higher level control providing mainly inhibitory input.

Tectospinal fibers are derived from deep layers of the superior colliculus. These fibers mediate reactive orienting head and eye movements that occur to a sudden visual, auditory, or somatosensory stimulus. Intentional movements of the head and eyes, however, are not mediated by this tract. The **vestibulospinal tracts** are active in helping maintain the antigravity tone responsible for the ability to sit, stand, and maintain any other posture that is not horizontal. When the center of gravity is not directly over the feet, this system also helps keep a person from falling, allowing corrective movements and altering muscle tone. The **rubrospinal tracts** descend from the red nucleus in the midbrain. Because these tracts share the same organization and many of the same functions as the corticospinal tracts, lesions affecting these tracts can rarely be delineated from corticospinal tract damage. Figure 6-3 illustrates the origins and paths of some of these extrapyramidal tracts.

CORTICONUCLEAR FIBERS

Before a recommended terminology change, the corticonuclear fibers of the pyramidal tract were called the *corticobulbar fibers*, a term that is still used in some quarters. Because that name erroneously implies that all fibers terminate in the medulla (the old term for the medulla was the bulb), the term corticonuclear replaced corticobulbar in the international terminology of neuroanatomic terms in 1998. The **corticonuclear fibers** of the pyramidal tract innervate the cranial

nerves and make up the voluntary pathway for the movements of all speech muscles, except those of respiration. They are the most important motor fibers for the speech-language pathologist.

Their course is not as direct as that of the corticospinal fibers (see Fig. 6-2). The corticonuclear fibers begin with the corticospinal fibers at the cortex but terminate at the motor nuclei of the cranial nerves located at various points in the brainstem. Unlike the corticospinal fibers, the corticonuclear fibers have many ipsilateral (terminating in motor nuclei in the brainstem on the *same* side of the brain as the primary site from which the axon began) as well as contralateral fibers. After the axons of the corticonuclear fibers leave the cortical motor areas, they travel the same path that the corticospinal fibers do through the corona radiata and the internal capsule. The corticonuclear fibers, however, transverse the **genu**, or bend, of the internal capsule rather than the posterior limb. The corticospinal and corticonuclear fibers separate at the upper brainstem level. Each of the different cranial nerve axons terminates at its own designated nuclei at some point along

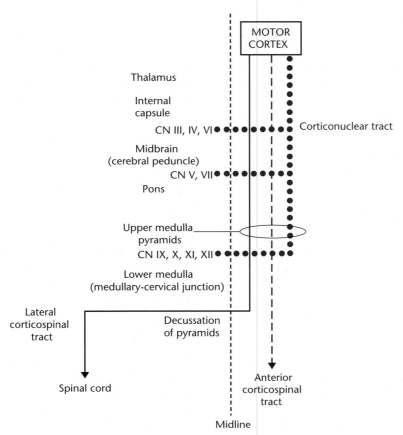

FIGURE **6-2**
The pyramidal tract, including both corticospinal and corticonuclear fibers.

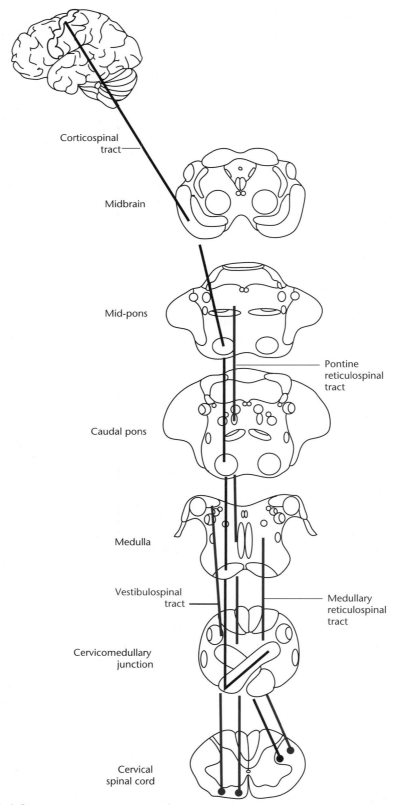

FIGURE **6-3**
The major descending motor tracts of the spinal cord, including the indirect activation pathways. The tectospinal and rubrospinal tracts are not shown. (Reprinted from Nadeau, S., et al. [2005]. *Medical neuroscience*. Philadelphia: Saunders/Elsevier.)

the brainstem. Some decussate and others primarily travel ipsilaterally. If they cross, they decussate at various levels of the brainstem. The general location of each of the nuclei for the cranial nerves most important to speech is discussed in Chapter 7.

UPPER AND LOWER MOTOR NEURONS

Upper Motor Neurons

A useful concept in clinical neurology has been the notion of **upper motor neurons** and lower motor neurons. All the neurons of the anterior and lateral corticospinal tracts, which send axons from the cerebral cortex to the anterior horn cells of the spinal cord, are considered upper motor neurons. The neurons of the corticonuclear tracts that send axons from the cerebral cortex to the nuclei in the brainstem also are upper motor neurons. No upper motor neurons leave the neuraxis. In other words, they are contained within the brain, brainstem, and spinal cord. The pyramidal tract, with its upper motor neuron activation, can be thought of as the direct activation pathway, or direct motor system, because of its direct connection and major activating influence on the lower motor neurons.[7]

Lower Motor Neurons

Lower motor neurons are all the neurons that send motor axons into the peripheral nerves: the cranial and spinal nerves. They are designated second-order neurons. Sherrington[16] called the lower motor neuron the "final common pathway." By this he meant that the peripheral nerves, both cranial and spinal, serve as a final route for all the complex motor interactions that occur in the neuraxis above the level of the lower motor neurons. The final muscle contraction is the product of all the interactions that have occurred in the central nervous system.

The concept of the **motor unit** helps explain the lower motor neuron pathway (Fig. 6-4). A motor unit is a structural and functional entity that can be defined as (1) a single anterior horn cell or cranial nerve neuron, (2) its peripheral axon and its branches, (3) each muscle fiber innervated by these branches, and (4) the myoneural juncture. Lesions may occur at many points within the motor unit and produce lower motor neuron signs.

BILATERAL SYMMETRY

Because the movements of limbs and digits would not be efficient or effective if the movement of one side mirrored the other, the corticospinal system allows for control of one side of the body to come from only one

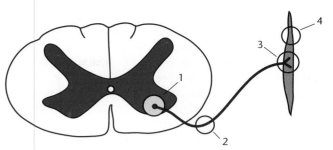

FIGURE **6-4**
The motor unit and typical lesion sites producing different signs and symptoms of lower motor neuron damage. *1*, Cell body, motor neuron disease; *2*, nerve axon, denervation produces neuropathy; *3*, myoneural juncture, neuromyopathy; *4*, muscle fiber, myopathy or dystrophy.

source (for 90% of the fibers), the opposite hemisphere's cortical motor areas. Because the oral musculature movements on one side of the face are mirrored by the same movements on the other side, the majority of the midline speech muscles work in **bilateral symmetry**, making speech more efficient. This is the result of the **bilateral innervation** to the cranial nerve nuclei that the corticonuclear fibers provide. If a cranial nerve's nuclei are said to be bilaterally innervated, the nuclei on the right side of the brainstem (in this example) receive axons from the primary motor cortices of *both* hemispheres. If that cranial nerve's nuclei were only contralaterally innervated, the axons providing innervation would come only from the left hemisphere's cortical motor areas. All but a few of the paired muscles of the face, palate, vocal folds, and diaphragm work together in synchrony much of the time in wrinkling the forehead, smiling, chewing, swallowing, and talking. This bilateral innervation of the speech muscles has important implications for the degree of speech muscle involvement in cases of dysarthria.

In corticonuclear lesions, the bilateral innervation provides a safety valve or compensatory mechanism for speech production. Assuming the left corticonuclear fibers coming from the motor cortex to the nuclei of a cranial nerve are damaged, the motor nuclei of that nerve will still receive impulses by way of the intact right corticonuclear tract, and paralysis of the muscle will not be severe. The innervation of the limbs, on the other hand, is primarily contralateral rather than bilateral, so lesions to the corticospinal fibers may produce severe unilateral limb paralysis. Unilateral lesions to corticonuclear fibers do not produce as severe weakness because of redundancy provided by the bilateral innervation.

Contralateral and Unilateral Innervation

Even though the cranial nerve nuclei are primarily bilaterally supplied, much variation among the nuclei exists regarding the amount of **unilateral innervation** versus contralateral innervation each receives. Areas with a more unilateral supply are more paralyzed after a unilateral lesion. Because of their primarily **contralateral innervation**, the muscles of the lower face and the trapezius muscles are most affected by unilateral damage. An intermediate paralytic effect is found in the tongue with a unilateral lesion. The diaphragm, ocular muscles, upper face, jaw, pharynx, and muscles of the larynx show little paresis with a unilateral lesion.

The nuclei for the facial nerve are complex. The facial nucleus is made up of a ventral and a dorsal component and combines bilateral innervation with contralateral innervation. The muscles of the upper half of the face, supplied by the ventral portion, are far more bilaterally innervated than the muscles of the lower half of the face, which are supplied by the dorsal portion of

the motor nucleus and receive more contralateral innervation. In practical terms, among the healthy population most people can wrinkle the forehead or lift both eyebrows together. Only a few people, with more contralateral fibers, are able to lift their eyebrows one at a time. The muscles of the midface receive a more equal combination of bilateral and contralateral innervation. Most, but not all, people can wink one eye at a time because of the increase of contralateral fibers to eyelid muscles compared with forehead muscles.

In the lower face the innervation is primarily contralateral. Most people are able to retract one corner of the mouth alone when asked to do so because of the limited bilateral innervation of the lower face muscles. Figure 6-5 shows the difference in effect on facial movement of an upper motor neuron lesion compared with a lower motor neuron lesion as a result of this unusual

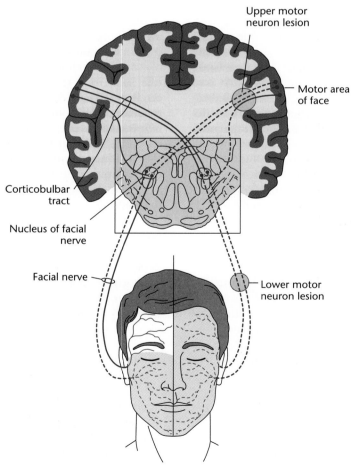

FIGURE **6-5**
Upper versus lower motor neuron facial paralysis. The *shaded areas* of the face show the distribution of the facial muscles paralyzed after an upper motor neuron lesion and a lower motor neuron lesion. (Reprinted from Gilman, S., Winans, S. S. [1982]. *Manter and Gatz's essentials of clinical neuroanatomy and neurophysiology* [6th ed.]. Philadelphia: F. A. Davis.)

TABLE 6-2	
Corticonuclear Innervation in the Cranial Nerves for Speech	
NERVE	INNERVATION
Trigeminal (V)	Bilateral innervation
Facial (VII)	Mixed bilateral and contralateral innervation
Glossopharyngeal (IX)	Bilateral innervation (motor innervation of IX is only to a single muscle)
Vagus (X)	Bilateral innervation
Spinal accessory (XI)	Contralateral innervation
Hypoglossal (XII)	Primarily bilateral innervation with contralateral innervation of one muscle (genioglossus)

TABLE 6-3	
Signs of Upper and Lower Motor Neuron Disorders	
UPPER MOTOR NEURON DISORDERS	LOWER MOTOR NEURON DISORDERS
Spastic paralysis	Flaccid paralysis
Hypertonia	Hypotonia
Hyperreflexia	Hyporeflexia
Clonus	No clonus
Babinski sign	No Babinski sign
Little or no atrophy	Marked atrophy
No fasciculations	Fasciculations
Diminished abdominal and cremasteric reflexes	Normal abdominal and cremasteric reflexes

innervation pattern. The principles of bilateral and contralateral innervation are practically applied when a speech cranial nerve examination is performed to determine if lesions are present affecting the corticonuclear fibers, cranial nerve nuclei, or the cranial nerves themselves. These principles are summarized for the cranial nerves in Table 6-2.

The concepts of bilateral symmetry and contralateral independence are of crucial clinical utility when analyzing and understanding muscle involvement in dysarthria. This is explained further in Chapter 7 in the discussion of testing the cranial nerves involved in speech.

INDICATORS OF UPPER VERSUS LOWER MOTOR NEURON DAMAGE

Once an understanding has been grasped of the anatomy of the pyramidal tract and the final common pathway, the concepts of upper and lower motor neurons, and the concept of bilateral versus contralateral innervation, it is important to understand and be able to identify the signs of upper versus lower motor neuron damage.

Lesions of the upper and lower motor neurons produce fairly different sets of signs and symptoms. Table 6-3 presents a contrast of the signs of damage to these two systems. This distinction provides the neurologist with a powerful tool in neurologic examination for deciding where a lesion is located in the nervous system. The most striking sign of a lesion in both upper and lower

motor neurons is paralysis. The type of paralysis, however, is quite different depending on the site of the lesion that produces the paralysis. The neurologist would note paresis or paralysis and proceed by assessing muscle tone, muscle strength, and reflexes. Understanding the differences in the type of paralysis, tone, and other confirmatory signs is a large step toward establishing a correct diagnosis of a neurologic disease involving motor disturbance.

Paralysis, Paresis, and Plegia
A gross limitation of movement is called **paralysis**, and an incomplete paralysis is known as **paresis**. A complete or near-complete paralysis of one side of the body is **hemiparalysis** or, more commonly, **hemiplegia**. The presence of right-sided hemiplegia or hemiparesis is an extremely important sign for the speech-language pathologist. Paralysis or paresis on the right side of the body suggests left hemisphere involvement. As previously noted, the left hemisphere is the primary site of brain mechanisms for language, so right hemiplegia is often associated with language disorders. Lesions of the bilateral motor strip or the pyramidal tract alone may produce the motor speech disorder of dysarthria.

Upper Motor Neuron Signs and Symptoms
Damage to the corticospinal tract anywhere along its course produces spastic paralysis. Spastic muscles display increased tone, or resistance to movement, a condition called **hypertonia**. Spastic hypertonicity can be identified by moving a limb through its full range of motion so that the joint is flexed or bent. The neurologic examiner puts an increased stretch on the muscles during range-of-motion testing. He or she thereby elicits a muscle stretch reflex, an increase in tone or tension that resists the flexion of the joint. The examiner

can feel this increased resistance to movement. (The muscle stretch reflex controls the degree of contraction in a normal muscle and provides muscles with tonus, or tone.) When an injury occurs to the corticospinal or corticonuclear tract, such as in a vascular stroke, this spasticity may take several days to weeks to develop and stabilize. Temporary flaccid hemiplegia may initially be present, with a more permanent spastic paralysis developing over time. The increasing spasticity of the muscles after a corticospinal injury may be caused by a buildup of collagen in the muscles as well as biochemical changes.[10]

A "clasp knife" reaction occurs in a spastic muscle when the neurologist feels increased tone or resistance to movement in the muscle after the joint has been briskly flexed and then feels the resistance fade. This reaction, which identifies spastic hypertonicity, is analogous to the resistance felt when a knife blade is first opened, followed by the reduction of resistance when the blade is straightened. This reaction occurs more typically in extension rather than in flexion of the elbow. A short span of no tone is usually present, then a rapid buildup of tone and a sudden release as the joint is moved, just as with opening a clasp knife.

Spasticity also is associated with exaggerated muscle stretch reflexes, resulting in **hyperreflexia**. Reflex action is tested at joints by putting stretch on tendons. This elicits the exaggerated muscle stretch reflex. Spastic paralysis, hypertonia, and hyperreflexia have most often been associated with pyramidal tract damage, particularly lesions of the corticospinal tract. However, the corticonuclear tracts are often also involved when a lesion interrupts the corticospinal tract, and signs of spasticity may be found in the midline speech muscles as well as in the distal limb muscles. Therefore the clinical signs of **spasticity**, or upper motor neuron lesion, are of equal interest to the speech-language pathologist and the neurologist. Spastic speech muscles may be weak, slow, and limited in range or movement. Hypertonia may decrease muscle flexibility of the articulators and limit the ability to achieve a full range of motion of the speech muscles.

Other Confirmatory Signs

Several signs, in addition to a clinical demonstration of clasp knife spasticity, hypertonia, and hyperreflexia, are used by the neurologist to help verify the diagnosis of spasticity and localize the lesion to the pyramidal tract.

The **Babinski sign**, or extensor plantar sign, in particular has been identified as an abnormal reflex sign that develops with corticospinal damage. It is the result of the release of cortical inhibition from a lesion. The sign has achieved considerable status in the diagnosis of upper motor neuron lesions because it is a highly reliable

abnormal reflex, is new behavior released by the presence of a lesion, and is clearly associated with a relatively specific lesion site—the cortex or the corticospinal tract. The speech-language pathologist is not directly interested in it because it does not involve the midline speech muscles, but its presence as a confirmation of an upper motor neuron lesion of the spastic type is important to all who manage neurologic patients.

The Babinski sign is observed as a reflex toe sign. It is elicited by stimulating the sole of the foot with a strong scratching maneuver. The normal response to stimulation of the sole, or plantar portion of the foot, is a slight withdrawal of the foot and downward turning or curling under of the toes. With a corticospinal lesion, the great toe extends upward and the other toes fan as the foot withdraws slightly. Physicians test this response several times to convince themselves that the upturning great toe sign can be repeatedly and automatically elicited. Automatic repetition of a given response such as this defines it as a reflex. The presence of a repeatable abnormal reflex sharply increases the probability of predicting with accuracy the possible site or sites of a neurologic lesion, though it may not be present if the patient with a vascular lesion is tested early after onset of the insult.

The Babinski sign is more reliable in adults than in infants and children. Normal infants are highly variable in display of the sign. The explanation usually given for this variability is that the immature nervous system and the damaged nervous system often show similar symptoms and signs. Damage to the nervous system often releases early reflex behavior that has become inhibited by development of higher centers, so signs of damage at that point in time are signs of immaturity at an earlier time. Clinical neurologists believe that the extensor plantar sign usually reaches stability by the age of 2 years. Other signs, such as a persisting asymmetrical tonic neck reflex and the Moro reflex, can be tested to suggest an upper motor neuron lesion in young children.

Another confirmatory sign of spasticity is **clonus**. Hyperactive muscle stretch reflexes associated with spasticity may show a sustained series of rhythmic beats or jerks when a neurologic examiner maintains one tendon of a muscle in extension. To test for clonus, the Achilles tendon in the ankle is often put under extension. If an upper motor neuron lesion is present, the ankle and the calf show sustained jerks. A few clonic jerks, called abortive clonus, are not clinically significant, but if the clonus is sustained over time, it is considered pathologic and an indicator of hyperreflexia. This sign is part of the clinical syndrome resulting from an upper motor neuron lesion.

With bilateral upper motor neuron lesions, a characteristic dysarthria may be present. This motor speech disorder, called spastic dysarthria, is discussed in Chapter 8.

Lower Motor Neuron Signs and Symptoms

If a lesion is in a cranial or peripheral nerve, or in the cell bodies of the anterior horn cell in the spinal cord or the nuclei of cranial nerves in the brainstem, neural impulses will not be transmitted to the muscles. This condition is called **denervation**. The result is that the muscles innervated by the cranial or spinal nerve become soft and flabby from a loss of muscle tone. This is a lower motor neuron paralysis.

The loss of muscle tone is called **hypotonia**. Hypotonia results in flaccid muscles. Thus lower motor neuron paralysis is called flaccid paralysis. Hypotonia may be an acquired condition, with disease or injury affecting the peripheral nervous system pathway, but it may also be a condition found at birth or developing shortly after birth. Infantile hypotonia may result from conditions such as chromosome disorders (e.g., Prader-Willi syndrome), genetic defects, spinal cord disorders, spinal muscular atrophy, muscular dystrophy, metabolic myopathies, or other problems that affect the peripheral pathways.[9] Figure 6-6 shows the posture, the frog-leg position, typically assumed by an infant with hypotonia.

Lower motor neuron paralysis also is sometimes associated with loss of muscle bulk, a condition called **atrophy**. Muscles undergoing atrophy display some degree of degeneration because they become denervated. Signs of this degeneration can be observed clinically. Atrophic muscles show fibrillations and fasciculations. These signs are caused by electrical disturbances in muscle fibers resulting from denervation. Fibrillations are fine twitches of single muscle fibers. These generally cannot be seen on clinical examination, except perhaps in the tongue, but must be detected by electromyographic examination. Fasciculations, on the other hand, are contractions of groups of muscle fibers that can be identified, with training, in skeletal muscles through the skin.

As muscle bulk is lost through atrophy in motor neuron disease, fasciculations may be seen in the muscles of the head and neck as well as other parts of the body. These muscle twitches may be particularly observed in the relatively large muscle mass of the tongue if the bulbar muscles are involved. Fasciculations have no direct effect on speech itself but serve as a sign of lower motor neuron disease.

Interruption of a peripheral nerve by a lower motor neuron lesion also damages the reflex arc involved with that nerve. The result is that normal reflex responses

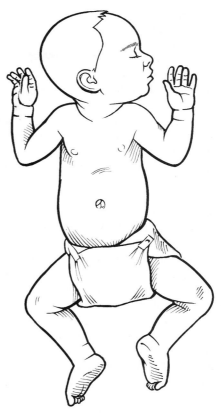

FIGURE 6-6
Typical frog-leg position assumed at rest by an infant with hypotonia. The thighs are fully abducted and the arms lie in a flaccid position next to the head.

mediated through the sensory and motor limbs of the arc become diminished. Reduced reflex response is called **hyporeflexia**. Complete lack of reflex is known as **areflexia**. Hyporeflexia and areflexia, however, are also associated with lower motor neuron disease.

Referring back to Figure 6-4 with some explanations of typical disorders can help the reader understand damage caused by more typical types of lower motor neuron disorders. The most obvious example of disorder is a lesion or cut in the spinal nerve (point 2). This damage paralyzes the muscle innervated by the nerve. In addition, the denervated muscle becomes hypotonic, areflexic, and atrophic. Finally, fasciculations appear. If a cranial nerve is denervated, weakness of speech muscles results from hypotonia and loss of muscle bulk.

A lesion may also occur in the cell body itself and produce paralysis and related lower motor neuron signs (see point 1 of Fig. 6-4). An example is acute bulbar poliomyelitis, which attacks the high cervical anterior horns as well as the cranial nerve nuclei of the bulbar muscles controlling speech. Speech muscles again may become weak and atrophic.

Lesions of the lower motor neuron type may also directly occur in muscles (point 4). An example of this type of disorder is seen in muscular dystrophy. Speech muscles lose strength and show disturbances of muscle bulk. This lower motor neuron disease within a muscle is called a myopathy, as opposed to a disease of the peripheral nerves, which is called a neuropathy. Lesions may also occur at the neuromuscular junction (point 3), as seen in myasthenia gravis. Speech muscles show fatigue and weakness in this myoneural disorder.

NEUROMUSCULAR CONTROL

In the final analysis, motor control of speech muscles, or any other musculature, is brought about by muscle contraction. At one time it was believed that the only route for control of voluntary muscle contraction was by way of the several descending motor pathways in the nervous system that end in nerve cells called alpha motor neurons. In the spinal cord these motor neurons are called anterior horn cells and are in the largest cells in the spinal cord. Homologous motor neurons are the cranial nerve neurons of the brainstem. Along with gamma motor neurons, the alpha motor neurons supply skeletal muscles. They discharge impulses through the spinal nerves to contract muscles of the trunk and limbs in the corticospinal system. Most motor commands for a given articulatory act, other oral-motor act, or facial movement are transmitted by the alpha motor neuron system through contraction of muscles innervated by cranial nerves.

Alpha Motor Neurons

The **alpha motor neuron** innervates fibers within the muscle called extrafusal fibers. The axon of each neuron branches to supply the fibers. An axon may supply only a few fibers, as in the case of a small muscle with precisely controlled contraction, or it may control several hundred fibers, as in the case of large muscles with strong, crude movements.

Three types of extrafusal fibers are found in skeletal muscle. All muscles contain all three types of fibers, but all muscle fibers in a motor unit are of the same type. The type is determined by the trophic influences of the innervating neuron. The neuron supplies the trophic or nutritional factors that direct the differentiation of the fibers and keep the muscle healthy. These substances are called myotrophic factors. The motor neuron also supplies the acetylcholine that stimulates contraction of muscle. The first of the three types of fibers are slow twitch (type I) fibers that contract slowly and are resistant to fatigue. These fibers predominate in sustaining postural activities, including standing. Fast twitch (type II) fibers contract faster but fatigue more rapidly. They exert a more powerful force and are primarily found in superficial muscles. An intermediate fiber has properties between the other two types in terms of speed of contraction and amount of force; they are considered fast twitch fibers, however.

Muscle Spindles

More recently another level of neuromuscular control has been identified at the level of the **muscle spindle**. Muscle spindles serve as sensory, or afferent, receptors within some striated muscles. They provide sensory information on the status of the normal stretch mechanisms in muscle. In muscles that have muscle spindles, the spindle is the mechanism by which, in passive stretch, the muscle contraction is elicited. The spindles are also innervated by efferent neurons called gamma motor neurons. Because they serve as afferent receptors yet they themselves receive efferent innervation, they are considered more complex sensory receptors than those found in the tendons and joints. Muscle spindles are most commonly found in the slow twitch fibers and are plentiful in the muscles along the vertebral column, the muscles of the neck, and the intrinsic muscles of the hand. They have been found to be present in large numbers in the muscles that close the jaws as well. Figure 6-7 illustrates the structure of a muscle spindle.

The muscle spindle is encapsulated, containing a limited number of short fibers that are parallel to other muscle fibers. Fibers of the muscle spindle are called intrafusal fibers, and the number of intrafusal fibers within a spindle varies. Two types of fibers within the intrafusal fibers are nuclear chain and nuclear bag fibers.

Two types of afferent axons arise from the intrafusal fibers. Primary endings, or annulospiral endings, are rapidly conducting afferent fibers that wrap around the center of the intrafusal fiber. Secondary, or "flower spray" endings, are more slowly conducting afferents and are found for the most part on nuclear chain fibers.

Both primary and secondary afferents are stimulated by the lengthening of the intrafusal fibers and the rate of change of their length. As the muscle fibers are shortened in response to the muscle contraction, the spindle afferents convey information to the alpha motor neurons, which control the neural discharge to extrafusal fibers. The primary afferents are large neurons with a rapid rate of conduction, up to 120 m/sec.

Gamma Motor Neurons

The efferent innervation to the muscle spindle is supplied by **gamma motor neurons**. As with the alpha

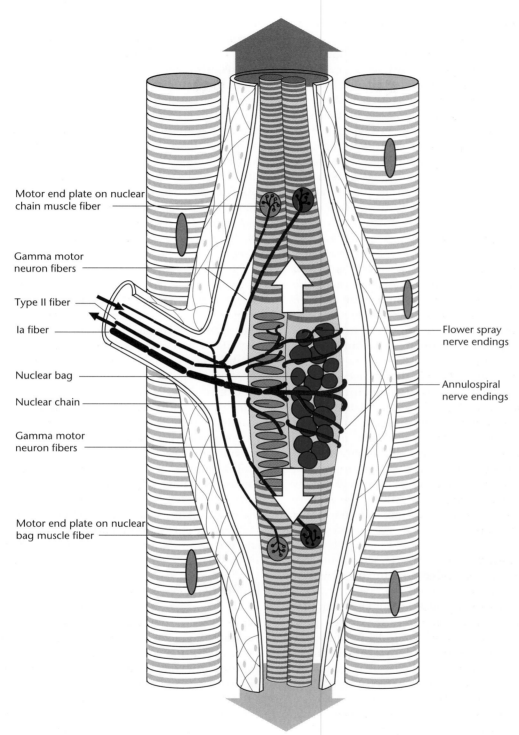

FIGURE **6-7**

The muscle spindle (simplified). *Large arrows* indicate passive stretch of the annulospiral endings produced by lengthening of the relaxed muscle as a whole. *Medium arrows* indicate active stretch of annulospiral endings produced by activity of gamma motor neuron fibers. *Small arrows* indicate directions of impulse conduction to and from the spindle when the parent muscle is in use. Muscle spindles are plentiful in jaw-closing muscles of the oral mechanism but are less plentiful or not present in lip, tongue, and jaw-opening muscles. (Reprinted from FitzGerald, M. J. T., & Folan-Curran, J. [2002]. *Clinical neuroanatomy and related neuroscience* [4th ed.]. Philadelphia: Saunders/Elsevier.)

motor neurons, these are part of a motor nerve. They are relatively small in size compared with the alpha efferents, but they make up approximately 30% of the motor neurons leaving the spinal cord.

The gamma motor neurons innervate the muscle spindle at each end. The firing of the gamma motor neuron causes the muscle spindle's intrafusal fibers to contract. This shortening of the fibers is detected by the annulospiral endings, and afferent impulses are sent to the spinal cord or brainstem where a synapse with an alpha motor neuron occurs. This synapse causes an efferent impulse to be sent to the extrafusal fibers of the muscle. A contraction of the fibers occurs until they are the same length as the fibers of the muscle spindles. Once this equalization takes place, the sensory receptor becomes silent and the process is terminated. This functional contractile process is known as the gamma loop system. Through this system the gamma motor neurons form an important muscle stretch reflex mechanism that acts in conjunction with the alpha motor neurons. This sensitivity to stretch provides fine compensations of muscle length and velocity and helps maintain muscle tone.

The speed with which the spindles convey sensory feedback information to the central nervous system would seem to mark them as likely candidates for the neural mechanisms controlling the fine and rapid movements of speech muscles. Evidence from the speech science laboratory indicates that rapid compensatory motor behavior is necessary for intelligible speech. Motor speech acts are rarely performed exactly the same way twice, but in most cases motor speech production meets the broad specifications of the motor commands in such a way that the listener can recognize an individual speech sound, or phon, as a member of a phoneme class. However, evidence for a significant role of the muscle spindle in oral-motor function has not been forthcoming.

Over the last 2 decades, clinical treatments targeting neuromuscular **facilitation** techniques have been published and have had some anecdotal evidence of success with children and adults with oral-motor speech, feeding, and swallowing problems.[2,3] This has increased interest in more accurately defining the exact muscle fiber composition of the muscles of the oral mechanism. In the case of density of muscle spindles, the jaw-closing muscles have been found to be rich with muscle spindles, but lip, tongue, and jaw-opening muscles are devoid of or have very few muscle spindles and do not demonstrate normal stretch reflex patterns. Therefore neuromuscular facilitation techniques targeting the peripheral nerve and muscle will not likely benefit from many of the techniques designed to reduce tone or increase muscle stretch reflexes to increase tone or stability.[4,5]

Golgi Tendon Organs

Beyond the muscle spindle system are joint receptors and special tendon receptors called **Golgi tendon organs**, which are involved in sensorimotor control of some of the muscles of the body. The Golgi tendon organs are directly attached to the tendons of muscles. They respond when either stretching or contraction places tension on the tendon, and they signal the force of muscle contraction. The Golgi tendon organs temper motor activity and inhibit activity in muscles when high levels of tension are placed on the tendon. Golgi tendon organs dampen oscillation of the limbs, at times producing joint stiffness. If these afferents allow too much freedom (such as in Parkinson's disease), the tendency to oscillate is not inhibited and tremor is seen.

The Extrapyramidal System

The pyramidal system is the primary pathway for voluntary movement (i.e., as the direct activation pathway). A subdivision of that system, the corticonuclear tracts, is the primary pathway for the voluntary control of most speech muscles. Still another motor system, the extrapyramidal system, plays a significant role in speech and its disorders.

The **extrapyramidal system** is composed of subcortical nuclei called the basal ganglia, together with the subthalamic nucleus, substantia nigra, red nucleus, brainstem, reticular formation, and the complex pathways that interconnect these nuclei. This text includes in the extrapyramidal system, as some neuroanatomists do, the descending vestibulospinal, rubrospinal, tectospinal, and reticulospinal tracts.

INDIRECT ACTIVATION PATHWAY

In his excellent summary of the anatomy of the motor pathways for speech production, Duffy[8] discusses the concept of the indirect activation pathway of the extrapyramidal system and its contribution to the control of movement. He differentiates between these pathways and those of the control circuits of the basal ganglia and cerebellum. The basal ganglia and the cerebellum are not sources of direct input to the lower motor neurons, whereas the structures of the indirect activation pathways do have direct input to the lower motor neurons of the spinal cord and to some of the cranial nerve nuclei. The input of the indirect activation pathways to the cranial nerve nuclei, and thus to speech production, is currently poorly understood, although projections to some of the nuclei have been documented.

TABLE 6-4
Major Components of the Indirect Activation Pathway of the Extrapyramidal System

COMPONENTS (NUCLEI OR TRACTS)	FUNCTIONAL ROLE IN MOTOR CONTROL
Reticular formation or reticulospinal tracts	Excitation or inhibition of flexors and extensors; facilitation or inhibition of reflexes and ascending sensory information
Vestibular nuclei or vestibulospinal tract	Facilitation of reflex activity and spinal mechanisms controlling muscle tone
Red nucleus or rubrospinal tract	Facilitation of flexor and inhibition of extensor neurons

Modified from Duffy, J. R. (2005). *Motor speech disorders: Substrates, differential diagnosis and management.* St. Louis: Mosby/Elsevier.

According to Duffy,[7] the components of the indirect activation pathway consist of many short pathways and interconnections with structures between the origin of the pathway in the cortex and its termination at the lower motor neuron. The nuclei and tracts considered to be components of the indirect activation system are listed in Table 6-4.

The primary function of the indirect activation pathway is motor control to regulate reflexes and maintain posture and tone. The control is subconscious and requires integration of many muscles. Its effect seems to be inhibitory, whereas the direct activation system facilitates movement. In speech, the indirect activation system probably inhibits interference with the movements of specific muscles so that appropriate speed, range, and direction of movement can be maintained. In general, damage to the indirect activation system affects muscle tone and reflexes. It usually is manifest in combination with damage to the direct activation system, the pyramidal tract.

BASAL GANGLIA

The term extrapyramidal system has clinical utility in that it is widely used to refer to a group of subcortical nuclei and related structures known as the basal ganglia (see Chapter 2, Figs. 2-15 and 2-16). The terminology used to describe the basal ganglia is not always agreed on and is generally confusing. However, the basal ganglia does have three major agreed-upon parts: the caudate nucleus, the putamen, and the globus pallidus (see Table 6-5). Other structures include the subthalamic nucleus and substantia nigra.[17]

The caudate nucleus lies just medial to the anterior limb of the internal capsule. The putamen and globus pallidus lie anterior to the genu of the internal capsule. The caudate nucleus lies adjacent to the wall of the lateral ventricle, close to the thalamus, which is part of the diencephalon. The structure is divided into a head, body, and tail by some neurologists, but others divide the caudate into only a head and tail. The caudate and the putamen together make up what is known as the striatum. Converging excitatory input comes into the striatum from almost the entire cortex, but especially the sensorimotor and frontal cortex.

The putamen and globus pallidus together comprise the lentiform nucleus, a thumb-sized structure wedged against the internal capsule. The globus pallidus, which is divided into an external and an internal part, is crossed by myelinated fibers, which give it a pale cast in its fresh state. The lentiform nucleus (i.e., the putamen and the globus pallidus), combined with the caudate nucleus, comprise what is known as the corpus striatum (Table 6-5).

Other structures related in function to the basal ganglia are found near the reticular formation of the mesencephalon. These include the subthalamic nucleus, substantia nigra, and red nucleus. The reticular formation itself is also thought of as part of the subcortical extrapyramidal system. The extrapyramidal system is concerned with coarse stereotyped movements. It has more influence over proximal (midline) than distal (peripheral) muscles. It maintains proper tone and posture. Even with destruction of the pyramidal tract, it can allow a person to eat and walk.

Most of the output of the basal ganglia is through the internal portion of the **globus pallidus** (**GPi**). These output nuclei project, via various nuclei in the thalamus, to most cortical areas of the frontal lobe. This forms an important circuit referred to as the basal ganglia–thalamocortical circuit.[1] Figure 6-8 illustrates in a simplified

TABLE 6-5
Major Extrapyramidal Nuclei

Basal ganglia
Globus pallidus ⎤ Lentiform nucleus ⎤
Putamen   ⎦   ⎬ Corpus striatum
Caudate nucleus   Striatum ⎦

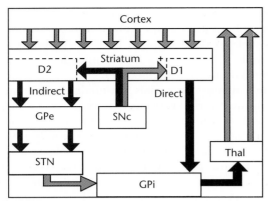

FIGURE 6-8

Simplified diagram of basal ganglia–thalamocortical circuitry (motor circuit). *Shaded arrows* are excitatory; *black arrows* are inhibitory. *GPe*, External segment of globus pallidus; *GPi*, internal segment of globus pallidus; *STN*, subthalamic nucleus; *SNc*, substantia nigra pars compacta; *Thal*, thalamus. The striatum projects to the GPi in a direct and an indirect pathway. The activity in these pathways is modulated by dopamine from the SNc; D1 receptors activate the striatal neurons forming the direct pathway, whereas D2 receptors inhibit the striatal neurons in the indirect pathway. (Adapted from Mink, J.W. and Thach, W.T., (1993). Basal ganglia intrinsic circuits and their role in behavior. *Current Opinion in Neurobiology 3*, pp. 950–957.; Graybiel, A.M.,(2000). The basal ganglia. *Current Biology 10*, pp. R509–R511.; DeLong, M. R. (2000). The basal ganglia. In E. R. Kandel, J. H. Schwartz, & T. M. Jessel (Eds.), *Principles of neural science* (4th ed., pp. 853–867). New York: McGraw-Hill.

manner the excitatory and inhibitory connections of this circuit.

The output nuclei receive projections from the striatum by two pathways, a direct and indirect pathway. The indirect pathway projects to the subthalamic nucleus, which then provides excitatory activation of the internal GPi. The striatal neurons projecting directly to the GPi, on the other hand, are inhibitory to its function. Critical to this difference in the nature of the input is the substantia nigra and its release of dopamine through both pathways. Targeting different receptors in the striatum, the substantia nigra provides both inhibition and excitation to the striatal neurons.

In the basal ganglia–thalamocortical circuitry, all projections from the striatum and the GPi are inhibitory, whereas projections from the cortex, subthalamic nucleus, and thalamus are excitatory. The output of the GPi is inhibited by striatal neurons projecting through the direct pathway using the neurotransmitter **gamma-aminobutyric acid (GABA)**. Thus through the direct pathway, the action of the thalamic neurons is disinhibited, allowing excitation of cortical neurons. In contrast, the activation of the indirect pathway of this circuit

provides activation or excitation of the GPi, providing more inhibition of the thalamic neurons and consequently inhibiting the cortex. Through the action of these two pathways, a balance is achieved in normal brain function and cortical motor activity is modulated by the circuitry (see Fig. 6-8).

In addition to the basal ganglia, the cerebellum and the cerebral cortex interact in a series of feedback loops, suggesting complex interaction of motor subsystems to coordinate everyday speech motor performance. Fibers from the GPi ascend to the level of the internal capsule, where they join cerebellothalamic fibers and synapse in the thalamus. Other fibers from the GPi synapse in the subthalamic nucleus, and another set terminates in the midbrain.

Fitzgerald and Folan-Curran[10] cite four different functional circuits that appear to operate in motor control and involve the basal ganglia: (1) a motor loop for learned movements, (2) a limbic loop pertaining to emotional aspects of movement, (3) a cognitive loop relating to motor intentions, and (4) an oculomotor loop concerned with voluntary eye movements. The substantia nigra, through its connections to the striatum (nigrostriatal pathways) and eventually to the SMA, appears to be important for facilitation, allowing the SMA to become active immediately before movement. This dopaminergic pathway is thought to help the SMA organize the sequence of cell column excitation in the motor cortex. Learned movement sequences may be stored in the putamen, assembled in sequence, and transmitted to the SMA by these pathways. Failure of the compact part of the substantia nigra to produce dopamine for facilitation along this nigrostriatal pathway results in Parkinson's disease. The classic dysarthria, hypokinetic dysarthria, which is associated with Parkinson's disease and parkinsonism, is discussed in Chapter 8.

Lesions of the basal ganglia generally produce two major types of movement disorders: poverty of movement (**akinesia**) and excessive involuntary movement (dyskinesia).[17] Akinesia is often accompanied by muscular rigidity, as in Parkinson's disease. The symptoms of these movement disorders suggest that basal ganglia disorders result in deficits in the initiation of movement (akinesia), difficulty in continuing or stopping an ongoing movement (dyskinesia), abnormalities of muscle tone (rigidity), and the development of involuntary movements (chorea, tremor, athetosis, and dystonia). Thus the basal ganglia are thought to participate heavily in motor control, particularly in the initiation of movement and the maintenance of ongoing movement. The basal ganglia particularly influence movements related to posture, automatic movements, and skilled voluntary movements.

Marsden[14] argues that the basal ganglia are responsible for the automatic execution of learned motor plans. This involves subconscious selection, sequencing, and delivery of the motor programs of a learned or practiced motor strategy, such as playing an instrument or writing by hand. When the basal ganglia are damaged, the individual appears to revert to slower, less automatic, and less-accurate cortical mechanisms for motor behavior. Alm[1] provides an excellent review of studies that support the possibility that the basal ganglia–thalamocortical circuit plays an important role in the pathophysiology of stuttering.

DYSKINESIA

Damage to other parts of the basal ganglia produce motor disturbances usually classified as involuntary movement disorders. The most commonly used technical term for them is **dyskinesia** (*dys*, meaning disorder, and *kinesia*, meaning movement). These disorders encompass a full range of bizarre postures and unusual movement patterns. The dyskinesias have long been described by such terms as tremor, writhing, fidgeting, flailing, restlessness, jerking, and flinging. Often the unusual movements that dominate the trunk and limbs of the dyskinetic patient are also reflected in the face and speech mechanism. The result is a serious and typical dysarthria classified under hyperkinetic dysarthria (see Chapter 8). In general, the dysarthria reflects the specific symptoms of each specific type of dyskinesia.

The term dyskinesia typically is used to indicate movement disorders associated with extrapyramidal lesions, but the term may be used in a broader sense to include any excess of movement (hyperkinesia) or reduction in movement (akinesia). **Hyperkinesia** has been used to indicate dyskinesias that present too much movement. **Hypokinesia** and akinesia, on the other hand, refer to too-little movement and reduced movement, respectively. In actual clinical use, the terms may not always be strictly applied to a person with extrapyramidal lesions. For instance, neurologists may apply hyperkinesia to the well-known extrapyramidally based twitching or fidgeting of Huntington's chorea as well as the abnormal hyperactivity of children in whom there may not be evidence of an organic lesion in the nervous system, let alone knowledge of a lesion localized to the extrapyramidal system.

Hypokinesia may be used to describe the reduced activity level of a depressive patient with no suspected neurologic lesion. By tradition, neurologists do not apply hypokinesia to limitations in movement resulting from lesions of the pyramidal tract or peripheral nerves. In other words, lesions that paralyze voluntary movement are not labeled hypokinetic. Thus hemiplegia, quadriplegia, and **paraplegia** are not considered hypokinetic disorders.

Dyskinetic Types

The responsibilities of speech-language pathologists do not extend to the identification of lesion sites in the complex circuitry of the extrapyramidal motor system, but they should attempt to recognize the standard dyskinesias of extrapyramidal origin and determine the effect of the symptoms of specific dyskinesias on the accompanying dysarthria. Undiagnosed cases of dyskinesia demand referral to a neurologist. Dyskinesia has several distinct patterns, but not all of them are related to the dysarthrias. Described are only those motor signs that produce motor speech symptoms.

Tremors

Tremors are defined as purposeless movements that are rhythmic, oscillatory, involuntary actions. Normal (or physiologic) and abnormal (or pathologic) tremors are usually distinguished. Tremors are pathologic if they occur in a disease and are characteristic of that disease. Normal tremor is called physiologic tremor. Several classifications of tremor are in use today. The speech-language pathologist should be familiar with three types of tremor associated with vocal performance in normal and pathologic conditions.

Rest Tremor. **Rest tremor** designates a tremor that occurs in Parkinson's disease. A tremor of three to seven movements per second occurs in the patient's limbs and hands at rest. The tremor is temporarily suppressed when the limb is moved, and it sometimes can be inhibited by conscious effort. The voice may be affected by the tremor. Tremulous voice has been described in approximately 14% of a large sample of parkinsonian patients. It is a salient vocal deviation that is easily recognized among the other vocal deviations of the hypokinetic dysarthria of parkinsonism.

Physiologic, or Action, Tremor. Healthy people demonstrate a fine tremor of the hands when maintaining posture. The rate may vary with age but usually falls within the range of 4 to 12 cycles per second. An **action tremor** may affect the laryngeal muscles and produce an organic or essential vocal tremor, the mechanism for which is unknown. This normal tremor is distinguished from pathologic tremors associated with known neurologic diseases such as Parkinson's and cerebellar disorders.

Intention Tremor. **Intention tremor** refers to a tremor that occurs during movement and is intensified at the termination of the movement. Intention tremor has been associated with the ataxic dysarthria seen in cerebellar disease. It is often seen in cerebellar disorders but is not exclusive to cerebellar dysfunction.

Chorea

Chorea refers to quick, random, hyperkinetic movements simulating fragments of normal movements. Speech, facial, and respiratory movements, as well as movements of the extremities, are affected by choreic symptoms in this dyskinesia. The movement is close to what is popularly described as fidgets. Chorea is one symptom of a hereditary disorder known as Huntington's disease, or Huntington's chorea, and is seen in other extrapyramidal disorders as well.

Athetosis

The hyperkinesia of **athetosis** is a slow, irregular, coarse, writhing, or squirming movement. It usually involves the extremities as well as the face, neck, and trunk. The movements directly interfere with the fine and controlled actions of the larynx, tongue, palate, pharynx, and respiratory mechanism. As with most other involuntary movements, the involuntary movements of athetosis disappear in sleep. In congenital athetosis, the most common type of spastic paralysis may also be observed, indicating involvement of both pyramidal and extrapyramidal systems. Lesion sites in pure athetosis are often in the putamen and the caudate nucleus. Hypoxia, or lack of oxygen at birth, is a common cause, producing death of brain cells before or during birth. Choreoathetotic movements have also been described; they appear to be a dyskinesia that lies somewhere between choreic and athetoid movements in terms of rate and rhythm of movement or that includes both types of movement. In fact, many of the involuntary movement disorders appear to blend one or more of the different clinical dyskinesias, as the term choreoathetosis implies.

Dystonia

In **dystonia** the limbs assume distorted static postures resulting from excess tone in selected parts of the body. The dyskinetic postures are slow, bizarre, and often grotesque, involving writhing, twisting, and turning. Dysarthria and obvious motor involvement of the speech mechanism are common. Often differential motor involvement occurs in the speech muscles, and some dysarthrias have been observed that primarily affect the larynx. Others affect the face, tongue, lips, palate, and jaw. A rare dystonic disorder of childhood is called dystonia musculorum deformans. It may be accompanied by dysarthria in its later stages.

Fragmentary, or focal, dystonias have been described, and some neurologists assert that they contribute to spastic or spasmodic dysphonia, a bizarre voice disorder that mixes aphonia (lack of voice) with a strained, labored whisper. The etiology of spastic dysphonia is unclear. Injections of botulinum are effective in reducing the dystonia.

Myoclonus

Myoclonus has been used to describe differing motor abnormalities, but basically a myoclonic movement is an abrupt, brief, almost lightning-like contraction of muscle. An example of a normal or physiologic myoclonic reaction occurs when a person is drifting off to sleep but suddenly awakened by a rapid muscle jerk. This muscle jerk is myoclonus.

Pathologic myoclonus is most common in the limbs and trunk but also may involve the facial muscles, jaws, tongue, and pharynx. Repetitive myoclonus in these muscles, of course, may affect speech. Myoclonic movements in the muscles of speech have been described as having a rate of 10 to 50 per minute, but they can be more rapid. The pathology underlying these movements has been debated, but because they have been associated with degenerative brain disease, the cerebral cortex, brainstem, cerebellum, and extrapyramidal system have all been considered as possible lesion sites.

A special myoclonic syndrome involving speech muscles called palatal myoclonus has been described. It involves rapid movements of the soft palate and pharynx and sometimes includes the larynx, diaphragm, and other muscles. The symptoms most often present in later life and are characteristic of several diseases. This myoclonus has a specific pathology in the central tegmental tract of the brainstem, but the etiology can be varied. The most common cause is a stroke, or cerebrovascular accident, in the brainstem.

Facial Dyskinesia (Tardive Dyskinesia)

In facial dyskinesia (**tardive**) **dyskinesia** bizarre movements are limited to the mouth, face, jaw, and tongue. This movement includes grimacing, pursing of the mouth and lips, and writhing of the tongue. These dyskinetic movements often alter articulation of speech. The motor speech signs of orofacial dyskinesia usually develop after the prolonged use of powerful tranquilizing drugs, the most common class of which are phenothiazines. Drug-induced dyskinesias associated with the phenothiazines and related medications may even produce athetoid movements or dystonic movements of the body. Parkinsonian signs and other symptoms associated with extrapyramidal disorders are also caused by these drugs. Orofacial dyskinesia also occurs in elderly patients without drug use. A rare disorder that includes dyskinesia of the eyelids, face, tongue, and refractory muscles is called Meige syndrome.

Other dyskinesias are included in the spectrum of extrapyramidal disorders but generally do not include motor involvement of the speech mechanism. These include hemiballismus, which causes forceful, flinging unilateral movements and may involve half of the body. Akathisia refers to motor restlessness or the inability to sit still. Restless leg syndrome is an example of this dyskinesia. Box 6-1 summarizes the extrapyramidal dyskinesias.

The Cerebellar System

The third major subcomponent of the motor system that affects speech is the cerebellum. Interacting with the pyramidal and extrapyramidal systems, the cerebellum is known to provide significant coordination for motor speech. As previously noted, the cerebellum is located dorsal to the medulla and pons. The occipital lobes of the cerebral hemispheres overlap the top of the cerebellum. The anatomy of the cerebellum is complex, and the speech-language pathologist need only understand it in a gross sense to see the relation of the cerebellum to speech performance.

ANATOMY OF THE CEREBELLUM

The cerebellum can be divided into three parts. The thin middle portion is called the vermis because of its serpentine, or snakelike, shape. The vermis lies between two large lateral masses of the cerebellum, the cerebellar hemispheres (Fig. 6-9). The vermis connects these two hemispheres. The vermis and hemispheres are divided by fissures and sulci into lobes and also into smaller divisions called lobules. The division into lobes and lobules is helpful in clarifying the physiologic function of the cerebellum. Although the lobes and lobules have been classified differently by different investigators, this text uses a classification system that divides the cerebellum into three lobes.

Three Cerebellar Lobes

The three cerebellar lobes are the anterior lobe, the posterior lobe, and the flocculonodular lobe. The anterior lobe, which is modest in size, is superior to the primary fissure. This part of the cerebellum roughly corresponds to what is known as the paleocerebellum, the second oldest part of the cerebellum in a phylogenetic sense. The anterior lobe receives most of the proprioceptive impulses from the spinal cord and regulates posture.

The posterior lobe, the largest part of the cerebellum, is located between the other two lobes. It comprises the major portion of the cerebellar hemispheres. It is the newest part of the cerebellum and is therefore also known as the **neocerebellum**. The posterior lobe

---

BOX 6-1

Common Extrapyramidal Dyskinetic Types

- *Tremors:* Purposeless movements that are rhythmic, oscillatory, involuntary actions. Designated as either normal (physiologic) or abnormal (pathologic).
  - Rest tremor: Designated tremor caused by Parkinson's disease. Presenting signs include tremor when affected limb is at rest and may include tremulous voice. Range of three to seven movements per second.
  - Action (physiologic) tremor: Fine tremor of hands while maintaining posture. Can affect laryngeal muscles, causing voice tremor. Range of 4 to 12 cycles per second.
  - Intention tremor: Tremor intensified at termination of movement. Associated with ataxic dysarthria and other cerebellar disorders.
- *Chorea:* Quick, random, hyperkinetic movements simulating fragments of normal movement. Movements are close to what is commonly described as "fidgets" and present as a symptom of Huntington's disease.
- *Athetosis:* Slow, irregular, coarse, writhing, or squirming movement. Involves extremities and can also directly interfere with fine and controlled actions of the swallowing and respiratory mechanisms.
- *Dystonia:* Limbs assume distorted, static postures resulting in excess tone in selected body parts. Movements include slow, bizarre, and often grotesque writhing, twisting, and turning motions.
- *Myoclonus:* Abrupt, brief, almost lightning-like contraction of muscle. Pathology is still debatable. Has been associated with degenerative brain disease, cerebral cortex, brainstem, cerebellum, and the extrapyramidal system. Palatal myoclonus is a special type involving rapid movements of the soft palate and pharynx, commonly caused by stroke or cerebrovascular accident in the brainstem.
- *Facial (tardive) dyskinesia:* Bizarre movements limited to mouth, face, jaw, and tongue characterized by grimacing, pursing of mouth and lips, and writhing of the tongue. Shown to develop from prolonged use of tranquilizing drugs, especially phenothiazines. A dyskinesia called Meige syndrome affects the eyelids, face, tongue, and refractory muscles.
- *Nonspeech-related dyskinesias:*
  - Hemiballismus: Forceful, flinging, unilateral movements that may involve the whole body.
  - Akathisia: Motor restlessness or the inability to sit still (e.g., restless leg syndrome).

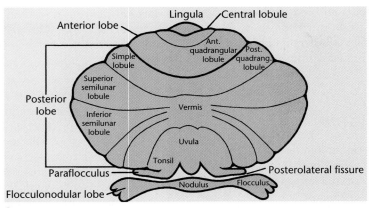

FIGURE 6-9
A schematic illustration of the cerebellum showing hemispheres, lobes, and lobules. *Ant.*, Anterior; *Post.*, posterior; *Quadrang.*, quadrangular.

receives the cerebellar connections from the cerebrum and regulates coordination of muscle movement.

The flocculonodular lobe consists of two small wispy appendages, known as **flocculi**, in the posterior and inferior region of the cerebellum. The flocculi are separated by the nodulus, the inferior part of the vermis. The flocculonodular lobe, the oldest portion of the cerebellum, contains the fastigial nucleus, which is composed of fibers that travel from the nucleus to the four vestibular nuclei in the upper medulla. The cerebellum mediates equilibrium by way of these fibers.

Synergy and Asynergy

The connections that the cerebellum has with other parts of the central nervous system are important to its function. Through these connections the cerebellum sends and receives afferent and efferent impulses and executes its primary function: a synergistic coordination of muscles and muscle groups. **Synergy** is defined as the cooperative action of muscles. Ensuring the smooth coordination of muscles is the prime task of the cerebellum. Specifically, the cerebellum, along with other structures of the nervous system, maintains proper posture and balance in walking and in the sequential movements of eating, dressing, and writing. It also guides the production of rapid, alternating, repetitive movements such as those involved in speaking and smooth pursuit movements. Voluntary movement, without assistance from the cerebellum, is clumsy, uncoordinated, and disorganized. Motor defect of the cerebellar system has been called asynergia or dyssynergia. **Asynergia** is a lack of coordination in agonistic and antagonistic muscles and is manifested as deterioration of smooth, complex movements.

Cerebellar Peduncles and Pathways

The cerebellum is connected to the rest of the nervous system by three pairs of **peduncles**, or feet. The cerebellar peduncles anchor the cerebellum to the brainstem. All afferent and efferent fibers of the cerebellum pass through the three peduncles and the pons to the other levels of the nervous system. The pons, which means bridge, is aptly named; it is literally a bridge from the cerebellum to the rest of the nervous system (Fig. 6-10).

The inferior cerebellar peduncle, or restiform body, carries primary afferent fibers from the structures close to it: the medulla, spinal cord, and cranial nerve VIII. Thus spinocerebellar, medullocerebellar, and vestibular fibers pass through the inferior peduncle.

The middle cerebellar peduncle, or brachium pontis, connects the cerebellum with the cerebral cortex by the pathways that traverse it. The middle peduncle is easily recognized; it is the largest of the three peduncles and also conveys the largest number of fibers from the cerebral cortex and pons. It carries pontocerebellar fibers as well as the majority of the corticopontocerebellar fibers. These fibers convey afferent information from the temporal and frontal lobes of the cerebrum to the posterior lobe of the contralateral cerebellum.

The superior cerebellar peduncle, or brachium conjunctivum, conveys the bulk of efferent fibers that leave the cerebellum. The primary efferent fibers arise from an important nucleus deep in the cerebellum called the dentate nucleus. The rubrospinal and dentatothalamic pathways, along with several other tracts, leave by way of the superior peduncle and terminate in the contralateral red nucleus and ventrolateral nucleus of the thalamus. From here impulses are relayed to the cerebral cortex.

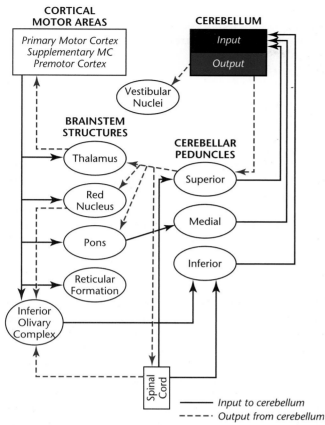

FIGURE 6-10
Major pathways of the cerebellum. *MC*, Motor cortex.

CEREBELLAR ROLE IN SPEECH

The major pathways and structures of the cerebellum have been outlined to suggest a rough schematic of the feedback nature of the afferent and efferent connections of the structure. Basic as the presentation is, it still highlights the fact that the cerebellar motor subsystem significantly influences the function of the other motor systems in the production of motor speech. The fact that the cerebellum plays an important part in the synergy of rapid alternating movements and the fine coordination of muscles suggests that it interacts in a crucial way with the corticonuclear fibers to provide the specialized rapid and precise motor control needed for ongoing connected speech.

Auditory, tactile, and visual areas also exist in the cerebellum. These centers in the cerebellum, both cortical and subcortical, project to similar areas in the cerebrum, which in turn project back to corresponding cerebellar areas. The cerebellum therefore is neither completely vestibular, proprioceptive, nor motor in function. Rather, it serves to reinforce or diminish sensory and motor impulses, acting as a critical modulator of neuronal function. Through its afferent and efferent feedback circuits, the cerebellum ensures a desired level of neural activity in the motor parts of the nervous system.

CLINICAL SIGNS OF CEREBELLAR DYSFUNCTION

Cerebellar or cerebellar pathway lesions manifest themselves by affecting coordination of **volitional** movements and often volitionally maintained postures. Clinical signs usually appear on the same side of the body as the cerebellar lesion. Upper motor neuron lesions of pyramidal pathways yield contralateral effects, whereas the cerebellum and its pathways manifest ipsilateral effects. Several classic signs of cerebellar disorders follow and are summarized in Table 6-6, along with tests used to determine the abnormality.

Ataxia

Ataxia is the prime sign of a cerebellar lesion (taxis means "ordering in rank and file"). The term ataxia is often used in several senses. It may refer to the general

TABLE 6-6	
Cerebellar Dysfunction Signs and Tests	
ABNORMALITY	SIGNS AND TESTS
Gait ataxia	Broad-based gait seen on tandem walking test
Arm ataxia	Finger to nose test, hand pronation to supination test results in overshooting of nose and slowed pronation and supination
Overshooting	Rebound noted on arm-pulling test
Hypotonia	Flaccid muscle tone noted on passive movement testing; pendular reflexes elicited on reflex testing; "rag doll" postures observed
Nystagmus	Pupil oscillation seen when patient attempts to follow finger through field of gaze
Dysarthria	Ataxic dysarthria with disturbance in speech rate and prosody; often associated with left cerebellar hemisphere lesion

incoordination of motor acts seen with cerebellar system lesions. In this sense it often describes a staggering or reeling gait and abnormal posture seen with cerebellar lesions. The patient compensates for the ataxic gait by standing and walking with feet wide apart in what is called a broad-based gait.

Decomposition of Movement

Decomposition of movement is also related to ataxia. The patient breaks a complex motor act into its components and executes the act movement by movement so that the act seems as if it were being performed by a robot. Decomposition of movement is considered an ataxic movement.

Dysmetria

Dysmetria is the inability to gauge the distance, speed, and power of movement. A patient may stop before the movement is performed or may overshoot the motor goal.

Adiadochokinesia or Dysdiadochokinesia

Adiadochokinesia, or **dysdiadochokinesia**, is the inability to perform rapid alternating muscle movements. Often the rate of alternating movement may be recorded in a neurologic examination. This measure is called an alternate motion rate. Diadochokinetic rate measures of the muscles of the oral mechanism during speech and nonspeech activities have long been used as an assessment task by the clinical speech-language pathologist. These rates, however, are used as measures of the integrity of the oral muscles in speech pathology and have not specifically been related to cerebellar function.

The neurologist may test alternating movements in many muscle groups in persons suspected of cerebellar disorders. Successive pronation or supination of the hands, rapid tapping of the fingers, and rapid opening and closing of the fists are all diadochokinetic diagnostic tests. During the testing of diadochokinesis or alternate motion rates, awkwardness or clumsiness of alternate movements may be seen.

Rebound

The rebound phenomenon is the inability to check the contraction of the flexors and rapidly contract the extensor. It may account for the lack of smooth diadochokinetic movements.

Hypotonia

Hypotonia (or muscle flaccidity) with a decrease in resistance to passive movement is seen in cerebellar dysfunction. The muscles of the body are flabby and lack normal tone.

Tremor

Tremor is seen as part of cerebellar disease. It is usually an intention or kinetic tremor not present at rest.

Nystagmus

Nystagmus involves oscillatory abnormalities of the pupil of the eye often seen in cerebellar disorders. The rhythmic oscillations may be vertical, horizontal, or rotary.

Muscle Stretch Reflexes

Muscle stretch reflexes are normal or diminished. Pendular reflexes often may be seen in cerebellar disease. When the knee jerk reflex is elicited, a series of smooth to-and-fro movements of the limb often occur before it comes to rest, as seen with a pendulum. This pendular reflex differs from a normal knee-jerk response.

Dysarthria

Dysarthria associated with damage to the cerebellum is called **ataxic dysarthria**. Its characteristics are discussed in Chapter 8.

Servomechanism Theory and Speech Motor Control

FEEDBACK

Several fruitful engineering concepts have been applied to neuronal transmission problems in the nervous system. These concepts have been particularly useful in explaining the possible control of neural impulses in the speech mechanism. The basic concept, known as the theory of **servomechanism control systems**, implies the concept of **feedback**. Feedback describes the functioning principle in self-regulating systems, either mechanical or biologic. Feedback assumes that the output of any self-regulating system, such as a thermostat, is fed back into the system at some point to control or regulate the output of the system. This concept of self-monitoring is most appropriate for understanding the biologic system known as the speech motor control system. For instance, the questions of how a speaker monitors speech and what neuronal feedback mechanisms are available to control speech movements seem likely ones for explanation by servomechanism theory.

OPEN AND CLOSED CONTROL SYSTEMS

Two types of bioengineering control systems have been described as applicable to neuronal transmission in speech production: closed-loop and open-loop control systems. A closed-loop system uses positive feedback in which output is returned as input to control further output. For example, when copying a complex and delicate drawing, the sensory input to the visual system guides the motor output of the hand. Similarly, hearing one's own speech while talking may at times control the motor speech output as one continues to talk more. In these two examples, motor output by hand or speech is assumed to be guided by the sensory input of vision or audition. Furthermore, if the sensory feedback were blocked, the drawing or speech would be assumed to go awry.

In an open-loop system, the output is generally preprogrammed, and the performance of the system is not matched with the system. For instance, if a person has learned a short poem by heart and has practiced it repeatedly, that person may be able to say the phonemes of the words in the poem without error even though his or her ears are stuffed with cotton. In an open-loop system the notion of **feedforward**, rather than feedback, is important. Once a phrase of a well-learned poem has been uttered, it cues the next preprogrammed phrase of speech without the need to hear what was said through auditory feedback. An open-loop system thus typically generates another input by its output system. The term negative feedback is also used in control systems of the servomechanism type. That term implies that when errors are fed back into the system, the error information acts to keep a given output activity within certain limits. Correcting an articulation error on hearing it is an example of the use of negative feedback in speech activity.

Much speech research has viewed speech motor control as the product of a closed-loop feedback system with sensory monitoring from hearing, touch, and deep muscle sense guiding the movements of the speech muscles. Circumstantial evidence for this position has come from studies of sensory dysfunction in some speech disorders. Yet evidence exists that much of speech motor control is preprogrammed by the brain and that feedforward control is also important. Neurologic control of speech may well involve combinations of both open and closed loops in a multiple-pathway, hierarchical system that provides the necessary flexibility, speed, and precision to program and execute the everyday movements of speech with such complexity and ease.

Synopsis of Clinical Information and Applications for the Speech-Language Pathologist

- The motor system has a hierarchy. It becomes progressively more sophisticated as the paths ascend and progressively less sophisticated as the paths descend.
- The lower levels of the motor system are partially constrained by the upper levels, but all have a certain autonomy.
- The levels of the motor system can be enumerated as Broca's area and the motor association cortex areas, the pyramidal system, the spinal cord and the brainstem nuclei (lower motor neuron), the cerebellum, and the extrapyramidal tract, including basal ganglia and the indirect activation pathway tracts.
- Motor speech commands are organized in the premotor and SMA (motor association areas) and Broca's area as well as the insula. Apraxia of speech is the disorder associated with damage to the motor speech programming areas.
- The pyramidal system includes the corticospinal tract for motor control of limbs and the corticonuclear tract, which provides motor control for muscles of the face, tongue, pharynx, and larynx.
- The corticospinal tract is a primarily contralateral innervation system, with 90% of the fibers decussating at

the level of the pyramids of the medulla and terminating in the opposite side of the spinal cord.
- The corticonuclear tract provides primarily bilateral innervation for the majority of the musculature innervated, with the decussation occurring at various levels of the brainstem. Although most of the nuclei receive both unilateral and contralateral fibers, the amount of unilateral versus contralateral innervation varies.
- Upper motor neurons are the first-order neurons in the corticospinal and corticonuclear tracts. The upper motor neurons send axons to the nuclei of the spinal cord or the cranial nerves in the brainstem. They comprise the first fiber pathway of the direct activation pathway that is the pyramidal tract.
- Lower motor neurons are the second-order neurons in the direct activation pathway. They send axons out of the spinal cord or brainstem and become the peripheral nerves. Sherrington called the lower motor neuron the final common pathway because it is the final route for all the complex motor activity occurring above the level of the lower motor neurons.
- The motor unit is a useful concept when studying the lower motor neurons. The motor unit consists of

Continued

Synopsis of Clinical Information and Applications for the Speech-Language Pathologist—cont'd

the cell body, the axon (the nerve itself), the junction of the nerve and muscle fiber (neuromuscular juncture), and the muscle fiber.

- The facial nerve (cranial nerve VII) is unusual in that it has a dorsal and ventral component to its nucleus. The ventral portion, supplying the upper face, is far more bilaterally innervated than the dorsal part, which supplies the lower part of the face. The clinical implication of this is that a unilateral upper motor neuron lesion affecting this nerve results in paresis or paralysis of the opposite side of the lower face, whereas the upper half of the face is relatively unaffected because of its bilateral innervation.

- Lesions of the upper motor neuron tract produce different clinical symptoms than lesions of the lower motor neuron tract. The speech-language pathologist must be able to recognize these signs. Damage to the two different pathways produces different types of dysarthria as well.

- Alpha motor neurons are the nerve cells that comprise the lower motor neuron. They are found in the anterior horn cells in the spinal cord and in the nuclei of the cranial nerves in the brainstem. They supply skeletal muscles through innervation of the extrafusal fibers of the muscles.

- The muscle spindle is present in many skeletal muscles and provides the sensory feedback to the muscle regarding length. This feedback results in the muscle stretch reflex. With the exception of the jaw-closing muscles, muscle spindles are few and scattered in the muscles concerned with speech and swallowing.

- The extrapyramidal system is composed of the descending indirect activation pathways (vestibulospinal, reticulospinal, rubrospinal, and tectospinal tracts), basal ganglia, subthalamic nucleus, substantia nigra, and reticular formation.

- The primary structures of the basal ganglia are the caudate nucleus, GPi, and putamen. The substantia nigra and subthalamic nucleus are also included. Four different functional circuits seem to operate in the basal ganglia system: a motor loop, a limbic loop, a cognitive loop, and an oculomotor loop.

- Basal ganglia disease can cause movement disorders and associated dysarthrias. The dysarthria of Parkinson's disease is an example of a hypokinetic dysarthria, and the motor speech disorder associated with Huntington's chorea is an example of hyperkinetic dysarthria. Both result from damage to parts of the basal ganglia.

- The small hemispheres at the base of the brain are the lobes of the cerebellum. The cerebellum, like the basal ganglia, serves as a "consultant" to the motor system and provides coordination needed for smooth, synergistic movement. Signs of cerebellar damage include ataxia, nystagmus, dysmetria, dysdiachokinesis, and sometimes an ataxic dysarthria.

- Speech motor control seems to be a product of both an open-loop and a closed-loop feedback system according to servomechanism theory. The open-loop system contains feedforward control, with the brain partially preprogramming movements that will be made to accomplish certain productions. The concept of speech motor control as a product of a closed-loop system has been generally accepted as the prime system controlling speech output, meaning that sensory monitoring from hearing, touch, and deep muscle sense guides production. Sufficient evidence exists that feedforward occurs, and both types of systems are probably in operation.

 ## CASE**STUDY**

A 63-year-old man awoke in the early morning with disorientation, inability to speak, and inability to move his right side. He was admitted through the emergency department with a preliminary diagnosis of acute left hemisphere cerebrovascular accident (also known as a stroke). A computed tomography scan was done early to rule out hemorrhage but did not show a lesion site. He was put on blood-thinning medication and began to show some movement of the right lower extremity and some ability to speak, although speech was very hesitant, non-fluent, and difficult to understand. He was able to answer yes/no questions accurately and could read fairly well. Further testing during the next few days revealed difficulty following body movement commands involving facial and oral movements and found him "awkward and slow" in following commands involving movements of the left hand. He was diagnosed with mild Broca's aphasia with accompanying

CASE**STUDY**—cont'd

apraxia of speech, right hemiparesis, mild right facial weakness affecting the movement of the right side of the lips, and "clumsy hand syndrome" (sympathetic apraxia) on the left side. He was discharged to an acute rehabilitation center, where he participated in occupational therapy, physical therapy, and speech therapy. He did well in treatment. At discharge 3 weeks later, he was walking with a cane, and movement and use of the right arm had improved, providing some gross functional use. Speech was still effortful with simple sentence structure and was distorted though intelligible.

QUESTIONS FOR CONSIDERATION:
1. Considering the right hemiparesis, mild Broca's aphasia, apraxia of speech, and sympathetic apraxia, what are the likely structures damaged by this stroke?
2. How might the presence of a sympathetic apraxia in the left hand greatly complicate the speech-language pathologist's treatment of a person with right hemiparesis and limited speech output?

REFERENCES

1. Alm, P. A. (2004). Stuttering and the basal ganglia circuits: a critical review of possible relations. *Journal of Communication Disorders, 37,* 4, 325-369.
2. Beckman, D. (1988). *Beckman oral motor interventions.* Course pack accompanying oral motor assessment and intervention workshop, Charlotte, NC: August 2001.
3. Boshart, C. (1998). *Oral-motor analysis and remediation techniques,* Temecula, CA: Speech Dynamics, Inc.
4. Clark, H. M. (2003). Neuromuscular treatments for speech and swallowing: a tutorial. *American Journal of Speech-Language Pathology, 12,* 4, 400-415.
5. Clark, H. M. (2005). Clinical decision making and oral motor treatments. *The ASHA Leader, June* 14, 8-9, 34-35.
6. Dronkers, N. F. (1996). A new brain region for coordinating speech articulation. *Nature, 384,* 159-161.
7. Duffy, J. R. (1995). *Motor speech disorders: Substrates, differential diagnosis and management.* St. Louis: Mosby–Year Book, Inc.
8. Duffy, J. R. (2005). *Motor speech disorders: Substrates, differential diagnosis and management* (2nd ed.). St. Louis: Mosby/Elsevier.
9. Fenichel, G. M. (1993). *Clinical pediatric neurology: A signs and symptoms approach.* Philadelphia: W. B. Saunders.
10. Fitzgerald, M. J. T., & Folan-Curran, J. (2002). *Clinical neuroanatomy and related neuroscience* (4th ed.). Edinburgh: W. B. Saunders.
11. Geschwind, N. (1975). The apraxias: Neural mechanisms of disorders of learned movements. *American Scientist, 63,* 188-195.
12. Guenther, F. H., Ghosh, S. S., & Tourville, J. A. (2006). Neural modeling and imaging of the cortical interactions underlying syllable production. *Brain and Language, 96,* 280-301.
13. Leiguardia, R. C., & Marsden, C. D. (2000). Imaging aphasia: The coming paradigm shift. *Brain and Cognition, 42,* 60-63.
14. Marsden, C. D. (1982). The mysterious function of the basal ganglia. *Neurology, 32,* 514-539.
15. Ogar, J., Willock, S., Baldo, J., Wilkins, D., Ludy, C., & Dronkers, N. (2006). Clinical and anatomical correlates of apraxia of speech. *Brain and Language, 97,* 3, 343-350.
16. Sherrington, C. S. (1926). *The integrative action of the nervous system.* New Haven: Yale University Press.
17. Weiner, W. J., & Lang, A. E. (1989). *Movement disorders: A comprehensive survey.* Mount Kisco, NY: Futura Publishing.

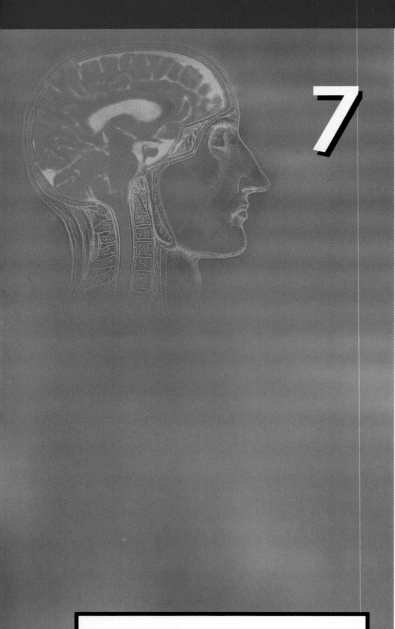

7

The Cranial Nerves

To those I address, it is unnecessary to go further than to indicate that the nerves treated in these papers are the instruments of expression from the smile of the infant's cheek to the last agony of life.

Charles Bell, 1824

CHAPTER**OUTLINE**

KEYTERMS

abduction
abducens
branchial set
central pattern
  generator
cranial nerves
diplopia
extraocular
internuncial
genioglossus
glottal coup
hyoglossus

lacrimal
palpate
parasympathetic nuclei
primary olfactory
  cortex
ptosis
secretomotor
styloglossus
sublingual
tinnitus
transitory

This chapter is intended to help the speech-language pathologist understand one of the most important parts of the nervous system regarding the acts of speaking and swallowing. The **cranial nerves** comprise a part of the peripheral nervous system that provides crucial sensory and motor information to the oral, pharyngeal, and laryngeal musculature. The speech-language pathologist should be familiar with the names, structure, innervation, testing procedures, and signs of abnormal function of the cranial nerves. This information is vital when working with the dysarthric and/or dysphagic adult and child.

Origin of the Cranial Nerves

NAMES AND NUMBERS

Twelve pairs of cranial nerves leave the brain and pass through the foramina of the skull. They are referred to by their numbers, written in Roman numerals, and by their names. The names sometimes give a clue to the function of the nerves, but the number, name, and concise descriptions of the various functions should all be learned (Table 7-1). Many students use a suggested mnemonic device to help them remember the cranial nerves (e.g., "On Old Olympus' Towering Top A Finn And German Vend At Hops") or create their own to aid their memory.

EMBRYOLOGIC ORIGIN

The nuclei of the cranial nerves are of three different types. The motor nuclei are distinguished by the embryologic origin of the muscles they innervate. The development of the body wall in the embryo is from blocks of mesoderm called somites. Cranial nerves III, IV, VI, and XII are derived from this somatic segmentation and thus are called the somatomotor, or somitic, set.

TABLE 7-1
The Cranial Nerves

NUMBER	NAME	SUMMARY OF FUNCTION
I	Olfactory	Smell
II	Optic	Vision
III	Oculomotor	Innervation of muscles to move eyeball, pupil, and upper lid
IV	Trochlear	Innervation of superior oblique muscle of eye
V	Trigeminal	Chewing and sensation to face, teeth, anterior tongue
VI	Abducens	Abduction of eye
VII	Facial	Movement of facial muscles, taste, salivary glands
VIII	(Vestibular) acoustic	Equilibrium and hearing
IX	Glossopharyngeal	Taste, swallowing, elevation of pharynx and larynx, parotid salivary gland, sensation to posterior tongue, upper pharynx
X	Vagus	Taste, swallowing, elevation of palate, phonation, parasympathetic outflow to visceral organs
XI	Accessory	Turning of head and shrugging of shoulders
XII	Hypoglossal	Movement of tongue

In the development of the embryo, the branchial (gill) arches are responsible for the structure, muscles, and nerves of the face and neck. Cranial nerves V, VII, IX, X, and XI are thus known as the **branchial set**.

The somites and branchial arches are transverse segments of the embryo. In contrast, the viscera, including the neuraxis, are developed from longitudinal tubes. The elaboration, or diverticulation, of the hollow tubes gives rise to three cranial nerves (I, II, and VIII) known as the solely special sensory set. Some branchial and somatic cranial nerves have a visceral component: III, VII, IX, and X. Cranial nerves V, VII, IX, and X also have a general sensory component (i.e., they participate in sensation of pain, pressure touch, vibration, and proprioception).

THE CORTICONUCLEAR TRACT AND THE CRANIAL NERVES

The cranial nerves consist of efferent motor fibers that arise from nuclei in the brainstem and afferent sensory fibers that originate in the peripheral ganglia. The motor, or efferent, parts are axons of the nerve cells within the brain. These nerve cells with their processes are part of the lower motor neurons. Groups of these nerve cells form the nuclei of origin for the cranial nerves.

The motor nuclei of origin of the cranial nerves receive impulses from the cerebral cortex through the corticonuclear tracts. The tracts begin in the pyramidal cells in the inferior part of the precentral gyrus and also in the adjacent part of the postcentral gyrus. The tracts then follow the path illustrated in Figure 6-2. They descend through the corona radiata and the genu of the internal capsule; they pass through the midbrain in the cerebral peduncles; and they then synapse either with the lower motor neuron directly or indirectly through **internuncial** neurons, a chain of neurons situated between the primary efferent neuron and the final motor neuron.

The majority of the corticonuclear fibers to the motor cranial nerve nuclei cross the midline, or decussate, before reaching the nuclei. All the cranial nerve motor nuclei have bilateral innervation except for portions of the trigeminal, facial, and hypoglossal fibers, which are discussed later.

The motor parts of the cranial nerves are formed by axons of nerve cells within the brain, but the sensory, or afferent, parts of the cranial nerves are formed by axons of nerve cells outside the brain. They are situated on the nerve trunks or in the sensory organ itself (e.g., the nose, ear, or eye). The central processes of these cells enter the brain and terminate by synapsing with cells grouped together to form the nuclei of termination. These cells have axons that cross the midline and ascend and synapse on other sensory nuclei, such as the thalamus. The axons of the resulting cells then terminate in the cerebral cortex.

Cranial Nerves for Smell and Vision

Cranial nerve I, the olfactory nerve, is a plexus of thin fibers that unite in approximately 20 small bundles called fila olfactoria. The olfactory receptors are situated in the mucous membrane of the nasal cavity. The nerve fibers synapse with other cells in the olfactory bulb and finally end in the olfactory areas of the cerebral cortex, the periamygdaloid and prepiriform areas. Together these are known as the **primary olfactory cortex**, and they also send fibers to many other centers within the brain to establish connections for automatic and emotional responses to olfactory stimulation.

Cranial nerves II, III, IV, and VI are concerned with vision. The optic nerve (II) is the primary nerve of sight. Its nerve fibers are axons that come from the retina, converge on the optic disk, and exit from the eye on both sides. The right nerve joins the left to form the optic chiasma. In the optic chiasma, fibers from the nasal half of the eye cross the midline, and fibers from the temporal half continue to run ipsilaterally. Most of the fibers synapse with nerve cells in the lateral geniculate body of the thalamus and then leave it, forming optic radiations. The optic radiations formed by these fibers terminate in the visual cortex and the visual association cortex.

Cranial nerve III is the oculomotor nerve, the nucleus of which is located at the level of the superior colliculus. Cranial nerve III has a somatomotor component that innervates the **extraocular** muscles to move the eyeball and a visceral component responsible for pupil constriction. Dysfunction of the third cranial nerve causes **ptosis** (drooping) of the eyelid. The eye may also be in **abduction** and turned down. If the visceral component is impaired, the pupillary reflex is lost and the pupil is dilated. Figure 7-1, *A*, illustrates a complete paralysis of the left oculomotor nerve.

Cranial nerve IV is the trochlear nerve, the nucleus of which is at the level of the inferior colliculus. This nerve innervates the superior oblique muscle. Confirmed lesions cause **diplopia** (double vision).

Cranial nerve VI, the **abducens**, has its nucleus on the floor of the fourth ventricle. Dysfunction prevents lateral movements of the eyeball. Figure 7-1, *B*, shows a complete paralysis of the left cranial nerve VI.

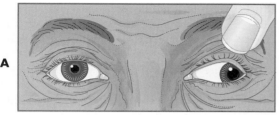
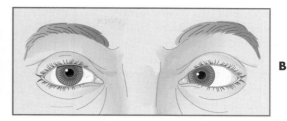

FIGURE **7-1**
A, Complete left III (oculomotor) nerve paralysis with a fully abducted eye, which is also depressed. The pupil of the eye is nonreactive and fully dilated. The ptosis of the left eye requires the examiner to lift the lid to examine movement. **B,** Complete left VI (abducens) nerve paralysis showing a fully adducted eye resulting from the unopposed pull of the medial rectus. (Reprinted from FitzGerald, M. J. T., & Folan-Curran, J. [2002]. *Clinical neuroanatomy and related neuroscience* [4th ed.]. Philadelphia: Saunders/Elsevier.)

The remaining seven cranial nerves are vital for the production of normal speech and thus are given more attention below, focusing on the pathway, structures innervated, functional purpose, signs of dysfunction, and testing procedure for each nerve. Learn them one by one. Test yourself on them until you are firmly acquainted with each nerve. Review Figure 3-2 for attachment sites of the cranial nerves to the brainstem.

Cranial Nerves for Speech and Hearing

CRANIAL NERVE V: TRIGEMINAL

Anatomy
Both the motor and sensory roots of the trigeminal nerve are attached to the lateral edges of the pons. The motor nuclei are restricted to the pons, but the sensory nuclei extend from the mesencephalon to the spinal cord.

Innervation
The motor part of the trigeminal nerve innervates the following muscles: masseter, temporalis, lateral and medial pterygoids, tensor tympana, tensor veli palatine, mylohyoid, and the anterior belly of the digastric muscle. The sensory fibers have three main branches:

1. The ophthalmic nerve, which is sensory to the forehead, eyes, and nose
2. The maxillary nerve, which is sensory to the upper lip mucosa, maxilla, upper teeth, cheeks, palate, and maxillary sinus
3. The mandibular nerve, which is sensory to the anterior two thirds of the tongue, mandible, lower teeth, lower lip, part of the cheek, and part of the external ear

Figure 7-2 shows a sensory map of the trigeminal nerve supply to the areas of the face and oral structures.

Function
Cranial nerve V is primarily responsible for mastication and for sensation to the face, teeth, gums, and anterior two thirds of the tongue. Innervating the tensor velar palatine, cranial nerve V is partially responsible for flattening and tensing the soft palate and for opening the eustachian tube. Innervating an extrinsic laryngeal muscle (the anterior belly of the digastric), it also assists in the upward and anterior movement of the larynx.

Testing
The jaw-closing and grinding lateral movements of chewing are the result of the function of the masseter and temporal, medial pterygoid, and lateral pterygoid muscles. The first three contribute to closure of the jaw,

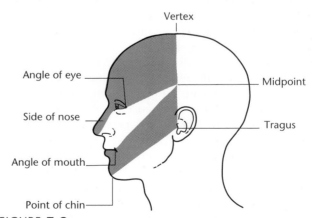

FIGURE **7-2**
Trigeminal nerve sensory map. (Reprinted from FitzGerald, M. J. T., & Folan-Curran, J. [2002]. *Clinical neuroanatomy and related neuroscience* [4th ed.]. Philadelphia: Saunders/Elsevier.)

but only the masseter can be directly tested. To evaluate the masseter, **palpate** the area of the muscle (2 cm above and in front of the angle of the mandible) as the patient bites down as hard as possible and then relaxes. As the patient bites, the bulk of the muscle can be felt. Try this to become familiar with the masseter. The muscle body should feel firm and bulky. The temporal muscle cannot be well palpated; however, if it is atrophied (shrunken) from a lower motor neuron lesion, the temple of the face will be sunken.

The strength of jaw closure should also be evaluated. To do so, place your hand on the tip of the patient's mandible as the jaw is held open. Place the other hand on the forehead to prevent neck extension. Ask the patient to bite down hard against the resistance of your hand. The patient should be able to close the jaw against a moderate resistance.

The lateral pterygoids enable the jaw to lateralize in chewing. To evaluate these muscles, ask the patient to open the jaw against resistance of your hand and note how the tip of the mandible lines up with the space between the upper medial incisors. Ask the patient to move the jaw from side to side and observe the facility of movement.

Finally, ask the patient to lateralize the jaw against resistance. Have him or her move the jaw to one side and hold it while you try to push it toward the center. Place your other hand against the opposite cheekbone so the patient cannot use the neck to help.

The patient with a unilateral paralysis of cranial nerve V shows a deviation of the jaw to the side of the lesion and an inability to force the jaw to the side opposite the lesion. Atrophy may also be noted after a period. These problems result from lower motor neuron lesions. Upper motor neuron lesions that are unilateral do not affect cranial nerves as much because the nuclei receive so many axons from the other hemisphere. Therefore the paresis is usually **transitory** or mild unless bilateral upper motor neuron lesions are present.

Bilateral upper motor neuron lesions result in an observable limitation of jaw movements. Opening and closing movements of the jaw, though possible, are restricted. Gross chewing movements are seen, but chewing and biting may lack vigor and are performed slowly.

To evaluate the sensory component of the trigeminal nerve, sensation to the face may be tested. The patient is asked to close the eyes, and a cotton swab is used to stroke the face in the three different distribution areas of the nerve. The examiner should stay in the central part of the face because, as shown in Figure 7-2, considerable overlap exists on the periphery. The ophthalmic division may therefore be tested by stroking above the eyebrows; the maxillary division by stroking the upper lip in an upward movement toward the cheekbone; and the mandibular division by stroking between the lower lip and the chin in an upward movement toward the cheekbone. Left and right sides should be done separately and compared. Stroking should be done with firm pressure and kept consistent across all trials.

Sensation to the anterior two thirds of the tongue may also be tested during the examination, especially if chewing and swallowing are a concern. The two sides of the tongue may be compared for sensitivity to the touch of a cotton-tip swab on the anterior as well as medial portion of the tongue.

CRANIAL NERVE VII: FACIAL

Anatomy

The facial nerve is a complex nerve carrying two motor and two sensory components. It involves several different nuclei, all lying within the pons near the reticular formation.

The special sensory component of the facial nerve involves the taste fibers for the tongue and palate. These fibers have their primary sensory neurons in the geniculate ganglion. They enter the brainstem in the sensory root of the facial nerve, called the nervus intermedius. They run in a bundle, or fasciculus, called the tractus solitarius and are joined in that bundle by the taste fibers from cranial nerves IX and X.

The taste fibers split off from the facial nerve in the middle ear as the chorda tympani. This joins the lingual branch of cranial nerve V. The taste fibers then terminate in the nucleus of the tractus solitarius. The fibers are distributed to the taste buds of the anterior two thirds of the tongue. Some fibers also terminate in the taste buds in the hard and soft palates. Ascending fibers from the nucleus solitarius run to the ventroposterior thalamus and then project to the cortical area for taste located at the lower end of the sensory strip in the parietal lobe.

The general sensory component of VII is a small cutaneous component whose nerve cells are found in the geniculate ganglion in the temporal bone. Impulses travel in the nervus intermedius, descending in the spinal tract of the trigeminal nerve and synapsing in the spinal nucleus of the trigeminal nerve located in the upper medulla. This sensory component may supplement the mandibular portion of cranial nerve V, providing sensation from the wall of the acoustic meatus and the surface of the tympanic membrane.

The visceral motor component of cranial nerve VII is composed of cell bodies that are preganglionic autonomic motor neurons. These cell bodies are collectively called the superior salivatory nucleus and the **lacrimal** nucleus. The fibers from the nucleus travel in the nervus intermedius and divide in the facial canal, becoming the greater petrosal nerve and the chorda tympani. The petrosal nerve fibers follow a complicated path and join fibers of the trigeminal to reach the lacrimal and mucosal glands of the nasal and oral cavities, where they stimulate secretion.

The branchial motor component of the facial nerve is of critical importance to the speech-language pathologist. The fibers of the motor nucleus extend to the floor of the ventricle, curve around the nucleus of the abducens (cranial nerve VI), and exit the brainstem near the inferior margin of the pons. These fibers then join those from the nucleus of the tractus solitarius and the autonomic or parasympathetic nuclei and enter the internal auditory meatus as they extend through the facial canal of the petrosal bone. They leave the skull through the stylomastoid foramen. While coursing through the facial canal, the facial nerve travels through the tympanic cavity, innervating the stapedius muscle. The facial nerve can therefore be involved in pathologic conditions related to the ear. Surgeons removing acoustic tumors must be mindful of the location of the facial nerve.

The dorsal motor nucleus that innervates the lower part of the face receives most of the corticonuclear fibers from the opposite hemisphere; thus innervation to these structures is primarily contralateral. The ventral motor nucleus that supplies the upper part of the face receives fibers from both cerebral hemispheres (i.e., receives crossed and uncrossed fibers), and innervation is bilateral.

Innervation

The **parasympathetic nuclei** are also known as the superior salivatory and the lacrimal nuclei. The superior salivatory nucleus receives afferent information from the hypothalamus and olfactory system as well as taste information from the mouth cavity. It supplies the submandibular **sublingual** salivary glands and the nasal and palatine glands.

The lacrimal nucleus solitarius receives information from afferent fibers from the trigeminal sensory nuclei for reflex response to corneal irritation. The sensory nucleus receives information concerning taste from fibers from the anterior two thirds of the tongue, the floor of the mouth, and the soft and hard palates.

The motor nucleus gives the face expression by innervation of the various facial muscles (i.e., the orbicularis oculi, zygomatic, buccinator, orbicularis oris, and labial muscles). Other muscles innervated are the platysma, stylohyoid, and stapedius and the posterior belly of the digastric.

Function

Most important to the speech-language pathologist is the fact that the facial nerve is responsible for all movements of facial expression. All facial apertures are guarded by muscles innervated by the facial nerve: the eyes, the nose, the mouth, and the external auditory canal. Cranial nerve VII enables the actions of wrinkling the forehead, closing the eyes tightly, closing the mouth tightly, pulling back the corners of the mouth and tensing the cheeks, and pulling down the corners of the mouth and tensing the anterior neck muscles.

Beyond these important movements in speech and swallowing, the facial nerve also helps pull the larynx up and back (through the belly of the digastric muscle). It provides motor innervation to the sublingual and submaxillary salivary glands, and it guards the middle ear by innervating the stapedius muscle, which dampens excessive movement of the ossicles in the presence of a loud noise. Finally, the facial nerve also is partially responsible for taste.

Testing

Tests of facial expression are the primary tests in the oral-motor exam for cranial nerve VII. Before any motor testing, however, the patient's face at rest should be noted, especially the symmetry. Then begin movement testing at the upper part of the face, focusing first on the forehead, then the eyes, and finally the mouth. Box 7-1 outlines what to observe and note before commencing with speech testing.

The patient with a lower motor neuron lesion of cranial nerve VII has involvement of the entire side of the face on the side of the lesion (ipsilateral). Figure 7-3 is an example of unilateral facial paralysis. Although speech may be distorted, it is usually not significantly hindered by peripheral involvement of cranial nerve VII. The patient with an upper motor neuron lesion shows complete involvement of the contralateral lip and neck muscles, some degree of involvement of the area around the eyes, and little difficulty with the forehead or frontalis muscle. It should be noted that the paralysis occurs on voluntary movement. The patient may have almost normal movement for emotionally initiated movements such as a true smile but be unable to lateralize the lips on the affected side when asked to do so voluntarily.

Because the facial nerve innervates the stapedius muscle, it may be paralyzed by a lesion. If this occurs, the patient may report that ordinary sounds seem uncomfortably loud.

The sensory component of the facial nerve may be assessed by testing the patient's sense of taste on the anterior two thirds of the tongue. Sensitivity of the two

BOX 7-1

Facial Assessment

Forehead

Ask the patient to wrinkle the forehead and look up at the ceiling. Note the symmetry of the wrinkling on both sides. Keep in mind that this ability or inability is diagnostic for localization. Because the upper part of the face is innervated bilaterally, only a lower motor neuron lesion would cause complete paralysis of this function. An upper motor neuron lesion causes some weakness on the opposite side, but it will not be nearly as perceptible because of the ipsilateral fiber innervation.

Eyes

Ask the patient to close the eyes as tightly as possible. Note the contraction of the orbicularis oculi and the consequent wrinkling around the eyes. Bilateral innervation is also present in this part of the face, though not to the degree that the forehead displays. The lower motor neuron–upper motor neuron difference holds true for dysfunction of this part of the face.

Mouth

Take a close look at mouth movements. First ask the patient to smile or pull back the corners of the lips. It helps to tell the patient to show the teeth when doing this, exaggerating the smile somewhat. Again, observe the symmetry of the two sides. Then ask the patient to pucker the lips; observe the symmetry of constriction. Finally, ask him or her to pull down the corners of the lips (as in pouting) or try to wrinkle the skin of the neck. Inspect for symmetry. Also test for the strength of movement against resistance and compare the two sides of the mouth.

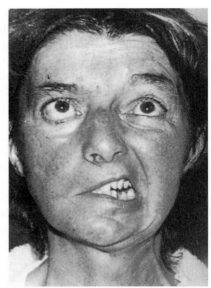

FIGURE **7-3**
Patient with complete facial nerve paralysis on the right side. The patient was asked to show her teeth and look up at the ceiling. Note the inability to raise the eyebrow, drooping of the lower eyelid, inability to retract the mouth, and lack of webbing on the neck (effect on the platysma muscle). This patient also was unable to abduct the eye because of involvement of the abducens. The patient was found to have demyelination affecting the facial nerve and abducens nerve, resulting from multiple sclerosis. (Reprinted from FitzGerald, M. J. T., & Folan-Curran, J. [2002]. *Clinical neuroanatomy and related neuroscience* [4th ed.]. Philadelphia: Saunders/Elsevier.)

sides of the tongue should be compared. The patient should be able to identify the four primary tastes (salty, sour, bitter, and sweet) if the sensory pathways are intact.

CRANIAL NERVE VIII: ACOUSTIC-VESTIBULAR OR VESTIBULOCOCHLEAR

The following explanation assumes the reader has studied the anatomy of the ear and is well versed in the structure and function of the cochlea and semicircular canals. A good working knowledge of the anatomy

of the ear is imperative; review of the information provided in Chapter 5 on the auditory system is suggested.

Anatomy

As can be ascertained from its name, the acoustic-vestibular, or vestibulocochlear, nerve consists of two distinct parts: the vestibular nerve and the cochlear, or acoustic, nerve. Both take afferent information from the internal ear to the nervous system, but as their names imply, they carry different types of information.

The vestibular nerve consists of nerve cells and their fibers, which are located in Scarpa's ganglion located in the internal acoustic meatus. The fibers enter the brainstem in a groove between the lower border of the pons and the upper medulla oblongata in a sulcus called the cerebellopontine angle. This location is the site of one of the most common brain tumors, a vestibular schwannoma, also known as an acoustic neuroma. A few of the axons terminate in the flocculonodular lobe of the cerebellum. Most axons enter the vestibular nuclear complex, which consists of a group of nuclei located in the floor of the fourth ventricle.

The cochlear nerve consists of nerve cells and fibers located in the spiral ganglion located around the modiolus of the cochlea. Nerve fibers wrap around each other in the modiolus, with a layering effect. Fibers from the apex, carrying low-frequency information, are found on the innermost part of the core, whereas fibers from the basal part of the cochlea, carrying high-frequency information, are found on the outermost layers. The nerve fibers from these cell bodies enter the brainstem at the lower border of the pons on the lateral side of the facial nerve. They are separated from the facial nerve fibers by the vestibular nerve. Figure 7-4 illustrates the relation of cranial nerve VIII to the inner ear.

When the cochlear fibers enter the pons, they divide into two branches. One branch enters the dorsal cochlear nucleus (high frequencies), and the other enters the ventral cochlear nucleus (low frequencies). Both nuclei are situated adjacent to the inferior cerebral peduncle.

From this point the axons take varied and complex paths. The system is largely contralateral. Most fibers decussate after the cochlear nuclei, though there are a few ipsilaterally projected fibers. The fibers form a tract called the lateral lemniscus as they ascend through the posterior portion of the pons and midbrain. All ascending fibers terminate in the medial geniculate body and from there project to the auditory cortex by way of the auditory radiations. Between the cochlear nuclei and the medial geniculate body the fibers take one of several pathways, including synapses at one or more of the following structures: the superior olives, the trapezoid body, the inferior colliculus, and the nucleus of the lateral lemniscus.

Innervation

Both portions of the vestibulocochlear nerve are primarily sensory in nature. The vestibular nerve receives afferent information from the utricle, saccule, and semicircular canal of the inner ear and from the cerebellum. The vestibular nerve also sends out efferent fibers that pass to the cerebellum through the inferior cerebellar peduncles and also to the spinal cord, forming the vestibulospinal tract. Efferent fibers are also sent to the nuclei of cranial nerves III (oculomotor), IV (trochlear), and VI (abducens) through the medial longitudinal fasciculus. As previously outlined, the cochlear nerve carries afferent fibers from the cochlea to the auditory cortex.

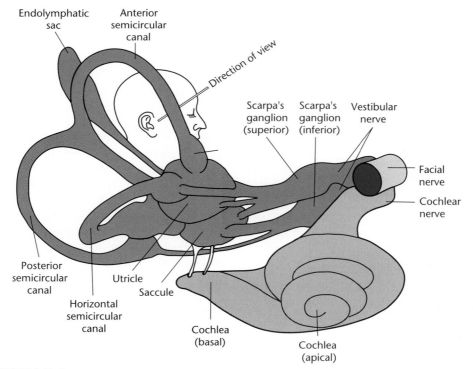

FIGURE 7-4
Relation of the vestibular, cochlear, and facial nerve to the inner ear. (Reprinted from Nadeau, S.E., Ferguson, T.S., Valenstein, E., Vierck, C.J., Petruska, J.C., Streit, W.J. & Ritz, L.A. [2005]. *Medical neuroscience*. Philadelphia: Saunders/Elsevier.)

Function

Cranial nerve VIII takes afferent information from the internal ear to the nervous system. It is responsible for sound sensitivity and innervates the utricle and the saccule of the inner ear, which are sensitive to static changes in equilibrium. In addition, innervation of the semicircular canals takes place through this nerve, controlling sensitivity to dynamic changes in equilibrium.

Testing

Although the speech-language pathologist may perform hearing threshold screening or testing that may provide information about the cochlear nerve, the audiologist usually is responsible for thorough assessment of hearing and cochlear function. Neurologists often perform simple tuning fork tests for acuity and sound lateralization, and some prefer to use whispered words.

Testing the vestibular function is also not in the purview of the speech-language pathologist. Vestibular function usually is investigated with caloric tests that involve raising or lowering the temperature of the internal auditory meatus, thereby inducing current in the semicircular canals and stimulating the vestibular nerve for testing. Neurologists also use maneuvers of changing head position. Dynamic platform posturography is a technique developed in recent years to perform a functional assessment of how senses are used for balance.

The patient reporting reduced hearing acuity, **tinnitus** (ringing in the ears), or dizziness should always be seen by an otologist and receive an audiologic evaluation. The dizzy patient may be referred to a neurologist, who typically will also refer for audiologic testing.

CRANIAL NERVE IX: GLOSSOPHARYNGEAL

Anatomy

The glossopharyngeal nerve carries two motor components and three sensory components. It can be found emerging from the medulla between the olive and the inferior cerebellar peduncle. The main trunk of the nerve exits the skull through the jugular foramen. Three nuclei in the brainstem are concerned with the functions of the glossopharyngeal nerve: the nucleus ambiguus, the inferior salivatory nucleus, and the nucleus solitarius.

Innervation

The nucleus ambiguus receives corticonuclear fibers from both hemispheres and is the efferent innervation to the stylopharyngeus muscle, which contributes to the elevation of the pharynx and larynx. The inferior salivatory nucleus receives afferent information concerning taste from the hypothalamus, olfactory system, and mouth cavity. Efferent fibers supply the otic ganglion of the ear and the parotid salivary gland. The nucleus solitarius receives fibers arising from the inferior ganglia. Peripherally these visceral afferent fibers of cranial nerve IX mediate general sensation to the pharynx, soft palate, posterior third of the tongue, fauces, tonsils, ear canal, and tympanic cavity. The fibers decussate and travel upward to the opposite thalamic and some hypothalamic nuclei. From here the axons pass through the internal capsule and end in the lower postcentral gyrus.

Function

Cranial nerve IX is efferent to one muscle only—the stylopharyngeus. This muscle dilates the pharynx laterally and contributes to the elevation of the pharynx and larynx. It thereby serves to help clear the pharynx and larynx for swallowing. **Secretomotor** fibers are also provided for the parotid gland's production of saliva. Sensory fibers carry taste information from the posterior third of the tongue. The glossopharyngeal nerve mediates the sensory portion of the palatal and pharyngeal gag.

Testing

Most functions of cranial nerve IX cannot be tested separately from those of cranial nerve X because the vagus has predominant control over laryngeal and pharyngeal sensory and motor function. However, testing the sensory portion of the pharyngeal gag does provide information about the integrity of cranial nerve IX. To do this, the examiner should use a cotton-tipped applicator with a long wooden end (as used in medical clinics). The examiner carefully puts the cotton tip back against one side of the posterior pharyngeal wall, avoiding any contact with the base of the tongue or the velum. With a gentle poking of the wall, a gag should be elicited. Both sides of the pharynx should be tested. Testing the pharyngeal gag is not easily done in most people because getting so far back in the oral cavity without touching any other structure is difficult.

If the gag is successfully stimulated and cannot be elicited, the examiner should ask if the patient feels the pressure of the touch. If the stimulus is felt and no gag occurs, only the motor portion of the gag (mediated by the vagus) may be impaired. This situation is rare. Because sensation precedes motor activity, the absence of sensation and the gag implicates cranial nerve IX and gives the clinician information about the integrity of sensation to the upper pharynx, which can be important information in swallowing assessment.

CRANIAL NERVE X: VAGUS

Anatomy

Like the glossopharyngeal nerve, the vagus nerve also has three nuclei: the nucleus ambiguus, the dorsal nucleus, and the nucleus solitarius, also located in the medulla. The axon from the cell body of the nucleus ambiguus has two major branches: a pharyngeal branch and a laryngeal branch. The laryngeal branch then branches again into the recurrent laryngeal nerve and the superior laryngeal nerve. The superior laryngeal nerve has two branches, the internal laryngeal and the external laryngeal.

The recurrent laryngeal nerve arises considerably below the larynx and ascends to terminate at the larynx. The right recurrent nerve runs in a loop behind the common carotid and subclavian arteries. The left recurrent nerve leaves the vagus at a lower level and loops under and behind the aortic arch. It then ascends to the larynx in a groove between the trachea and esophagus and enters through the cricothyroid membrane. Damage to the recurrent laryngeal nerve sometimes occurs during surgery, especially heart and thyroid surgery.

Innervation

The nucleus ambiguus receives an approximately equal number of corticonuclear fibers from both hemispheres; these fibers are efferent to the constrictor muscles of the pharynx and the intrinsic muscles of the larynx. The efferent fibers of the dorsal or parasympathetic nucleus innervate the involuntary muscles of the bronchi, esophagus, heart, stomach, small intestine, and a portion of the large intestine. The afferent fibers of the nucleus of the tractus solitarius follow much the same path as those of the glossopharyngeal nerve and terminate in the postcentral gyrus.

Function

Vagus means wanderer, an appropriate name considering the many functions of the vagus nerve. It is motor to the viscera (heart, respiratory system, and most of the digestive system). It supplies primary efferent innervation to the palatal muscles (except for innervation of the tensor palatine by the trigeminal nerve). The vagus is also the primary efferent for the pharyngeal constrictors. On its own, the vagus innervates all of the intrinsic muscles of the larynx, primarily through the recurrent laryngeal branch. The cricothyroid, however, is innervated by the external laryngeal branch of the superior laryngeal nerve.

The vagus has both a visceral and a general sensory component in its afferent pathways. The visceral component carries visceral sensation that is not appreciated at a conscious level. Sensory information from the mucous membranes of the epiglottis, base of the tongue, aryepiglottic folds and the majority of the larynx is carried in the internal laryngeal branch of the superior laryngeal nerve. Visceral sensation from below the larynx is carried in the recurrent laryngeal nerve.

General sensation (pain, temperature, and touch) from the larynx, pharynx, skin of the external ear, and the external auditory canal is carried in the vagus as well. From the vocal folds and below the larynx, general sensation is carried in the recurrent laryngeal nerve. From above the vocal folds, sensation travels in the internal laryngeal division of the superior laryngeal nerve. Damage to one or both of these sensory components of these nerves could result in silent aspiration (aspiration with no reflexive cough) because of the decreased sensory input. The sensory information would normally cause a reflex to trigger or cause a tickle in the throat or airway, indicating that something foreign is on the membranes and needs to be coughed out.

Testing

Remember that evaluation of swallowing function involves testing cranial nerves IX and X. Palatal function is controlled primarily by cranial nerve X, with the tensor veli palatine innervated by V. Intrinsic laryngeal muscle function is covered solely by cranial nerve X.

Palatal function is tested by first observing the palate at rest as the patient opens the mouth to allow viewing. Look at the palatal arches and observe their symmetry. Note if one arch hangs lower than the other. Next ask the patient to phonate an "ah" and observe. The soft palate should elevate and move posteriorly and symmetrically. If the palate does not elevate, the palatal gag reflex, primarily innervated by cranial nerve IX, should be tested by touching the tongue blade against the palatal arches. The gag is a reflex activity, and it is preserved in an upper motor neuron lesion because the reflex arc is still intact. As in all reflexes, it may be lost acutely after an upper motor neuron lesion; then it may become hyperactive. If both volitional and reflex activities of the palate are diminished, a lower motor neuron lesion is evidenced. Bear in mind that palatal elevation also is reduced by a cleft palate, congenital oral malformations, and soft tissue palatal lesions. Do not overlook these vital facts in vigorously searching for an upper or lower motor neuron lesion.

Laryngeal function evaluation is adequately completed only by a direct or indirect laryngoscopy in which the vocal cords can be seen. A finer analysis of vocal cord movement patterns can be done by using laryngeal stroboscopy. Damage to the vagus nerve may cause paralysis or paresis of the vocal cord. Innervation is bilateral to the larynx, with the crossed and uncrossed fibers being approximately equal. Therefore complete paralysis of a vocal cord from an upper motor neuron lesion is rare.

Preliminary assessment of laryngeal function is performed by traditional clinical voice evaluation procedures. The patient is asked to phonate and prolong a vowel such as /a/. Maximum phonation time varies for normal adults. If the patient can phonate for a 7- to 8-second duration, laryngeal and respiratory control is presumed acceptable. Perceptual analysis of the voice is done by the clinician during this phonation and during conversation. The patient may be asked to demonstrate laryngeal function and control by raising and lowering the pitch of a prolonged vowel or singing up and down the scale. Remember that the ability to change pitch depends on proper function of the cricothyroid muscle, which is innervated by the superior laryngeal nerve rather than the recurrent nerve. Estimate of the strength of laryngeal closure can be made perceptually by asking the patient to perform the **glottal coup**, which is essentially to make a short, sharp grunting sound. A voluntary (as opposed to reflexive) cough should also be requested. The clinician listens for the sound made at the larynx in these two maneuvers to be strong and sharp. Stress testing of the vocal mechanism is done by asking the patient to count to 300 or to keep talking for a prescribed length of time. More sophisticated analyses of the voice may be performed with instrumentation for acoustical analysis.

In spastic dysarthria cases from an upper motor neuron lesion, a rough, harsh quality is heard on phonation. In bilateral upper motor neuron lesions (pseudobulbar palsy), a characteristic voice quality is heard, characterized by what Darley, Aronson, and Brown[3] describe as "strain-strangle." This voice is harsh, with a very strained, tense quality as if the person is fighting to push the air flow through the larynx and supralaryngeal areas.

A lower motor neuron lesion causes complete paralysis of the ipsilateral vocal cord, resulting in a hoarse, breathy voice. In some lower motor neuron diseases the voice will initially be strong; however, after the patient talks for a while, the voice becomes progressively weaker and more breathy. Transient hoarseness sometimes results from direct damage to the recurrent laryngeal nerve during carotid artery or thyroid surgery.

CRANIAL NERVE XI: SPINAL ACCESSORY

Anatomy
The spinal accessory nerve consists of a cranial and a spinal root. The nucleus of the cranial root is found in the nucleus ambiguus of the medulla. It receives corticonuclear fibers from both cerebral hemispheres.

These fibers then join the glossopharyngeal, vagus and spinal accessory nerves.

The spinal root's nucleus is located in the spinal nucleus of the anterior gray column of the spinal cord. The fibers pass through the lateral white column and eventually form a nerve trunk, which joins the cranial root to pass through the foramen magnum. The spinal root then separates from the cranial root, however, to find its way to the sternocleidomastoid and trapezius muscles.

Innervation
The cranial root joins the vagus to innervate the uvula and the levator palatine. As previously mentioned, the spinal root innervates the sternocleidomastoid and trapezius muscles.

Function
The spinal accessory nerve's primary function is as motor to the muscles (including the sternocleidomastoid) that help turn, tilt, and thrust the head forward or raise the sternum and clavicle if the head is in a fixed position. It provides innervation also to the trapezius muscle, which is responsible for shrugging the shoulders.

Testing
When testing cranial nerve XI, the spinal part is evaluated. The accessory part is accessory to the vagus and cannot be tested alone.

Initially, look at the size and symmetry of the sternocleidomastoid muscles and palpate them. (Do this on yourself and others to become familiar with normal muscle size and firmness.) Ask the patient to turn the head to one side and hold it there while you try to push it back to the middle. Put one hand on the patient's cheek and the other on the shoulder to brace the patient. Gently push against the cheek and observe and palpate the sternocleidomastoid on the opposite side of the neck.

Next have the patient try to thrust the head forward while you resist the movement with your hand against the forehead. Again, observe and palpate the sternocleidomastoid muscle.

Finally, ask the patient to shrug his or her shoulders while you press down on the shoulders. You should feel the shoulders elevate against your gentle resistance.

CRANIAL NERVE XII: HYPOGLOSSAL

Anatomy
The hypoglossal nerve runs under the tongue and controls tongue movements. The nucleus, called the hypoglossal nucleus, is located in the medulla beneath the lower part of the fourth ventricle. It receives fibers

from both cerebral hemispheres, with one exception. The cells serving the genioglossus muscle receive only contralateral fibers. The nerve fibers pass through the medulla and emerge in the groove between the pyramid and the olive. Other apparent branches of the hypoglossal are not connected with the hypoglossal nuclei but rather are derived from the ansa cervicalis of cervical vertebrae C1, C2, and C3. *Ansa* means loop, and some branches of these spinal nerves form a loop and join the hypoglossal nerve to help innervate the sternothyroid, sternohyoid, and omohyoid muscles.

Innervation

The hypoglossal nerve innervates the intrinsic muscles of the tongue. It also innervates four extrinsic tongue muscles: the genioglossus, hyoglossus, chondroglossus, and styloglossus.

With the branches from the ansa cervicalis, cranial nerve XII contributes to the innervation of the sternothyroid, sternohyoid, and omohyoid muscles, thus contributing to the elevation and depression of the larynx.

Function

The hypoglossal nerve innervates the muscles responsible for tongue movement. The four intrinsic muscles of the tongue control tongue shortening, concaving (turning the tip and lateral margins upward), narrowing, elongating, and flattening. The extrinsic muscles innervated account for tongue protrusion (**genioglossus**), drawing the tongue upward and backward (**styloglossus**), and retraction and depression of the tongue (**hyoglossus**). The hyoglossus also acts with the chondroglossus to elevate the hyoid bone, thus participating in phonation.

Testing

Ask the patient to open the mouth and let you look at the tongue at rest. Inspect it for signs of atrophy. With a unilateral lower motor neuron lesion, one side of the tongue will look shrunken or atrophied. This atrophy occurs on the same side as the lower motor neuron lesion. A lower motor neuron lesion may cause fasciculations or fibrillations, seen as tiny ripples under the surface of the tongue. Specialists disagree whether these movements in the denervated tongue are fasciculations or fibrillations.

Normal tongues may also show some ripples when they are not completely relaxed. Therefore, if fasciculations seem present, ask the patient to move the tongue around and then relax it; again observe the surface for fasciculations. Even in a normal tongue, however, ripples may still be present. Therefore, as DeMyer[4] points out, the clinician does better to rely on atrophy and weakness as signs of lower motor neuron damage.

The tongue should also be observed for tremor or random movements at rest.

Next ask the patient to protrude the tongue; evaluate the symmetry of this posture. The tongue tip should be at midline. If the patient has weak lip musculature on one side, that side may be lower, causing the tongue to look as if it deviates to that side. Therefore try to align the tip of the tongue with the midline of the jaw visually. That side of the lip can be pulled back so that it is symmetrical with the other side of the lip; then ask the patient to protrude the tongue. If the cranial nerve is dysfunctional, the genioglossus will not be able to push its side out; the stronger side will overcome the weaker and the tongue will deviate to the weaker side (Fig. 7-5).

In lower motor neuron damage the weakness is on the same side as the lesion. In upper motor neuron damage, because of the contralateral control, the tongue deviates to the side opposite the lesion. For example, in many stroke patients with left hemisphere damage to the area of the motor strip, the tongue shows a characteristic deviation to the right on protrusion. This is usually less marked than in lower motor neuron tongue weakness.

The patient who has bilateral XII nerve damage has weakness on both sides and is unable to protrude the tongue beyond the lips. Strength of tongue protrusion may be tested by asking the patient to push against a tongue blade held directly in front of the lips.

Other movements of the tongue must be evaluated to document precisely the range, rate, and strength of the tongue for follow-up in treatment and for diagnostic purposes. Ask the patient to lateralize the tongue (i.e., move it from one corner of the mouth to the other). The tongue should move the full range from corner to corner. Evaluate the strength of lateral movement by asking the patient to push the tongue against the inside of the cheek against your fingers placed for resistance on the outside of the cheek; ask the patient to make a ball in the cheek with the tongue. A tongue blade can also be placed along the side of the tongue, with the patient pushing against a light resistance.

The ability to elevate the tongue can be evaluated by having the patient open the mouth to a moderate degree while you hold down the mandible with your finger on it. Ask the patient to try to touch the top lip and also the alveolar ridge with the tongue. This should be done with full range of movement and little effort.

Strength of elevation of the tip, blade, or back of the tongue is difficult to assess with tongue blade resistance. Hearing is the better assessor of strength of elevation. The tip of the tongue should be able to make firm contact to produce /t/, /d/, /t͡ʃ/ (as in c*h*um), and /dʒ/ (as in *j*udge) and to elevate fully for /l/ and /n/. The blade of the tongue should elevate well to produce a

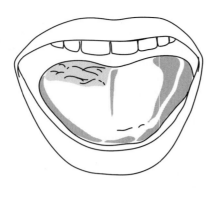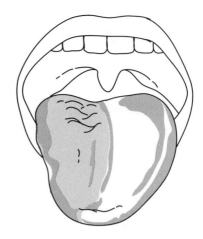

FIGURE **7-5**

Unilateral paresis of the tongue. *Left,* The resting tongue shows a smaller weak side (atrophy) with a corrugated surface suggesting fasciculations and the effects of atrophy. These tongue signs suggest denervation. *Right,* The protruded tongue deviates to the weak side. In a lower motor neuron lesion, the deviated tongue points to the side of the lesion. (Reprinted from Darley, F. et al. [1975]. *Motor speech disorders.* Philadelphia: W. B. Saunders.)

distinct /i/ (*e* as in *e*at) and /j/ (*y* as in *y*oung). Elevation of the back of the tongue is necessary for production of the velar consonants /k/ and /g/. Careful examination of the production of these consonants and vowels as well as others, in isolation and in context, provides the most information regarding tongue elevation and strength.

Table 7-2 summarizes the five cranial nerves (V, VII, IX, X, and XII) involved in the oral musculature.

Cranial Nerve Cooperation: The Act of Swallowing

The act of swallowing is highly complex and must be studied independently in regard to its cranial nerve innervation. Logemann[7] describes normal deglutition as consisting of four phases: the oral preparatory phase,

TABLE 7-2
Summary of Cranial Nerve Function for the Oral Musculature

CRANIAL NERVE	MUSCLES INNERVATED	MOVEMENTS AND SENSATION INNERVATED	TEST PROCEDURE	SIGNS OF LOWER MOTOR NEURON DAMAGE	SIGNS OF UPPER MOTOR NEURON DAMAGE
V: trigeminal	Masseter, tensor tympani, tensor veli palatine, mylohyoid, digastric (anterior belly)	Jaw closing, lateral jaw movement, contribution to laryngeal elevation, sensation to face and anterior tongue	Palpation of masseter, closing and lateralization against resistance, sensation on face and tongue	Weakness, jaw deviation to lesion side, atrophy	Mild, transitory weakness
VII: facial	Orbicularis oculi and oris, zygomatic, buccinator, platysma,	Forehead wrinkling, closing eyes, closing mouth, smiling, tensing cheeks, pulling	Observation of facial symmetry at rest; have patient wrinkle forehead,	Involvement of entire side of face, weakness, limited range	Complete involvement of lips and neck muscles, less involvement of

TABLE 7-2
Summary of Cranial Nerve Function for the Oral Musculature—cont'd

CRANIAL NERVE	MUSCLES INNERVATED	MOVEMENTS AND SENSATION INNERVATED	TEST PROCEDURE	SIGNS OF LOWER MOTOR NEURON DAMAGE	SIGNS OF UPPER MOTOR NEURON DAMAGE
VII: Facial	stylohyoid, stapedius, portion of digastric (posterior belly)	down corner of mouth, tensing anterior neck muscles, moving stapedius to dampen ossicles; taste from anterior two thirds of tongue and hard and soft palates	close eyes tightly, smile, pucker, and pull down lip corners; identification of tastes	of movement, decreased taste sensation	eye area muscles, little difficulty with forehead muscles; weakness, limited range of movement of affected muscles; decreased taste sensation
IX: glossopha-ryngeal	Stylopharyngeus, otic ganglion, parotid salivary gland, part of the middle pharyngeal constrictor	Elevation of pharynx and larynx, pharyngeal dilation, salivation; taste from posterior third of tongue; sensation from posterior tongue and upper pharynx	Tested with cranial nerve X for motor; sensory test for pharyngeal gag	—	—
X: vagus	Inferior, middle, and superior pharyngeal constrictors; salpingopharyngeus, glossopalatine, pharyngopalatine, levator veli palatine, uvular, cricothyroid, thyroarytenoid, posterior and lateral cricoarytenoid, interarytenoid, and transverse and oblique interarytenoid muscles; various muscles of the viscera, esophagus, and trachea	Palatal elevation and depression, laryngeal movement, pharyngeal constriction, cricopharyngeal function; visceral and general sensation from base of tongue, epiglottis, larynx and pharynx	Observation of palatal movement, palatal gag reflex; laryngoscopic evaluation of vocal musculature; ability to change pitch; phonation time; assessment of swallowing	Absence of gag reflex, poor movement of palate or pharyngeal wall, absent or delayed swallow response, aspiration, breathy hoarse voice (may be improved by pushing effort)	Poor palatal or pharyngeal wall movement, harshness or strained-strangled voice quality, delayed or absent swallow reflex, aspiration
XII: hypoglossal	Superior longitudinal, inferior longitudinal, transverse	All tongue movements as well as some elevation of the hyoid bone	Observation for atrophy or fasciculations as well as symmetry	Atrophy, fasciculations, weakness, reduced range of	Weakness, reduced range of movement, deviation of tongue to

Continued

TABLE 7-2

Summary of Cranial Nerve Function for the Oral Musculature—cont'd

CRANIAL NERVE	MUSCLES INNERVATED	MOVEMENTS AND SENSATION INNERVATED	TEST PROCEDURE	SIGNS OF LOWER MOTOR NEURON DAMAGE	SIGNS OF UPPER MOTOR NEURON DAMAGE
XII: Hypoglossal	vertical, genioglossus, hyoglossus, and styloglossus		on protrusion; assessment for lateralization, protrusion, elevation, retraction (to observe range of movement); assessment of movement against resistance for strength testing on lateral, protrusion, and elevation movement; articulation testing	movement, deviation of tongue to side of lesion, decreased tone, consonant imprecision	contralateral side, increased tone, consonant imprecision

the oral phase, the pharyngeal phase, and the esophageal phase.

In the oral preparatory phase, the food is masticated, mixed with saliva, and formed into a cohesive bolus held against the hard palate. This stage is variable in duration depending on ease of mastication, oral motor efficiency, and individual preference in savoring taste. The oral stage begins when the lips seal and the back of the tongue begins moving the bolus posteriorly. The tongue forms a central groove that acts as a ramp or chute for the food. The oral stage is considered a voluntary part of the swallowing and typically takes less than 1 second. The pharyngeal phase, which also takes 1 second or less, begins with the triggering of the swallow response or pharyngeal response at the anterior faucial pillars. The triggering of the swallow causes several physiologic activities to occur in the pharynx simultaneously: velopharyngeal closure; laryngeal elevation; inversion of the epiglottis; closure of all sphincters (aryepiglottic folds, false vocal folds, and true vocal folds); initiation of pharyngeal peristalsis (squeezing); and relaxation of the cricopharyngeal sphincter to allow material to pass from pharynx to esophagus. If the swallow is not triggered this response does not occur, and none of these activities spontaneously occurs. The bolus may be pushed into the pharynx and come to rest in the valleculae or pyriform sinuses and

spill over into the airway (i.e., aspiration). Some of the maneuvers that usually occur reflexively can be put under voluntary control to help provide some protection, primarily the closure of the vocal folds if they are functional. Finally, in normal swallowing the esophageal phase occurs as the bolus enters the esophagus through the cricopharyngeus. A wave of contractions (peristalsis), innervated by cranial nerve X, is initiated in the esophagus and the bolus is passed through into the stomach. Normal esophageal transit time is 8 to 20 seconds. Box 7-2 outlines the four phases of deglutition, and Figure 7-6 illustrates the final three stages.

Efficient swallowing demands cooperation and coordination of the cranial nerves also involved in speech production. Figure 7-7 is a simplified summary of the actions that occur in swallowing and the cranial nerves that are responsible. The trigeminal nerve (V) plays an important part because of the efferent control of the muscles of mastication and the afferent control for general sensation to the anterior two thirds of the tongue. Cranial nerve VII, the facial nerve, controls taste for the anterior two thirds of the tongue and controls the lip sphincter and the buccal muscles, allowing food to be held inside the mouth.

The hypoglossal nerve (XII) controls the movement of the tongue. Through research using pharyngeal

Four Phases of Deglutition

1. **Oral preparatory phase:** Tongue forms the liquid or solid into a cohesive bolus after the solid has been chewed and mixed with saliva. Bolus is held as a cohesive unit against the hard palate.
2. **Oral phase:** Lips seal and tongue moves food to the back of the mouth.
3. **Pharyngeal phase:** Swallow response is triggered, causing several physiologic activities to occur simultaneously and pushing food from the pharynx into the esophagus.
4. **Esophageal phase:** Food passes, by peristaltic action, through the esophagus to the stomach.

manometry, it has been found that the tongue is the major force generating the driving pressure that pushes the bolus through the pharynx.[1] This action of the tongue has been compared with that of a plunger and is called the tongue driving force. Pharyngeal constriction, controlled by the vagus nerve, has been found to be much less of a force than originally believed. In the same study, a descending pharyngeal contraction was shown to be applied only to the residual bolus tail.[1] This constriction clears the bolus from the laryngeal vestibule. It is therefore called the pharyngeal clearing force.

The vagus also mediates the action of the cricopharyngeus, which relaxes to allow the bolus to pass from the hypopharynx to the esophagus. The movement of the intrinsic muscles of the larynx to close the entrance to the airway is also innervated by the vagus. The elevation and anterior movement of the larynx are significant mechanical forces contributing to the opening of the cricopharyngeus. Therefore cranial nerves V, VII, IX, X, and XII, all with efferent innervation to one or

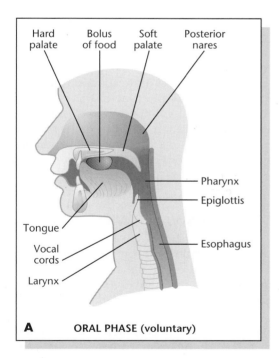

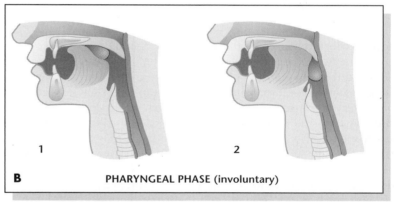

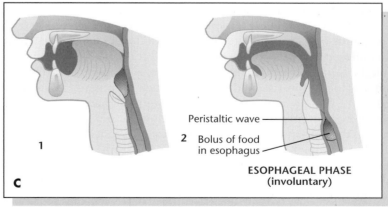

FIGURE **7-6**
The initial phase of swallowing, the oral preparatory phase (**A**), involves mastication and mixture of the food with saliva. It is then followed by oral (**B1**), pharyngeal (**B2** and **C1**), and esophageal (**C2**) phases. (Modified from Mahan, K. L., & Escott-Stump, S. [Eds.]. [2004]. *Krause's food, nutrition, & diet therapy* [11th ed.]. Philadelphia: Saunders/Elsevier.)

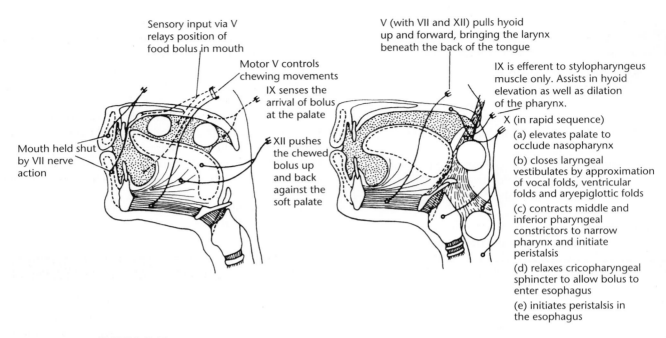

Sensory input via V relays position of food bolus in mouth

Motor V controls chewing movements

IX senses the arrival of bolus at the palate

Mouth held shut by VII nerve action

XII pushes the chewed bolus up and back against the soft palate

V (with VII and XII) pulls hyoid up and forward, bringing the larynx beneath the back of the tongue

IX is efferent to stylopharyngeus muscle only. Assists in hyoid elevation as well as dilation of the pharynx.

X (in rapid sequence)

(a) elevates palate to occlude nasopharynx

(b) closes laryngeal vestibulates by approximation of vocal folds, ventricular folds and aryepiglottic folds

(c) contracts middle and inferior pharyngeal constrictors to narrow pharynx and initiate peristalsis

(d) relaxes cricopharyngeal sphincter to allow bolus to enter esophagus

(e) initiates peristalsis in the esophagus

FIGURE **7-7**

The neurology of swallowing. (Reprinted from Patten J. [1977]. *Neurologic differential diagnosis*. London: H. Starke, Ltd.)

more extrinsic muscles of the tongue and larynx, are important to this aspect of swallowing. The study also indicated that the opening of the cricopharyngeus creates a negative pressure; thus a suction pump effect significantly increases the rate of bolus flow and contributes to the elimination of the bolus before the larynx reopens.[1]

The hypoglossal, glossopharyngeal, and vagus nerves are all major contributors to clearing the bolus through the pharynx. The tongue driving force and the pharyngeal clearing force, combined with the hypopharyngeal suction pump, produce a rapid transit through the pharynx once the swallow response has been triggered.

The glossopharyngeal nerve is thought to be the primary afferent of the swallow response, and the vagus is thought to be the secondary afferent. The swallowing center is located in the medulla in the nucleus solitarius, where the glossopharyngeus and vagus terminate. The sensory events stimulating the swallow response occur with stimulation to jaw, posterior tongue, faucial pillars, and upper pharynx. This stimulation is mediated through the glossopharyngeal, vagus, and trigeminal nerves. These afferent fibers converge on the nucleus solitarius in the medulla. They communicate with neurons in the nucleus ambiguus by way of interneurons, thereby stimulating the motor response. The medullary swallowing center is referred to as the **central pattern generator**.[6] Triggering of the swallow response and the timing and sequence of the muscle contractions that follow are hypothesized to be controlled by a network of neurons in the medulla. Sensory feedback may alter the detail of the central pattern generator to some extent.[9]

If swallowing is inefficient and aspiration occurs, a reflexive cough should occur as one of the respiratory system's defenses against foreign matter. The cough reflex is induced by irritation of the afferent fibers of the pharyngeal distribution of the glossopharyngeal nerve along with the sensory endings of the vagus nerve in the larynx, trachea, and larger bronchi.[2]

ASSESSMENT OF SWALLOWING

The cranial nerve examination is critical to the assessment of swallowing. Careful evaluation of the sensory component of the cranial nerves is probably more important in the swallowing evaluation than when the examination is for a speech disorder alone.

Taste, carried by cranial nerves VII and IX, should be tested with some of the primary tastes (salt, sweet, bitter, and sour). The testing must be done on both sides of the anterior two thirds of the tongue and on both sides of the posterior third of the tongue to include cranial nerves VII and IX.

General sensation to the tongue, carried by cranial nerves V and IX (posterior third), should be tested with the two sides compared regarding sensitivity to touch.

As previously mentioned, testing of the pharyngeal gag can be attempted.

The motor examination for swallowing should consist of the same maneuvers as for the speech examination. The clinician should assess swallowing, observing the patient's attempt at swallowing a liquid, a semisolid (e.g., pudding), and a solid. This swallowing should only be done if the clinician's judgment is that it will be safe to try in the clinic setting. If patient safety is a concern or if the cranial nerve examination has pointed to a likely pharyngeal-stage swallowing disorder, a modified barium swallow should be requested. This should be performed only by a speech-language pathologist or other professional with appropriate training and experience in the administration and interpretation of this radiologic procedure. The purpose of the examination should be to document problems and evaluate therapeutic alternatives that may improve oral intake. Fiberoptic endoscopic examination for swallowing is another instrumental procedure that may be helpful when a pharyngeal stage disorder is present.[5] Ultrasound has been used to examine the oral stage,[10] and manometry has been used to look at the pharyngeal and esophageal pressures.[8]

Synopsis of Clinical Information and Applications for the Speech-Language Pathologist

- The speech-language pathologist must be knowledgable regarding the function and assessment of the cranial nerves, which are vital for speech production and swallowing.
- Twelve pairs of cranial nerves can be found exiting the brainstem; seven are concerned with communication and/or swallowing.
- Cranial nerves I (olfactory), II (optic), III (oculomotor), IV (trochlear), and VI (abducens) are concerned with smell and vision as well as movement of the eyes.
- Cranial nerve VIII (vestibuloacoustic) is the auditory nerve carrying the sensation of sound to Heschl's gyrus. The vestibular portion of the nerve controls the sense of equilibrium.

- Cranial nerve XI (spinal accessory) contributes to movement of the uvula and the levator palatine through its cranial root. Testing of the spinal part of the nerve is the only possible test of the nerve's viability.
- The five remaining cranial nerves (V, trigeminal; VII, facial; IX, glossopharyngeal; X, vagus; and XII, hypoglossal) are main motor and sensory nerves for oral-motor and sensory function, enabling speech production, oral feeding, and swallowing.
- Table 7-2 summarizes pertinent clinical information on anatomy, innervation, testing, and signs of damage to these five cranial nerves.

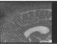

CASE**STUDY**

A 34-year-old female welder sought help from her physician for persistent ringing (medically known as *tinnitus)* and "wave crashing" sounds in her right ear. These symptoms were initially attributed to occupational noise exposure. However, a year later she continued to experience the same sounds but with additional symptoms that brought new concern. She now demonstrated a clumsy gait, had pain in her right ear, and reported dizziness. She also thought that her hearing in her right ear had decreased. Her symptoms worsened and she went to the emergency department. She reported in the emergency department that she had suddenly begun having difficulty seeing clearly out of her right eye, was having some difficulty with swallowing, and had some slurring of speech.

Examination showed moderate facial weakness and right-sided weakness of her mouth and tongue. Voice and speech production were notably weak. The physician diagnosed classic signs of a **flaccid** dysarthria.

QUESTIONS FOR CONSIDERATION:
1. What, if any, cranial nerves are involved here?
2. Could this patient's symptoms be explained as noise-induced hearing loss with cranial nerve damage?
3. The final diagnosis for this patient was a vestibular schwannoma (or acoustic neuroma). What are some of the characteristics of this tumor? (The answer to this question will involve some research.)

REFERENCES

1. Cerenko, D., McConnel, F. M. S., & Jackson, R. T. (1989). Quantitative assessment of pharyngeal bolus driving forces. *Otolaryngology Head and Neck Surgery, 100,* 1, 57-63.

2. Cherniack, R., Cherniack, L., & Naimark, A. (1972). *Respiration in health and disease* (2nd ed.). Philadelphia: W. B. Saunders.

3. Darley, F., Aronson, A., & Brown, J. (1975). *Motor speech disorders.* Philadelphia: W. B. Saunders.

4. DeMyer, W. (1980). *Technique of the neurologic examination: A programmed text* (3rd ed.). New York: McGraw-Hill.

5. Langmore, S., Schatz, K., & Olsen, N. (1988). Fiberoptic endoscopic examination of swallowing safety: A new procedure. *Dysphagia, 2,* 216-219.

6. Larson, C. (1985). Neurophysiology of speech and swallowing. *Semin Speech Lang, 6,* 275-289.

7. Logemann, J. A. (1984). *Evaluation and treatment of swallowing disorders.* San Diego: College Hill Press.

8. McConnel, F., Cerenko, D., Hersh, T., & Weil, L. (1988). Evaluation of pharyngeal dysphagia with manofluorography. *Dysphagia, 2,* 187-195.

9. Miller, A. J. (1982). Deglutition. *Physiol Rev, 62,* 129-184.

10. Sonies, B. (1990). Ultrasound imaging and swallowing. In Donner, M., & Jones, B. (Eds.). *Normal and abnormal swallowing: Imaging in diagnosis and therapy.* New York: Springer-Verlag.

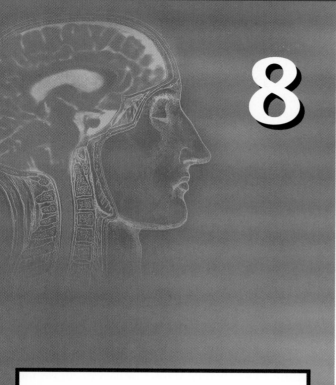

8 Clinical Speech Syndromes of the Motor Systems

Speech is deranged in a variety of ways by disease of the brain. The process of articulation is immediately affected by a mechanism of nerve nuclei situated in the pons and medulla, but these are excited to action by centers in the cerebral cortex. Thus there are higher and lower mechanisms; the former is cerebral, the latter is bulbar.

William R. Gowers, *A Manual of Disease of the Nervous System*, 1888

KEY TERMS

adduction
amyotrophic lateral
  sclerosis (ALS; Lou
  Gehrig's disease)
aphemia
apraxia of speech
articulary undershoot
ataxic dysarthria
athetosis
cerebrovascular
  accident (CVA)
childhood apraxia of
  speech
choreiform
cogwheel rigidity
diplegia
dysfluency
dysphagia
dystonia
essential tremor
excess and equal
  stress
explosive speech
fasciculations
flaccid
flaccid dysarthria

fricatives
Huntington's chorea
hypernasality
hypokinetic dysarthria
kernicterus
L-dopa
monoloudness
multiple sclerosis
myasthenia gravis
oral apraxia
palilalia
Parkinson's disease
parkinsonism
disease
pathologic tremor
plosives
pseudobulbar palsy
scanning speech
Shy-Drager syndrome
spastic dysarthria
spastic (spasmodic)
  dystonia (SD)
Sydenham's chorea
tardive dyskinesia
unilateral upper motor
  neuron dysarthria

CHAPTER OUTLINE

Speech-language pathologists must have an understanding of the function of the cranial nerves and the rest of the motor and sensory system for the treatment of motor speech disorders. Data kept at the Mayo Clinic between 1987 and 1990 and from 1993 to 2001 revealed that of the 10,444 people whose primary diagnosis was an acquired communication disorder, 58% were diagnosed with a motor speech disorder.[15] Figure 8-1 shows the distribution of the different categories of the acquired communication disorders found on evaluation. These data indicate that speech-language pathologists whose practice is primarily with adult clients must be well versed in the anatomy and physiology of the motor speech system and familiar with the clinical signs and symptoms of diseases and conditions producing them. This knowledge will be important to the treatment of children with motor speech disorders also, which will be discussed in Chapter 9.

Dysarthrias

In the classic Mayo Clinic study, Darley et al[11] define dysarthria as the speech disorder resulting from paralysis, weakness, or incoordination of the speech musculature that is of neurologic origin. Their definition encompasses any symptoms of motor disturbance of respiration, phonation, resonance, articulation, and prosody.

Damage to the motor system responsible for speech production may occur at any point along the pathway from the cerebrum to the muscle itself. In their classic studies of types of dysarthria resulting from certain sites of damage in the neural system, Darley et al[11,12] identified six different dysarthrias based on neuroanatomic and acoustic-perceptual judgments of speech. This chapter describes the classic dysarthrias according to

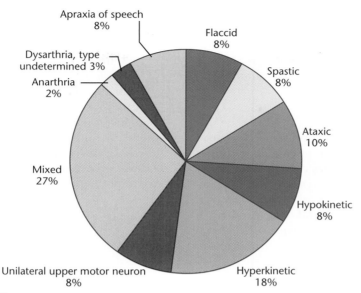

FIGURE **8-1**

Distribution of neurologic communication disorders, Speech pathology, Department of Neurology, Mayo Clinic, 1987-1990 and 1993-2001. (Reprinted from Duffy, J. [2005]. *Motor speech disorders: Substrates, differential diagnosis, and management* [2nd ed.]. St. Louis: Mosby.)

neuroanatomic site of dysfunction; associated disease processes; and the effects of these diseases on articulation, resonance, phonation, prosody, and swallowing. The following is not an exhaustive discussion of the diseases or of the types of dysarthrias resulting from neurologic disease. Keep in mind that any disease or trauma that affects the movement, coordination, and timing of the oral musculature may produce a dysarthria.

Upper Motor Neuron Lesions

Upper motor neuron damage may result in a spastic paralysis and hyperactive reflexes. The dysarthria associated with unilateral upper motor neuron lesions is called unilateral upper motor neuron dysarthria. The dysarthria associated with bilateral upper motor neuron lesions is known as spastic dysarthria. An overview of upper motor neuron lesions is found in Box 8-1.

UNILATERAL UPPER MOTOR NEURON DYSARTHRIA

As discussed by Duffy,[15] the dysarthria associated with unilateral upper motor neuron damage has been given scant attention in the literature, probably because the symptoms are usually mild and sometimes transitory.

BOX 8-1

Upper Motor Neuron Lesions

Unilateral Upper Motor Neuron Dysarthria

- Primarily caused by stroke but can also result from trauma or tumors
- Imprecise articulation; slow rate and irregular articulatory breakdown may also occur
- Harshness, reduced loudness, and hypernasality common
- Difficulty with oral stage transit

Spastic Dysarthria

- May be caused by stroke, head trauma, tumor, infection, degenerative disease, or inflammatory or toxic-metabolic disease
- Loss of skilled movement, hyporeflexia, positive Babinski sign, muscle weakness, loss of muscle tone
- Usually severe impairment of range of rate of movement of oral musculature
- Harsh voice with strained-strangled quality, low pitch, and monoloudness; often accompanied by hypernasality and imprecise consonant production
- Aspiration common, often with moderate to severe dysphagia

This section on upper motor neuron lesions is primarily devoted to a discussion of spastic dysarthria for the same reasons. However, a brief review of unilateral upper motor neuron dysarthria, as termed by Duffy, is warranted because it is as frequently encountered as the other types discussed in this chapter.

Etiology

The primary etiology of **unilateral upper motor neuron dysarthria** is stroke. Many other etiologies of upper motor neuron damage cause more diffuse brain injury and result more often in bilateral damage to the pyramidal pathways. Trauma and tumors can cause injury confined to a single hemisphere and can produce a unilateral upper motor neuron dysarthria. Unilateral upper motor neuron dysarthria can result from damage to either hemisphere.

Speech Characteristics

Only a small number of studies have looked at the speech characteristics of unilateral upper motor neuron dysarthria.[16,19] The collective findings of these studies indicate that the most prominent deviant characteristic of speech is imprecise articulation. Slowed rate and irregular articulatory breakdown were also noted in a number of cases. Other characteristics present in some cases were harshness, reduced loudness, and **hypernasality**. Most characteristics were described as mild to moderate in severity, although some patients had more severe dysarthria. Although many patients demonstrated significant recovery during the spontaneous recovery period, some dysarthrias persisted and required speech therapy for the reduced intelligibility.

Swallowing

Robbins[38] studied patients with left and right hemisphere strokes and showed that the patients differed from healthy individuals in increased oral-stage durations for liquid and semisolid swallows and the occurrence of laryngeal vestibule penetration. This difficulty with oral-stage transit was particularly true for left hemisphere–damaged patients. On further analysis, Robbins also found that patients with right-hemisphere **cerebrovascular accident (CVA)** demonstrated laryngeal penetration and aspiration significantly more often than patients with left-sided CVA. Silent aspiration (i.e., no coughing occurred reflexively) occurred with much greater frequency in patients with right-sided CVA. In addition, more aspiration occurred with anterior lesions than with posterior lesion sites.

Evatt et al[17] reported on a study of swallowing in 57 acute unilateral stroke patients. They found that aspiration in association with reduced pharyngeal clearance was present in 39% of the right hemisphere–damaged patients and 57% of the left hemisphere–damaged patients. The incidence of aspiration was also significantly greater in left hemisphere–damaged patients than in right hemisphere–damaged patients when analysis was performed on individuals older than 65 years. A study by Alberts et al[1] that used magnetic resonance imaging concluded that stroke patients should be individually evaluated for swallowing dysfunction regardless of the location or site of the lesion because even small-vessel strokes were associated with aspiration in greater than 20% of patients.

SPASTIC DYSARTHRIA

Etiology

Bilateral upper motor neuron damage may result from stroke, head trauma, tumor, infection, degenerative disease, and inflammatory or toxic-metabolic diseases. In most instances of **spastic dysarthria**, bilateral damage occurs to both the direct activation pathway (corticobulbar or corticospinal tract) and the indirect activation pathway (extrapyramidal pathways from cortex to brainstem and spinal cord). This usually occurs because the pathways are in close proximity from cortex to the termination at the cranial nerve or spinal nerve. The resulting oral-motor disorder from bilateral upper motor neuron damage to both systems is sometimes called **pseudobulbar palsy**. This name is derived from the resemblance of the oral-motor and speech characteristics to lower motor neuron damage and flaccid dysarthria (bulbar palsy).

Associated Neurologic Characteristics

Direct activation pathway damage results in the characteristic loss of skilled movement, hyporeflexia, a positive Babinski sign, and muscle weakness and loss of tone.

Damage to the indirect activation pathway causes increased muscle tone (spasticity) and hyperactive stretch reflexes. This hypertonicity and hyperreflexia dominate if both systems are damaged, which is usually the case. Although tone is increased, the muscles are weak, range of movement is limited, and rate of movement is slow because of the direct activation motor system damage.

Oral Musculature

In pseudobulbar palsy, the oral musculature usually shows severe impairment of range and rate of movement. The tongue may extend only to the lips on protrusion. The lips move slowly and excursion is limited. Palatal movement is severely reduced and sluggish on phonation. The gag reflex may be absent in the acute stages but later returns and may be hyperactive. Chewing and swallowing are both frequently affected, and drooling is present in most cases.

Speech Characteristics

The patient usually demonstrates a classic spastic dysarthria. Speech characteristics are as follows.

Phonation

The voice of the patient with spastic dysarthria is described as harsh, and many have a characteristic strained-strangled quality. An effortful grunt is often heard at the end of vocalizations. Excessively low pitch is frequently found, with pitch breaks in some cases. Very little variation in loudness (**monoloudness**) and reduced stress are also noted. Occasionally heard in spastic dysarthria is excess and equal stress (i.e., inappropriate stress on monosyllabic words and the usually unstressed syllables of polysyllabic words).

Resonance

Hypernasality is a frequent component of spastic dysarthria. Nasal emission is uncommon, however.

Articulation

As in most dysarthrias, imprecision of consonant production is a noticeable part of the speech disorder in spastic dysarthria. Vowel distortion has been noted in some cases. Zeigler and von Cramer's acoustic study[48] of 10 patients with spastic dysarthria revealed a disproportionate impairment of the back of the tongue compared with the blade of the tongue. Impaired acceleration of the moving articulators also accounted for part of the distortion and the increase in production time often noted in these speakers.

Swallowing

Horner et al[20] studied 70 patients with bilateral hemispheric strokes. By using videofluoroscopy, they found that 49% of the patients aspirated. The following symptoms associated with **dysphagia** are often observed in patients with bilateral upper motor neuron damage: reduced labial, lingual, and mandibular strength and sensation; delayed swallow response; reduced pharyngeal peristalsis; incomplete laryngeal elevation and closure; and cricopharyngeal dysfunction.[10] The dysphagia may be severe, and drooling may be noted. With mild dysphagia, the patient may unconsciously alter the eating pattern to eat more slowly and carefully, denying any difficulty.[15]

Lower Motor Neuron Lesions

FLACCID DYSARTHRIA

Damage to the lower motor neuron system impairs the final common pathway for muscle contraction. The muscles become hypotonic or **flaccid.** Thus every type of movement is affected (voluntary, automatic, and reflexive movement are all impaired), and **flaccid dysarthria** may be seen.

Etiology

Any disease that affects part of the motor unit—the cell body, its axon, the myoneural junction, or the muscle fibers themselves—may yield lower motor neuron symptoms. Thus viral infections, tumors, trauma to the nerve itself, or a brainstem stroke with involvement of the nerve fibers may be the cause of the dysarthria. Myasthenia gravis results from impairment of transmission across the myoneural junction or the synapse between the nerve and muscle. Bulbar palsy results from damage to the motor units of the cranial nerves. Möbius syndrome (congenital facial **diplegia**) involves bilateral sixth (abducens) and seventh (facial) nerve palsies of congenital origin rather than generalized bulbar palsy. Most patients with these palsies talk acceptably except for slurring. Direct muscle involvement is found in diseases such as muscular dystrophy, myotonia, and myositis.

Associated Neurologic Characteristics

Damage to the lower motor neuron system causes flaccid paralysis. Reflexes are reduced (i.e., hyporeflexia is present). The affected muscle usually becomes shrunken or atrophied over time. Many times the involved muscles, especially the tongue muscles, show **fasciculations**—tiny spontaneous muscle contractions of the motor unit or muscle fibers innervated by an axon. The fasciculations appear as spontaneous dimpling of the tongue, which may look as though tiny worms are moving just beneath its surface.

Oral Musculature

Because the cranial nerve nuclei are dispersed throughout the brainstem rather than being clustered together, the oral structures may be selectively impaired and should be carefully evaluated.

Muscle tone in lower motor neuron damage is flaccid or hypotonic. Muscles are weak. The affected side of the lips sags, and in some cases drooling may be present. In bilateral weakness the whole mouth may sag, and the lower lip may be so weak that habitual open-mouth posture results. The patient may have difficulty puckering the lips or pulling up the angles of the lips to smile.

Weakness of the mandibular muscles may not be readily evident in unilateral involvement. Careful observation reveals that the jaw deviates to the side of weakness. With bilateral damage the jaw obviously sags. With damage to any component of the motor unit supplying the tongue, the muscles become atrophied and shrunken over time, and the tongue is atonic or flabby. This tends to affect protrusion, lateralization, and elevation, particularly of the posterior portion of the tongue. Fasciculations are often observed after a period.

Palatal weakness or immobility may also be present, and the gag reflex is reduced or absent. Pharyngeal involvement may occur, causing swallowing difficulty and possibly nasal regurgitation of fluids.

Speech Characteristics

Speech-language pathologists are most likely to be consulted concerning patients with a bulbar palsy resulting from vascular disease, head trauma, or diseases such as amyotrophic lateral sclerosis (ALS). These patients may exhibit a flaccid dysarthria and show some of the following characteristics on speech testing.

Phonation

Unilateral vocal fold paralysis is relatively unusual in disease processes affecting the brainstem nuclei. If unilateral damage is present, the quality of phonation depends on the position of the vocal fold. If it is paralyzed in an adducted position, the voice is harsh and loudness is reduced. If it is in the abducted position, more breathiness is heard with reduced loudness.

More likely is bilateral vocal cord involvement. The characteristics of this are a breathy voice, inspiratory stridor (or audible inhalation), and abnormally short phrases. Monotony of pitch and loudness is distinctive in many patients as well.

Resonance

Hypernasality is noted as an outstanding characteristic of the patients with flaccid dysarthria. Nasal emission of air is also found in a high percentage of patients.

Articulation

Imprecise consonant production may be present in mild to severe (unintelligible speech) degrees. The consonants requiring firm contact from tongue tip elevation are particularly vulnerable. **Plosives** such as /p/, /t/, and /k/ and **fricatives** such as /f/ and /s/ are frequently affected because of the lack of intraoral pressure that results from palatal dysfunction.

Swallowing

A brainstem CVA can cause flaccid dysarthria with lesions affecting the motor nuclei. Robbins et al[39] studied 10 patients with brainstem CVAs and found that these patients aspirated more frequently than did the patients with left or right cortical CVAs. Aspiration usually occurred during the swallow because of reduced airway protection or after the swallow because of large amounts of stasis in the pharyngeal recesses, particularly in the piriform sinuses. Incomplete as well as delayed relaxation of the cricopharyngeal sphincter was also noted in these patients.

Myasthenia Gravis

Myasthenia gravis is a chronic autoimmune disease resulting from a reduction in available acetylcholine receptors at the neuromuscular junction. Changes in the eyes such as ptosis (drooping of the eyelid) or double vision typically occur. The muscles may be weak, with the jaw sagging accompanied by weak chewing. Swallowing difficulty, or dysphagia, is not uncommon, and myasthenia especially should be considered with a history of difficulty with swallowing that worsens in use and improves with rest.[25]

Voice symptoms can exist without other signs of dysarthria. The flaccid dysphonia of myasthenia should be suspected when, despite normal laryngoscopic findings, the voice nevertheless becomes progressively more breathy and reduced in intensity as the client speaks. Respiratory weakness, in addition to extremity weakness, may be present, and myasthenia can occur with no oral motor involvement. Box 8-2 summarizes the lower motor lesions.

BOX 8-2

Lower Motor Neuron Lesions

Flaccid Dysarthria

- May be caused by any disease that affects part of the motor unit (viral infections, tumors, nerve trauma, brainstem stroke)
- Selective impairment of a muscle or muscle group can occur, resulting in a flaccid paralysis, brainstem CVA, or bulbar palsy
- Damage resulting in flaccid paralysis, hyporeflexia, and shrunken or atrophied muscle
- Hypernasality and nasal emission common; selective consonants, plosives, and fricatives often affected
- Frequent aspiration
- Myasthenia gravis, a chronic autoimmune disease caused by reduced acetylcholine receptors at neuromuscular junctions results in a unique symptomatology
  - Ptosis, double vision, muscle weakness, and dysphagia common
  - Flaccid dysphonia, progressive breathiness, and reduced voice intensity common

Mixed Upper and Lower Motor Neuron Lesions

AMYOTROPHIC LATERAL SCLEROSIS

A common finding in clinical practice is a lesion or disease process that has not confined itself to one motor system but instead has affected both upper and lower motor neuron systems. The most frequently encountered example of this damage is **amyotrophic lateral sclerosis** (**ALS,** also known as **Lou Gehrig's disease**).

Etiology

ALS causes progressive degeneration of the neurons of the upper and lower motor neuron systems and is of unknown etiology. Onset is typically in the fifth decade, although it may be earlier or later, and early symptoms depend on which motor neurons initially are affected. If brainstem nuclei are the first to be affected, the initial signs may be slurring of speech or difficulty swallowing. Often only a slight change in voice quality is the first sign. The bulbar or brainstem symptoms are particularly devastating, and verbal communication and oral feedings usually become impossible over time. The patient with this type of ALS has a variable life expectancy but typically may survive only 1 to 3 years after onset. Pneumonia is frequently the cause of death. ALS has no known effective treatment or cure, although many palliative treatments are available, including physical therapy, drugs for reduction of muscle pain, and speech therapy in some cases.

Associated Neurologic Characteristics

Signs may be present from damage to both upper and lower motor neuron systems. Muscles are weak but reflexes are hyperactive. Spasticity is usually present unless the lower motor neuron damage is well advanced.

Oral Musculature

Oral peripheral examination yields indications of a pervasive weakness in lips, tongue, and palate. Range of movement is reduced, and sometimes one side is slightly more affected than the other. The tongue may show fasciculations and, in more advanced cases, atrophy. The patient may report and demonstrate difficulty swallowing, especially liquids, and, with progression, difficulty handling oral secretions.

Speech Characteristics

Signs of involvement of both upper and lower motor neuron systems are again present. It is unpredictable as to which signs will predominate in a given case and what changes may occur through the course of the disease.

A Mayo Clinic study involved 30 patients with ALS. The characteristics of the speech of this group were as follows.[13]

Phonation

Some patients showed symptoms similar to those shown by patients with pseudobulbar palsy, with much harshness and a strain-strangle quality associated with low pitch. The harshness associated with ALS may often have a wet, gurgly quality. Other patients showed signs more like those of the bulbar group, with poor vocal fold **adduction** resulting in breathiness and short phrases. Audible inspiration was also noted. Monotony of pitch and loudness as well as reduction of stress was present in most patients.

Resonance

Hypernasality was frequent in these cases. Nasal emission, though noted, was not prominent.

Articulation

Imprecise consonant production was a principal characteristic. Vowels were often distorted, as were consonants. The slow rate and reduced range of movement of the articulators greatly affected sound production. Hypernasality also contributed to phoneme distortion, and precision of articulation was often so poor as to render speech unintelligible.

Swallowing

The degree of dysphagia in patients with ALS varies greatly depending on the extent of involvement of the oral musculature and the type of motor system involvement predominating. Evidence of poor lingual control frequently is found, with lingual stasis and aspiration before the swallow. A delayed swallow response may also be present, causing aspiration before the swallow. Poor tongue propulsion, weak pharyngeal contractions, and/or cricopharyngeal dysfunction may also result in pharyngeal stasis and aspiration after the swallow. Airway protection may be significantly better in patients with predominantly spastic (upper motor neuron) symptoms than in those with more lower motor neuron symptoms. The amount of aspiration may thus be reduced in these patients despite a severe dysarthria.

Dysphagia usually parallels or follows the loss of speech. Managing secretions and maintaining appropriate amounts of fluid intake often are huge challenges for ALS patients. Feeding tube placement often is necessary during the final course of the disease.

Box 8-3 presents an overview of the most common example of mixed upper and motor neuron lesions, ALS.

Amyotrophic Lateral Sclerosis

- Most common example of mixed upper and lower motor neuron lesions; also known as Lou Gehrig's disease
- Causes progressive motor neuron degeneration; usually appears in fifth decade; etiology unknown
- Weak muscles, hyperactive reflexes, and spasticity common
- Weakness in lips, tongue, and palate with reduced range of movement and/or atrophy
- Mixed upper and lower motor neuron symptoms, frequent hypernasality, and imprecise consonant production
- Degree of dysphagia variable; usually follows or parallels degree of dysarthria

Basal Ganglia Lesions: Dyskinetic Dysarthrias

The basal ganglia control circuit contributes to complex movements by integrating and controlling the component parts of the movements and also helps inhibit unplanned movement. Lesions produce dyskinetic movements and may yield two types of dysarthria, hypokinetic and hyperkinetic, as summarized in Box 8-4.

HYPOKINETIC DYSARTHRIA: PARKINSONISM

The most common disease associated with **hypokinetic dysarthria** is **Parkinson's disease**. This disorder is characterized by degenerative changes in the substantia nigra, which cause a deficiency in a chemical neural transmitter known as dopamine in the caudate nucleus and putamen.

Etiology
Parkinson's disease usually is idiopathic (i.e., spontaneous, not caused by another disease), but parkinsonism (or Parkinson-like symptoms) is caused by carbon monoxide poisoning, arteriosclerosis, manganese poisoning, and some tranquilizing drugs (e.g., prochlorperazine [Compazine], trifluoperazine [Stelazine], and haloperidol [Haldol]).

Associated Neurologic Characteristics
The three cardinal features of **parkinsonism** are tremor, rigidity, and bradykinesia.[22] A tremor may be present at

Basal Ganglia Lesions

Hypokinetic Dysarthria: Parkinsonism

- Parkinson's disease: most common disease associated with hypokinetic dysarthria; usually idiopathic
- Three cardinal features: tremor, rigidity, and bradykinesia
- Slow rate of movement of tongue, lips, and palate
- Speech varies considerably with pathology, but hypophonia and accelerated speech rate are key features in most patients
- Dysphagic symptoms in all four stages of swallow

Hyperkinetic Dysarthria

Essential Tremor
- Encountered as organic voice tremor when larynx involved; may be pure with no other tremor present
- Regular alteration of pitch and loudness noted in mild cases; in severe cases, voice stoppage

Chorea
- Two major types: Sydenham's chorea (childhood disease) and Huntington's chorea (progressive and fatal genetic disease)
- Huntington's characterized by dementia and involuntary movements
- Variable presence of hypotonia and involuntary movement
- Harsh, strained-strangled voice quality common, along with transient breathiness, excessive loudness, and problems with pitch; often imprecise consonants and distorted vowels
- Dysphagia common in Huntington's; oral swallowing stages significantly affected

Dystonia and Athetosis
- Classified as the slow hyperkinesias; no well-established etiologies
- Dystonic (with excessive tone) trunk, neck, and proximal limb parts; athetotic (writhing) movements of arms, face, and trunk
- Dystonia: harsh, strained-strangled voice, imprecise consonants, vowel distortion, hypernasality, and velar control
- Athetosis: excessively loud or breathy; problems with jaw, tongue, and lip movement
- Limited information on dysphagia

Tardive Dyskinesia
- Caused by long-term use of phenothiazines and similar classes of drugs
- Choreiform, myoclonic, peculiar rhythmic movements and abnormal oral movement
- Usually mild speech disorders
- Possible poor coordination in any stage of swallow

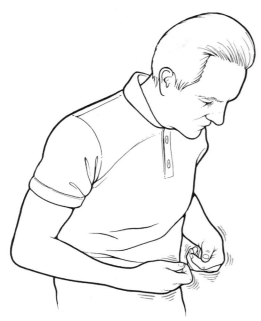

FIGURE **8-2**
Resting tremor and characteristic posturing of parkinsonism. A patient may have difficulty initiating movement (akinesia), or movement may be slow and lack spontaneity once initiated (bradykinesia). (Reprinted from Haines, D. [2006]. *Fundamental neuroscience* [3rd ed.]. Philadelphia: Churchill Livingstone.)

rest that tends to subside on movement and is absent during sleep. It is often called a pill-rolling tremor because of the pattern of movement of the fingers, as if rolling a small pill between the thumb and the fingers. Rigidity is a common characteristic and is elicited by passive movement of the limb, which induces involuntary contractions in the muscle being stretched. The rigidity may be smooth or intermittent (referred to as **cogwheel rigidity**). Bradykinesia is defined as reduced speed of movement of a muscle through its range. Hypokinesia, or reduced amplitude of movement, is a prime characteristic as well. Figure 8-2 depicts characteristic posturing and tremor of Parkinson's disease.

Dementia is a correlate of Parkinson's disease, with an incidence between 15% and 40%.[7] Language characteristics of this dementia include impaired receptive vocabulary, difficulty in comprehending the meanings of ambiguous sentences, impaired ability to describe objects verbally, and impaired ability to identify a speaker's intention. Discourse comprehension is certainly at risk.[34]

Other features of parkinsonism are referred to as minor, but at least one of these features should be present for the diagnosis to be made. These include micrographia, which is the tendency for the height of the

handwritten letters to get smaller as the person writes. Excessive salivation and a dysphonia, described later in this chapter, may be present. The parkinsonian facies is described as a masked facies, with very little movement used in facial expression. The parkinsonian posture is stooped and leaning slightly forward. A characteristic gait, called a festinating gait, may also be present that involves short, slow, shuffling steps.

Treatment for parkinsonism usually involves prescription of a dopamine agonist drug. Until recently, most drugs contained a chemical called **L-dopa** such as carbidopa/levodopa (Sinemet) or bromocriptine (Parlodel). Other dopamine agonists and other drugs that potentiate the effect of levodopa are now available. Surgical treatments, such as pallidotomy and deep brain stimulation, have been researched and have begun to be used clinically with a degree of success in controlling tremor as well as speech and voice symptoms in some patients.[43] Physical therapy and speech therapy are also often prescribed, and new techniques show promise for improving speech and voice production in selected patients.[37]

Oral Musculature

Frequently the standard oral examination yields only slow rate of movement of the lips and tongue as the major finding, with some reduced range of movement. Palatal movement may be sluggish.

Diadochokinetic rate testing may yield the most interesting information. When a patient is asked to execute the syllable repetition for the diadochokinetic testing, reduction of range of movement becomes more evident. The patient also tends to show an accelerated or rapid rate of speaking. As repetition continues, constriction for consonant production may lessen and syllables may seem to run together. Some patients may use so little movement, combined with a rapid rate, that no differentiation can be made between syllables and more of a humming or whirring sound is heard.

Speech Characteristics

The speech of patients with Parkinson's disease varies tremendously depending on the stage of the disease and the effectiveness of medication. A study of the vocal tract characteristics of 200 patients with Parkinson's disease helped quantify and describe certain features of this disorder.[28] Only 11%, or 22 of the patients, were found to have no vocal tract problems.

Phonation

Laryngeal disorders were found to be present in 89% of the patients in the study by Logemann et al.[28] Hoarseness was the major perceived characteristic, occurring in 45% of the patients. Roughness, breathiness, and tremulousness also occurred. All patients, except one who had articulation problems, also showed laryngeal dysfunction.

Duffy[15] notes that, even when not pervasive, a strained, whispered aphonia occasionally is noted in the midst of a breathy, harsh vocal quality; it occurs toward the end of a vowel-prolongation task and persists for several seconds. Dysphonia may, in fact, be the presenting and most debilitating speech feature in persons with hypokinetic dysarthria. Monopitch and monoloudness are also frequent characteristics of the vocal production of these patients. Maintaining adequate intensity is quite difficult for most patients.

Articulation

A detailed analysis of the articulatory errors of the 200 Parkinson's patients in the study by Logemann et al[28] showed that changes in the manner of articulation predominated over changes in the place of articulation.[27] Stop plosives, affricates, and fricatives were most affected, as were the features of continuance and stridency. Inadequate narrowing or constricting of the vocal tract as a result of inadequate tongue elevation appeared to be the reason for these changes. Netsell et al[35] have called the result of this phenomena **articulatory undershoot**.

Resonance

Ten percent of the patients in the study by Logemann et al[28] showed hypernasality. No regular pattern of hypernasality occurred with articulation or laryngeal disorders.

Prosody

Approximately 20% of the patients in the study by Logemann et al[28] showed what the authors called a rate disorder. Furthermore, 10% of the patients were judged as using syllables that were too short, whereas 6% used syllables that were too long. Abnormally long pauses occurred in 2% of those tested. In other descriptions of rate and prosody, variable rate, short rushes of speech, and inappropriate silences have been noted as characteristic. Patients with hypokinetic dysarthria are often described as showing prosodic insufficiency.

Compulsive repetition of phonemes and syllables, noted as **dysfluency**, has been frequently observed in patients with Parkinson's disease. The presence of **palilalia** has also been noted with Parkinson's disease. Palilalia is characterized by repetitions that usually involve words, phrases, or sentences and is usually associated with bilateral subcortical damage.

In summary, the typical patient with Parkinson's is expected to have a phonatory disorder characterized by monopitch, monoloudness, and decreased intensity.

Speech rate is likely accelerated, especially during alternate motion rate testing and within segments of conversational speech. Repeated phonemes as well as inappropriate silences are noted.

Swallowing

Dysphagic symptoms have been identified in all four stages of the swallow in patients with Parkinson's disease. The exact nature of the disorder is still not well understood.[26] The oral stage of the swallow may show a rocking pattern, with the anterior tongue repetitively moving the bolus upward and backward while the posterior tongue remains elevated against the palate, preventing the bolus from entering the pharynx and preventing initiation of the swallow response. Although this may last for several seconds and significantly lengthen the oral stages, many patients are unaware of the abnormality. Incoordination and tremulousness, with difficulty initiating tongue movement, are often a part of the oral stages in patients who do not demonstrate the rocking pattern.

Delay of the swallow response, causing aspiration before the swallow, often is noted in these patients. Other disorders include problems with soft palate function, poor laryngeal closure, and reduced pharyngeal peristalsis. Esophageal hypomotility or dysmotility may also be present.

Logemann[26] notes that it is not unusual to find patients with Parkinson's disease who have chronic aspiration, as demonstrated by videofluoroscopy study, but few indications of aspiration in their history or other examinations. These patients tend to aspirate silently, without cough or other external signs, and have not been diagnosed with an aspiration pneumonia. The exact mechanism of this phenomenon is not well understood neurologically or in terms of pulmonary function.[26]

Much variability exists among individuals regarding onset and degree of dysphagia, but progression of the disease results in a greater tendency toward development or worsening of dysphagic symptoms. Medication can have a positive effect, and consideration should be given to timing its administration with meals. Overmedication can cause increased problems, however. The effect of medication should be considered.[39]

HYPERKINETIC DYSARTHRIAS

Hypokinetic dysarthria and hypokinesia are related to reduction of movement from extrapyramidal system damage, but hyperkinetic dysarthria is related to increase in movement. The involuntary movement disorders of tremor, chorea, athetosis, and dystonia also result from extrapyramidal damage. The specific localization of the damage in these disorders is not well understood.

PATHOLOGIC TREMOR

Tremor can be classified as either normal or abnormal (i.e., pathologic) depending on whether it is associated with a disease state. Both normal and **pathologic tremor** may occur at rest, in static postures, or with movement.

Essential tremor (also called action, senile, or heredofamilial tremor) is the tremor most often encountered in speech-language pathology practice. Essential tremor of the voice is known in speech pathology as organic voice tremor. In this condition the extrinsic and intrinsic muscles of the larynx may show tremor either independently or along with tremor of other parts of the body, such as the hands, jaw, or head.

Speech Characteristics

In a pure organic voice tremor, articulatory and resonance characteristics are normal and only phonation is affected. On prolongation of a vowel, the mildly affected patient's voice has a regular tremor of altering pitch and loudness. With more severe disease the voice may simply stop, resembling the disorder known as spastic dysphonia. However, significant differences have been found between the two disorders in terms of regularity of voice arrest and accompanying characteristics. Patients with organic voice tremor also demonstrate excessively low pitch and monopitch, intermittent or constant strained-strangled harshness, and pitch breaks.

CHOREA

Two major diseases in the disorder group known as chorea are **Sydenham's chorea** and **Huntington's chorea**. Huntington's chorea is autosomal dominantly inherited, and a child of an affected individual has a 50% chance of developing the disease. Onset is typically in the fifth decade, although a so-called juvenile variant and senile variant also occur. The cause is unknown, and the disease is progressive and fatal. Pathologic changes documented usually include loss of neurons from the caudate nucleus, pallidum, and cerebral cortex, with less-constant changes in other areas.

Sydenham's chorea (called "Saint Vitus' dance" in ancient terminology) is a noninherited childhood disease that may follow strep throat, rheumatic fever, or scarlet fever. The symptoms usually clear up within 6 months.

Associated Neurologic Characteristics

Huntington's chorea is characterized by dementia and involuntary movements. Choreic movements are rapid and coordinated but purposeless. They occur unpredictably and may involve any group of muscles. Voluntary and automatic movements may be interrupted so that coordinated breathing and speech may be quite difficult. The limbs are hypotonic. Postures cannot be maintained.

Oral Musculature

The presence of hypotonia and involuntary movement of the oral musculature is variable in chorea. A common characteristic of Huntington's disease is the inability to keep the tongue protruded for more than a few seconds. Sydenham's chorea often involves involuntary movements of the mouth and larynx. Even if little involuntary movement of oral musculature is present, the speech probably will be affected by the movements of other parts of the body.

Speech Characteristics

In the Mayo Clinic study of 30 adults with chorea, the following problems were noted.[13]

Phonation

A harsh voice quality and/or a strained-strangled sound were found in many patients. Transient breathiness also occurred. Excess loudness variations were prominent as a result of the poor control of ancillary movement. Lower-than-average pitch levels, voice stoppages, and pitch breaks were other characteristics noted in various patients. Sudden forced inspiration or expiration was observed in some patients.

Resonance

Forty-three percent of the patients in the study by Darley et al[13] demonstrated hypernasality. The interference with resonance also contributed to articulatory problems, including imprecise consonants and short phrases.

Articulation

The difficulty of muscular adjustment yielded imprecise consonant production and, in 23 patients in the study by Darley et al,[13] distorted vowels. Misdirection of movement resulted in a feature called irregular articulatory breakdown. Reduced stress and short phrases were also displayed by many of the chorea patients. Prolonged intervals and variable rates were quite prominent and contributed to the perception of prosodic deviations.

Swallowing

Dysphagia is noted to be a frequent symptom in Huntington's disease.[23] The severity of dysphagia varies from patient to patient primarily because of the constantly changing postures and interpatient variability inherent in the clinical population. The oral stages of the swallow are significantly affected by the irregular and uncoordinated tongue movements and changes in facial tone. Aspiration before the swallow may occur because these random movements prematurely push the bolus over the base of the tongue.

Irregular and uncoordinated movements of the vocal folds and the respiratory musculature as well as neck hyperextension may compromise airway protection. Pharyngeal peristalsis may be weak, and esophageal dysmotility has been reported.

DYSTONIA AND ATHETOSIS

Dystonia and **athetosis** are movement disorders classified as the slow hyperkinesias. Movements are characteristically unstable and sustained, suggesting possible conflicts between flexion and extension of the muscles.

Etiology

Most of these disorders do not have well-established etiologies or focal lesion sites. Encephalitis, vascular lesions, birth trauma, and degenerative neuronal disease are often precipitating diseases. Most hyperkinesias show localized damage to the confines of the basal ganglia. Involuntary movement disorders are sometimes caused by the effects of drugs such as phenothiazine and related compounds, especially the more powerful tranquilizers.

Athetosis is a rare disorder usually seen as a form of congenital cerebral palsy. It is also seen as a rare progressive disease of adolescence, the cause of which is unknown, and as an accompanying residual deficit with hemiplegia after cerebral infarction. Localization of the lesion is difficult, but the putamen seems to be almost always involved.

Associated Neurologic Characteristics

Dystonia implies excess tone in selected parts of the body. Dystonia mainly affects the trunk, neck, and proximal parts of the limbs. The slow movements are usually sustained for a prolonged period. The movements usually build up to a peak, are sustained, and then recede, although they occasionally begin with a jerk. Athetotic movements are slow and writhing and are predominantly of the arms, face, and tongue. The movements tend to be exaggerated by attempts at voluntary activity, which make voluntary movements clumsy and inaccurate.

Speech Characteristics
Phonation

The dystonic patient usually has a harsh or strained-strangled voice quality. Other patients, though fewer in number, may demonstrate intermittent breathiness and audible inspiration. Monopitch and monoloudness are also seen in these patients. Because of the involuntary movements, dystonic patients often have voice stoppages and periods of inappropriate silence. Excess loudness variations accompany the excessive movement. Voice tremor also is found among dystonic patients.

Phonation in athetosis is often significantly affected. The patient often has poor respiratory reserve and respiratory patterns. Both dilator and constrictor spasms have been noted in laryngeal functioning. Voicing is often excessively loud or excessively breathy, and it is unpredictable and frequently poorly coordinated with articulation.

Spastic or **spasmodic dysphonia (SD)** is a chronic phonation disorder of unknown etiology. It is included here because its symptoms are found to occur in disorders of movement, and some researchers have postulated that it may be a form of focal dystonia.[4] Aronson and Hartman[3] discussed differential diagnoses for patients with essential tremor who had SD. The signs of SD also occur in cases that appear to be psychogenic or idiopathic. No single cause has been identified.

SD is characterized by a strained voice quality with voice arrests caused by laryngeal adductor spasm. It is frequently associated with pain in the laryngeal area. The interruptions to phonatory airflow are assumed to be caused by hyperadduction of the vocal folds, but indirect laryngoscopy usually reveals normal vocal fold movements.

Abductor laryngospasms also occur in some patients, as does a mixture of adductor and abductor spasms. These spasms may be different forms of SD. Rosenfield[41] postulates that voice production in SD can be viewed as a primary problem resulting from abnormal movements in the speech motor system. Furthermore, it may also be considered as resulting from an attempt to cope with the underlying movement disturbance. SD can also be a focal laryngeal dystonia.

Treatment of SD is controversial, and although various treatments have been shown to be successful, no single treatment has been discovered. Psychogenic SD necessitates careful differential diagnosis and may respond to behavioral therapy.[2] Recurrent laryngeal nerve resection has had varying success according to published clinical reports.[14] Patients must be carefully selected,[31] and symptoms may reappear after the procedure.[42,47] Active investigation and a clinical trial are ongoing of the use of botulinum, a toxin injection, which has been found to improve voice production dramatically for some SD patients.[6,32]

Articulation

As might be predicted, the articulation of patients with these involuntary movement disorders is highly variable, with a range of severity from slight distortion to unintelligible. The dystonic patients of the Mayo Clinic study demonstrated prominent articulation imprecision of consonant production.[11] Results also showed vowel distortion and irregular breakdown of articulation. Short phrases were noted with prolonged intervals. Prolongation of phonemes and variability of rate were also frequently observed. Reduction of stress was a relatively prominent characteristic of speech production.

Kent and Netsell[21] and Platt et al[36] have investigated the articulation of athetoid adults by using cinefluorographic and intelligibility measures. The studies found that athetoid speech is frequently reduced in intelligibility as a result of articulation problems. Kent and Netsell[21] found large ranges of jaw movement, inappropriate tongue positioning, prolonged transition time, and retruding of the lower lip. Platt et al[36] found particular difficulty with accuracy of anterior tongue placement, reduced precision of fricatives and affricatives, and inability to achieve extreme positions in vowel formation. They found place and voicing errors to be predominant, particularly in final consonants.

Resonance

Of the 30 dystonic patients studied by the Mayo Clinic, 11 were found to show hypernasality.[11] In the Kent and Netsell[21] cinefluorographic study of athetoid adults, all subjects had trouble achieving velopharyngeal closure. The most severe problem, however, was velar control. Instability of velar position was frequently noted. The velum sometimes moved inappropriately, causing a loss of closure, or in some cases the velum showed repetitive movements that were not related to respiration.

Swallowing

Dysphagia in dystonic patients has been described on a limited basis in the literature. Bosma et al[5] describe difficulty with lip control and lingual coordination in a patient with drug-induced bulbar and cervical dystonia. The patient had difficulty holding food in the mouth and controlling it to prevent premature entrance into the pharynx. The pharyngeal stage was normal in this group's patients.

Pharyngeal stage efficiency may depend on the posturing of the head and neck. A pulling of the neck to the side or a hyperextension often occurs, which may cause stasis and perhaps aspiration if the airway cannot be protected during the prolonged posturing.

TARDIVE DYSKINESIA

Another movement disorder resulting from extrapyramidal damage is **tardive dyskinesia**, which is attributable to the long-term use of phenothiazines and similar drugs. Symptoms include **choreiform**, myoclonic, and peculiar rhythmical movements, with a high incidence of abnormal movements in the oral region. Constant random movements of the lips and tongue may be found, with a frequent "fly catcher's" movement of the tongue in which the tongue involuntarily moves in and out of the mouth. Velar movement may also be involved. Intelligibility is variably affected, with some patients becoming unintelligible because of the random movements. Most patients, however, have only a mild speech disorder.

The random movements may result in poor coordination in any of the four stages of swallowing. Pocketing of food; pharyngeal stasis; and aspiration before, during, and after the swallow may be found on study of the dysphagia. Reflux of food may be a result of esophageal discoordination. Decreased sensation may also result in lack of reflexive cough or silent aspiration.

The Cerebellum and Cerebellar Pathway Lesions

ATAXIC DYSARTHRIA

As noted, the cerebellum serves as an important center for the integration or coordination of sensory and motor activities. It receives fibers from the motor and sensory cortex either directly or through intervening nuclei. Damage to the cerebellum and/or its pathways causes a disorder called ataxia, and the motor speech symptoms yield an **ataxic dysarthria**.

Etiology

Ataxic dysarthria is caused by damage at some point in the cerebellar control circuit. Damage may occur localized to the cerebellum alone or may be part of more generalized damage affecting several systems. Causes include degenerative diseases (Friedreich's ataxia, olivopontocerebellar atrophy, and multiple sclerosis), stroke, trauma, tumors, alcohol toxicity, drug-induced neurotoxicity (from such drugs as phenytoin [Dilantin], carbamazepine [Tegretol], lithium, or diazepam [Valium]), encephalitis, lung cancer, and severe hypothyroidism.

Associated Neurologic Characteristics

Ataxia is a disruption in the smooth coordination of movement with failure to coordinate sensory data with motor performance. The hand may overshoot its target when reaching for an object. If the outstretched arm is pushed aside, it swings past its former position and overcorrects. Abnormalities such as these are shown when the patient is asked to touch his or her nose or run the heel down the shin. Rapid alternating movements may be affected. Equilibrium is affected and gait may be impaired. Movement is slow to be initiated and slow through the range. Repetitive movements may be irregular and poorly timed, a condition called dysdiadochokinesia. Muscle tone is hypotonic. Intention or kinetic tremor (tremor during purposeful movement) is also present.

Speech Characteristics

Dysarthria with localized damage to the cerebellum has the following characteristics.

Phonation

The voice may be approximately normal or occasionally may show excessive loudness variations. Harshness similar to a coarse voice tremor may also be noted.

Resonance

Velopharyngeal functioning is usually intact, with normal resonance characteristics. Hypernasal resonance occasionally is found. Nasal emission is less frequently demonstrated.

Articulation

Imprecise consonant production, vowel distortion, and irregular articulatory breakdown mark the speech of ataxic dysarthria. Rate is usually slow, although some patients use normal rate.

Prosody

Prosodic changes are usually readily observable in ataxic dysarthria. A speech prosody characteristic termed **excess and equal stress** by Darley et al[11] is a predominant feature, although it is not found in all speakers with ataxic dysarthria. This description refers to the tendency to put excessive vocal emphasis on typically unstressed syllables and words using a slow, metered pattern. Duffy[15] postulates that in some patients the irregular articulatory breakdown may predominate, giving the speech an intoxicated, irregular character that overrides the measured aspect of excess and equal stress patterns.

Also contributing to the prosodic changes is the prolongation of phonemes and normal intervals in speech. The term **scanning speech** often is used in connection with ataxic dysarthria. This term was originated by Charcot[9] to describe the speech of a patient with multiple sclerosis. Charcot described the speech as being very

---

BOX 8-5

Ataxic Dysarthria

- Caused by damage to the cerebellum and/or its pathways (e.g., degenerative diseases, stroke, trauma, tumors, alcohol toxicity, drug toxicity, encephalitis, lung cancer, hypothyroidism)
- Failure to coordinate sensory data with motor performance, hypotonic muscle, and kinetic tremor
- Irregular articulatory breakdown, slow rate, and readily observable prosodic changes. Harshness, excessive loudness, and voice tremor possible.

---

slow, with a pause after each syllable as if the words were being measured or scanned. This seems to be almost equivalent to what Darley et al[11] describe as excess and equal stress. Others have used the term scanning speech to describe a different set of characteristics; therefore the term has not been found useful and is not recommended.

The term **explosive speech** also has been used to describe ataxic production. The Mayo Clinic study noted excess loudness variations with excessive effort in 10 of 30 ataxic speakers.[11] This forceful effort and increase in intensity, especially noted after pauses, give the impression of explosiveness.

Damage to the cerebellum resulting in ataxic dysarthria is summarized in Box 8-5.

Other Mixed Dysarthrias with Diverse Lesions

MULTIPLE SCLEROSIS

Etiology

The etiology of **multiple sclerosis (MS)** has not been discovered, although evidence suggests that a viral agent may initiate demyelination.[40] MS is a complex disease causing demyelination in various tracts of mainly white matter. Figure 8-3 shows a magnetic resonance image of a patient with MS. With MS, the lesions involve the entire central nervous system, but the peripheral nervous system is seldom involved.

Associated Neurologic Characteristics

Early signs are often mild or unnoticed. They may include transient paresthesias of the extremities, transient diplopia or blurring of vision, mild weakness or clumsiness, and mild vertigo. More severe signs of MS include marked difficulty with gait, dysarthria, significant

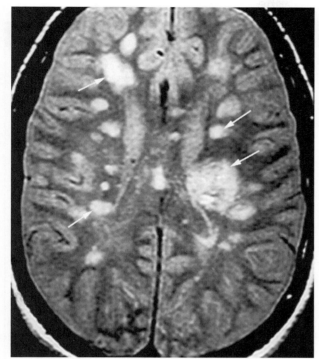

FIGURE **8-3**
Multiple demyelinated plaques *(arrows)* are seen in this magnetic resonance image of a patient with MS. (Reprinted from Nadeau, S. E., Ferguson, T.S., Valenstein, E., Vierck, C.J., Petruska, J.C., Streit, W.J. & Ritz, L.A. [2005]. *Medical neuroscience*. Philadelphia: Saunders.

weakness, visual disturbances, nystagmus, bladder disturbance, and personality change caused by frontal lobe involvement. Van den Burg et al[45] also noted impairments in perceptual motor functioning and mild deficiencies in intelligence, specifically in memory, in a group of 40 mildly disabled MS patients.

MS may take different forms. Some patients show a relapsing-remitting course in which they have attacks (or exacerbations) from which they recover completely, especially in the early stages of the disease. In the later stages these patients may accumulate disabilities with each new attack. Other patients may show a chronic progressive course, which usually involves progressive spinal cord dysfunction. This form may evolve from the relapsing form or be present from the onset of the disease.[46]

Speech Characteristics

Duffy[15] cautions that a mixed spastic-ataxic dysarthria may be the most common type of dysarthria associated with MS but should not be considered the only type found in MS. Because of the variable sites of damage in the disease, many different dysarthrias are possible. Spastic, ataxic, or a mixture of these dysarthrias occurs more frequently.

In a Mayo Clinic study of 168 patients diagnosed with MS, 59% were judged as having normal overall speech performance.[13] Twenty-eight percent showed minimal impairment, and 13% had more severe impairment. Darley et al[13] labeled the dysarthria they most often found as a mixed spastic-ataxic dysarthria.

Phonation
The most frequently encountered deviation was impairment of loudness control. Harsh voice quality also was frequently seen. Breathiness was noted in 37 patients. Pitch control and inappropriate pitch levels were also found.

Articulation
Approximately half of the patients were judged to have defective articulation. Although the cerebellar system is frequently involved in MS, only 9% of patients showed the irregular articulatory breakdowns characteristic of ataxic dysarthria.

Resonance
One quarter of MS patients demonstrated some degree of hypernasality.

Prosody
A characteristic called impaired emphasis ranked high in the speech of these subjects. Impaired features included judgments of rate, appropriateness of phrasing, pitch and loudness variation for emphasis, and increased stress on typically unstressed words and syllables. Only 14% of patients demonstrated the ataxic characteristic called excess and equal stress.

Swallowing
If corticobulbar tracts or lower brainstem nuclei are involved, dysphagia may result in patients with MS. Merson and Rolnick[33] report that dysphagia is common in MS. Because the types, severity, and rate of deterioration in MS are so variable, characterizing common symptoms is difficult. Careful examination is critical. Sensory changes, including abnormal taste, have been reported for some patients.[8]

SHY-DRAGER SYNDROME

Etiology
This syndrome was first described by Shy and Drager in 1960.[44] It usually appears after the fourth decade of life and affects men more often than women by a ratio of 3:2. It is a degenerative disease of the autonomic nervous system that may also affect several components of the central nervous system. Prognosis is usually poor, though progression is slow.

Associated Neurologic Characteristics

With this disease, involvement may include the pyramidal, extrapyramidal, or cerebellar system or some combination of the three systems. Early signs usually involve autonomic nervous system disorders, including bowel and bladder incontinence, impotence, reduction of perspiration, and difficulty maintaining blood pressure when standing (known as orthostatic hypotension). Later symptoms include a gait disturbance, weakness, tremor of the limbs, and dysphagia and dysarthria.

Speech Characteristics

A study by Ludlow and Bassich[30] comparing acoustic and perceptual analyses of Parkinson's disease and **Shy-Drager syndrome** documented the following characteristics for the speech of seven patients diagnosed as having Shy-Drager syndrome.

Phonation

Strained-strangled voice quality and breathiness were noted in the voice quality of these patients. A wet hoarseness was also identified in many cases. The voice was often judged too soft, and mean intensity level was below normal.

Resonance

Hypernasality may occur if the involvement of the pyramidal system produces elements of a spastic dysarthria.

Articulation

Imprecise consonants are a predominant part of this dysarthria. A variable rate was also ranked high in the deficiency ratings.

Prosody

Although patients with Shy-Drager syndrome were shown to have poorer-than-normal ability to change fundamental frequency, their ability was better than that of patients with Parkinson's disease. Acoustic analysis showed, however, that the patients with Shy-Drager use their retained ability to change pitch quite poorly. The results are acoustically perceived as monopitch and reduced stress.

The dysarthrias associated with MS and with Shy-Drager are summarized in Box 8-6.

Apraxias

Apraxia is a disorder of learned movement that is not caused by paralysis, weakness, or incoordination and cannot be accounted for by sensory loss, comprehension deficits, or inattention to commands, according to Geschwind.[18] It has also been defined as a disorder of

---

BOX 8-6

Other Mixed Dysarthrias with Diverse Lesions

Multiple Sclerosis
- Unknown etiology, although studies suggest a viral agent may be responsible
- Early signs mild; severe signs include gait difficulty, dysarthria, visual disturbances, nystagmus, bladder disturbances, and personality changes
- Mixed spastic-ataxic dysarthria most common; frequent problems with volume and pitch control
- Possible dysphagia with corticobulbar or lower brainstem involvement

Shy-Drager Syndrome
- Degenerative disease of the autonomic nervous system
- Early signs: Bowel and bladder incontinence, impotence, reduction of perspiration, difficulty maintaining blood pressure while standing
- Later signs: Gait disturbance, weakness, limb tremor, dysphagia, dysarthria
- Strained-strangled voice quality, wet hoarseness, hypernasality, imprecise consonants, and a poor ability to change pitch all possible

---

motor planning. Apraxia is a high-level motor disturbance of the integration of the motor components necessary to carry out a complex motor act. Review the section on motor planning and the apraxias in Chapter 6 while studying the description of the disorders of motor programming described below.

Apraxias are important to the speech-language pathologist because certain types of apraxia may directly affect the motor programs of the speech muscles. Other forms of apraxia often accompany the aphasias and other cerebral language deficits in the cortical motor association areas and the association pathways of the brain. The major apraxias were defined in Table 6-1 in Chapter 6.

Hugo Liepmann (1863-1925) is credited with elucidating the concept of apraxia around 1900, although John Hughlings Jackson described an apraxic disturbance of the tongue as early as 1866. Liepmann used early disconnection theory to explain apraxia and demonstrated lesion sites to support the variety of apraxias he described.[24] Because this chapter is concerned with clinical speech syndromes, the apraxias that affect movements of other parts of the body are discussed in Chapter 10. Remember, however, that a limb or ideomotor apraxia may also be present in patients with apraxia of speech. Features associated with oral apraxia and apraxia of speech are summarized in Box 8-7.

BOX 8-7

Apraxias

Oral Apraxia

- Inability to perform nonspeech movements with muscles of the larynx, pharynx, tongue, and cheeks
- Paralysis, significant weakness, or incoordination of oral musculature not noted on examination
- Affects voluntary and sometimes imitative movements. Reflexive preserved.

Apraxia of Speech

- Impaired ability to execute speech movements voluntarily in the absence of paralysis, weakness, or incoordination of speech musculature
- May appear independent or in conjunction with oral apraxia
- Most often associated with Broca's aphasia.
- Speech impaired by inconsistent initiation, selection, and sequencing of articulatory movements; no consistent disturbances of phonation, respiration, and resonance; no related neurologic impairments of oral musculature

Oral Apraxia

Speech-language pathologists recognize a nonspeech disorder of the oral muscles called **oral apraxia**, the inability to perform nonspeech movements with the muscles of the larynx, pharynx, tongue, and cheeks, although automatic and sometimes imitative movements of the same muscles may be preserved. This disorder is not the result of paralysis, weakness, or incoordination of the oral musculature, and it may be isolated or coexist with an apraxia of speech. Oral apraxia is usually called buccofacial apraxia by neurologists.

Oral praxic disturbance must be differentiated from disorders of the motor pathways involved in upper motor neuron and lower motor neuron systems. A careful cranial nerve examination usually indicates whether the disturbance is on the higher level of motor planning of praxis as opposed to being a lower level motor deficit associated with either supranuclear lesions or cranial nerve lesions. Motor involvement generally affects both voluntary and reflexive oral acts in lower level motor deficits of the central and peripheral nervous systems. Voluntary oral motor acts are limited by paralysis, weakness, and incoordination, and the more reflexive acts of mastication and deglutition are affected as well. Supranuclear lesions are associated with typical tongue deviation, hypertonic oral muscles, palatal paresis, hyperactive gag reflex, and lower facial paresis. Lower motor neuron lesions are associated with tongue deviation and atrophy, hypotonic oral muscles, palatal paresis, and a hyporeflexive gag reflex. Facial paresis is hypotonic. Extrapyramidal lesions produce involuntary movements of oral muscles, and ataxic movements of oral muscles are found in cerebellar disorders.

Oral apraxia testing is completed on a spontaneous level to verbal command and on an imitative level. Commands requiring oral-facial movements such as "lick your lips" or "clear your throat" may be used. Failure to perform appropriately on a number of similar commands suggests a diagnosis of oral apraxia in brain-injured adults. Love and Webb[29] used a 20-item informal test for assessing oral apraxia. Published tests of apraxia of speech usually include tasks for assessing nonverbal oral apraxia.

Apraxia of Speech

Apraxia of speech is an impaired ability to execute voluntarily the appropriate movements for articulation of speech in the absence of paralysis, weakness, or incoordination of the speech musculature. In 1900 Liepmann[24] discussed a form of apraxia that could be localized to the speech muscles; some 40 years earlier, Broca described elements of this disorder as part of aphemia. **Aphemia**, the defect in speech and language that Broca believed resulted from damage to the third left frontal convolution of the brain, has become known as Broca's aphasia. The disorder is marked by effortful groping for articulatory movements produced in an apparently trial-and-error manner. Articulation on repeated utterances is inconsistent. Speech is dysprosodic, often characterized by great difficulty in initiating utterances. A developmental form of verbal apraxia is known as **childhood apraxia of speech** (see Chapter 9). The current discussion concerns acquired apraxia of speech in adults.

Oral apraxia and speech apraxia may appear independently or coexist. Oral apraxia may be the basis of a speech apraxia. Speech apraxia may appear in a pure form but is most often accompanied by a language disorder, as seen in classic Broca's aphasia. Some neurologists and speech-language pathologists deny that what is called apraxia of speech is a pure disorder of praxis. They view the apraxic elements in Broca's aphasia as more of a linguistic problem than a motor problem. Evidence is not yet available to resolve the issue.

Pure apraxia of speech traditionally has been associated with the left frontal lobe, and the lesion is presumed to be localized specifically to Broca's area or deep to it. Apraxia of speech as an element of a classic Broca's aphasia with linguistic disorder implies a lesion extending beyond Broca's area into regions other than the frontal lobe. The issue of lesion site is not yet settled because sites beyond Broca's area have also been suggested as contributing to speech apraxic symptoms.

If the speech-language pathologist is presented with a case that appears to be a pure speech apraxia, it must be differentiated from dysarthria. In speech apraxia, articulation is impaired by inconsistent initiation, selection, and sequencing of articulatory movements; in dysarthria, articulatory movements are more consistent, with distortion errors predominating. Speech apraxias do not display consistent disturbances of phonation, respiration, and resonance, whereas persons with dysarthrias almost always display consistent phonatory, resonance, and respiratory disorders. With dysarthria there is impairment of nonspeech musculature, including paralysis, weakness, involuntary movement, and/or ataxia. Persons affected by apraxia of speech do not have these neurologic impairments of the oral musculature or if they are present, the apraxia is not the cause of these deficits.

Synopsis of Clinical Information and Applications for the Speech-Language Pathologist

- Of the acquired neurogenic communication disorders seen in large speech-language pathology practices, the majority are likely to be motor speech disorders.
- Dysarthria and apraxia of speech are the two primary classifications of motor speech disorders.
- Dysarthria implies true organically based paralysis, weakness, or incoordination of the oral musculature that results in distortion of speech and/or difficulty with feeding or swallowing.
- Apraxia of speech is a sensorimotor disorder of motor programming of the speech musculature for the production of speech. It is not caused by weakness, paralysis or incoordination of the oral musculature.
- The evaluation of a patient with suspected motor speech disorder should include assessment of hearing and language (to rule out other causes of the communication problem or to define accompanying problems), an oral-motor examination, speech-production tasks, and a screening or full assessment of feeding and swallowing.
- The Mayo Clinic classification system categorized the dysarthrias into six major classes: spastic, flaccid, hypokinetic, hyperkinetic, ataxic, and mixed. Unilateral upper motor neuron dysarthria has been added more recently as a separate type. Each of these dysarthrias is associated with disorders or diseases affecting certain parts of the motor system. Each has associated classic perceptual features that the student should learn.
- Apraxia of speech also is associated with damage to the motor speech planning areas of the motor cortex and also has certain perceptual features that should be learned.
- Other diseases and disorders produce dysarthrias but were not included in the discussion of the more common disorders. These can be found in Table 8-1.

TABLE 8-1

Other Neurologic Diseases Associated with Dysarthria

NAME	ETIOLOGY	SPEECH SYMPTOMS
Bell's palsy	Inflammation or lesion of cranial nerve VII	Slurring caused by unilateral weakness of labial muscles
Polyneuritis	Follows infections or may be caused by diabetes or alcohol abuse	Flaccid dysarthria
Hemiballismus	Lesions of subthalamic nucleus	Hyperkinetic dysarthria
Palatopharyngolaryngeal myoclonus	Brainstem lesions producing rhythmic myoclonic movements of the palate, pharynx, and/or larynx	Hyperkinetic dysarthria, which is sometimes only noted on vowel prolongation
Gilles de la Tourette's syndrome	No known etiology	Hyperkinetic dysarthria with spontaneous, uncontrolled vocalizations such as barking, grunting, throat clearing, snorting; echolalia and coprolalia (obscene language without provocation) may be present
Olivopontocerebellar atrophy	Degeneration of olivary, pontine, and cerebellar nuclei	Mixed dysarthria of hypokinetic, spastic, and ataxic types
Progressive supranuclear palsy	Neuronal atrophy in brainstem and cerebellar structures	Mixed dysarthria, which may include hypokinetic, spastic, and ataxic types

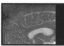

CASE**STUDY**

A 48-year-old accountant reported excess stress in his life. He often made presentations to various companies looking to hire his accounting firm. For the past several months, he reported to his physician that he had been having difficulty speaking and swallowing. He described his speech as "sounding like I am speaking through my nose." He also admitted to noticing mild tremors of his eyebrows and mouth. An oral peripheral mechanism examination revealed bilateral facial weakness, reduced tongue strength, and a hyperactive gag reflex, which was a new finding for him. After an extensive diagnostic workup, the physician diagnosed this patient with ALS.

QUESTIONS FOR CONSIDERATION:
1. What type of dysarthria is usually present for patients with ALS?
2. What parts of the motor system are impaired with this type of dysarthria?
3. What are some of the clinical signs of this type of dysarthria?

REFERENCES

1. Alberts, M. J., Horner, J., Gray, I., & Brazer, S. R. (1992). Aspiration after stroke: Lesion analysis by brain MRI. *Dysphagia, 7*, 170-173.

2. Aronson, A. E. (1985). *Clinical voice disorders* (2nd ed.). New York: Thieme-Stratton.

3. Aronson, A. E., & Hartman, D. E. (1981). Adductor spastic dysphonia as a sign of essential (voice) tremor. *Journal of Speech and Hearing Disorders, 46*, 52-58.

4. Blitzer, A., Lovelace, R. E., Brin, M. F., Fahn, S., & Fink, M. E. (1985). Electromyographic findings in focal laryngeal dystonia (spastic dysphonia). *Annals of Otology, Rhinology and Laryngology, 94*, 592-594.

5. Bosma, J., Geoffrey, V., Thach, B., Weiffenbach, J., Kavanagh, I., & Orr, W. (1982). A pattern of medication induced persistent bulbar and cervical dystonia. *International Journal of Orofacial Myology, 8*, 5-19.

6. Brin, M. F., Blitzer, A., Fahn, S., Gould, W., & Lovelace, R. E. (1989). Adductor laryngeal dystonia (spastic dysphonia): Treatment with local injections of botulinum toxin (Botox). *Movement Disorders, 4*, 287-296.

7. Brown, R. G., & Marsden, C. D. (1984). How common is dementia in Parkinson's disease? *Lancet*, ii, 1261-1265.

8. Bucholz, D., & Robbins, J. (1997). Neurologic diseases affecting oropharyngeal swallowing. In Perlman, A., & Schulze-Delrieu, K. (Eds.), *Deglutition and its disorders: Anatomy, physiology, clinical diagnosis, and management.* San Diego: Singular Publishing Group, Inc.

9. Charcot, J. M. (1877). *Lectures on the diseases of the nervous system.* Vol. 1. London: The New Sydenham Society.

10. Cherney, L. R. (1994). *Clinical management of dysphagia in adults and children.* Gaithersburg, MD: Aspen Publishers.

11. Darley, F., Aronson, A., & Brown, J. (1969a). Differential diagnostic patterns of dysarthria. *Journal of Speech and Hearing Research, 12*, 246-269.

12. Darley, F., Aronson, A., & Brown, J. (1969b). Clusters of deviant speech dimensions in the dysarthrias. *Journal of Speech and Hearing Research, 12*, 462-496.

13. Darley, E, Aronson, A., & Brown, J. (1975). Motor speech disorders. Philadelphia: W. B. Saunders.

14. Dedo, H. H. (1976). Recurrent laryngeal nerve surgery for spastic dysphonia. *Annals of Otology, Rhinology and Laryngology, 85*, 451-459.

15. Duffy, J. R. (2005). *Motor speech disorders: Substrates, differential diagnosis, and management.* (2nd ed.). St. Louis: Mosby.

16. Duffy, J. R., & Folger, W. N. (1986). *Dysarthria in unilateral nervous system lesions.* Presented at the annual convention of the American Speech-Language-Hearing Association, Detroit, MI.

17. Evatt, M. L., Reus, C. M., Brazer, S. R., Massey, E. W., & Horner, J. (1993). Dysphagia following unilateral ischemic stroke. *Neurology, 43* (supplement), A159 (Abstract).

18. Geschwind, N. (1975). The apraxias: Neural mechanisms of disorders of learned movements. *American Scientist, 63*, 188-195.

19. Hartman, D. E., & Abbs, J. H. (1992). Dysarthria associated with focal unilateral upper motor neuron lesions. *European Journal of Disorders of Communication, 27*, 187.

20. Horner, J., Massey, E. W., & Brazer, S. R. (1993). Aspiration in bilateral stroke patients: A validation study. *Neurology, 43*, 430-433.

21. Kent, R., & Netsell, R. (1978). Articulatory abnormalities in athetoid cerebral palsy. *Journal of Speech and Hearing Disorders, 43*, 353-374.

22. Kirshner, H. S. (2002). *Behavioral neurology: Practical science of mind and brain,* (2nd ed.). Boston: Butterworth-Heinemann.

23. Leopold, N. A., & Kagel, M. C. (1985). Dysphagia in Huntington's disease. *Archives of Neurology, 42*, 57-60.

24. Liepmann, H. (1900). Daskrankheitshid Apraxia (motorishen). *Asymbolie Mtschr Psychiat, 8*, 15, 44, 102-132, 182-197.

25. Logemann, J. A. (1983). *Evaluation and treatment of swallowing disorders.* San Diego: College Hill Press.

26. Logemann, J. A. (1988). Dysphagia in movement disorders. In Janokovic, J., & Tolosa, E. (Eds.), *Advances in neurology.* Vol. 49. Facial dyskinesias. New York: Raven Press.

27. Logemann, J. A., & Fisher, H. B. (1981). Vocal tract control in Parkinson's disease: Phonetic feature analysis of misarticulations. *Journal of Speech and Hearing Disorders, 46*, 348-352.

28. Logemann, J. A., Fisher, H. B., Boshes, B., & Blonsky, E. R. (1978). Frequency and co-occurrence of vocal tract dysfunction in the speech of a large sample of Parkinson patients. *Journal of Speech and Hearing Disorders, 43*, 47-57.

29. Love, R. R., & Webb, W. G. (1977). The efficacy of cueing techniques in Broca's aphasia. *Journal of Speech and Hearing Disorders, 42*, 170-178.

30. Ludlow, C., & Bassich, C. J. (1983). The results of acoustic and perceptual assessment of two types of dysarthria. In Berry, W. R. (Ed.), *Clinical dysarthria*. San Diego: College Hill Press.

31. Ludlow, C. L., Naunton, R. F., & Bassich, C. J. (1984). Procedures for the selection of spastic dysphonia patients for recurrent laryngeal nerve section. *Otolaryngology Head and Neck Surgery, 92*, 24-31.

32. Ludlow, C. L., Naunton, R. F. Fulita, M., & Sedory, S. E. (1990). Spasmodic dysphonia: Botulinum toxin injection after recurrent nerve surgery. *Otolaryngology Head and Neck Surgery, 102*, 122-131.

33. Merson, R. M., & Rolnick, M. I. (1998). Speech-language pathology and dysphagia in multiple sclerosis. *Physical Medicine & Rehabilitation Clinics of North America, 9*, 631-641.

34. Murray, L. L., & Stout, J. C. (1999). Discourse comprehension in Huntington's and Parkinson's diseases. *American Journal of Speech-Language Pathology, 8*, 137-148.

35. Netsell, R., Daniel, G., & Celesia, G. G. (1975). Acceleration and weakness in parkinsonian dysarthria. *Journal of Speech and Hearing Disorders, 40*, 467-480.

36. Platt, L. J., Andrews, G., & Howie, P. M. (1980). Dysarthria of adult cerebral palsy: II. Phonemic analysis of articulation errors. *Journal of Speech and Hearing Disorders, 23*, 41-55.

37. Ramig, L. O., & Dromey, C. (1996). Aerodynamic mechanisms underlying treatment-related changes in vocal intensity in patients with Parkinson's disease. *Journal of Speech and Hearing Research, 30*, 798-807.

38. Robbins, J. (1989). *Swallowing and brain imagery in asymptomatic normals and stroke patients*. Presented at Swallowing and Swallowing Disorders: From Clinic to Laboratory, Northwestern University, Evanston, IL.

39. Robbins, J., Webb, W. G., & Kirshner, H. S. (1984). *Effects of Sinemet on speech and swallowing in parkinsonism*. Presented at American Speech-Language-Hearing Association Convention, San Francisco, CA.

40. Rodriguez, M. (1989). Multiple sclerosis: Basic concepts and hypothesis. *Mayo Clinic Proceedings, 64*, 570.

41. Rosenfield, D. B. (1988). Spasmodic dysphonia. In Jankovic, J., & Tolosa, E. (Eds.), *Advances in neurology*. Vol. *49. Facial dyskinesias*. New York: Raven Press.

42. Rosenfield, D. B., Miller, R. H. Jankovic, J., & Nudelman, H. (1984). Persistence of spasmodic dysphonia symptoms following recurrent laryngeal nerve surgery: An electrodiagnostic evaluation. *Neurology, 34* (supplement 1), 291 (Abstract).

43. Schultz, G. M., & Grant, M. K. (2000). Effects of speech therapy and pharmacologic and surgical treatments on voice and speech in Parkinson's disease: A review of the literature. *Journal of Communication Disorders, 33*, 59-88.

44. Shy, G., & Drager, G. (1960). A neurological syndrome associated with orthostatic hypotension: A clinical pathologic study. *Archives of Neurology, 2*, 511-527.

45. van den Burg, W., van Zomeren, A. H., Minderhoud, J. M., Prange, A. J. A., & Meifer, N. S. A. (1987). Cognitive impairment in patients with MS and mild physical disability. *Archives of Neurology, 44*, 494-501.

46. Weiner, H. L., & Levitt, L. P. (1994). *House officer series: Neurology* (5th ed.). Baltimore: Williams & Wilkins.

47. Wilson, F. B., Oldring, D. I., & Mueller, K. (1980). Recurrent laryngeal dissection: A case report involving return of spastic dysphonia after initial surgery. *Journal of Speech and Hearing Disorders, 45*, 112-118.

48. Zeigler, W., & von Cramer, D. (1986). Spastic dysarthria after acquired brain injury: An acoustic study. *British Journal of Communication Disorders, 21*, 173-187.

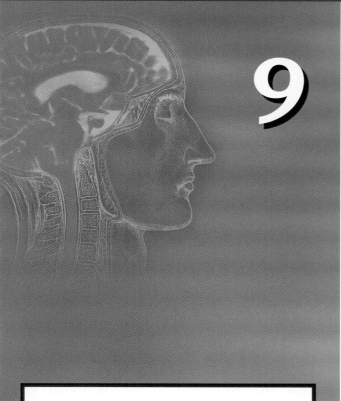

9

Pediatric Clinical Speech Syndromes: The Developing Brain

An examination of infant behavior is an examination of the central nervous system.

—Arnold Gesell and Catherine S. Amatruda,
Developmental Diagnosis, 1947

KEY**TERMS**

anoxia
asymmetric tonic neck
  reflex (ATNR)
ataxic cerebral palsy
athetoid cerebral
  palsy
bite reflex
cerebral palsy
congenital childhood
  suprabulbar palsy
deglutition
developmental
  anarthria
developmental
  apraxia of speech
developmental
  dysarthria
developmental motor
  speech disorders
Duchenne dystrophy
fluency disorders
fluent
gag reflex
Galant reflex
mastication

modified feeding
Moro reflex
monoplegia
muscular dystrophy
neurolinguistics
obligatory
positive support
  reflex
prematurity
prone
pseudohypertrophy
rooting reflex
segmental rolling
  reflex
spastic cerebral palsy
suckling reflex
supine
swallowing reflex
symmetric tonic neck
  reflex
tongue reflex
tonic labyrinthine
  reflex (TLR)
topologic involvement
triplegia

CHAPTER**OUTLINE**

Developmental Motor Speech Disorders
  Cerebral Palsy
    Spastic cerebral palsy
      Spastic hemiplegia
      Spastic paraplegia and diplegia
      Spastic quadriplegia
    Athetoid cerebral palsy
    Ataxic cerebral palsy
  Childhood Suprabulbar Paresis
  Muscular Dystrophy
**Diagnosis of Neurologic Disorder with
  Primitive Reflex**
  Asymmetric Tonic Neck Reflex
  Symmetric Tonic Neck Reflex
  Positive Support Reflex
  Tonic Labyrinthine Reflex
  Segmental Rolling Reflex
  Galant Reflex
  Moro Reflex
Oral and Pharyngeal Reflexes
  Rooting Reflexes
  Suckling Reflex
  Swallowing Reflex
  Tongue Reflex
  Bite Reflex
  Gag Reflex

Developmental Motor Speech Disorders

Early cerebral injury to speech mechanisms of the developing brain result in conditions classified as **developmental motor speech disorders**. Included in a classification of the motor speech disorders are the developmental dysarthrias, developmental anarthrias, and developmental apraxias of speech. **Developmental dysarthria** is a speech disorder resulting from damage to the immature nervous system; it is characterized by weakness, paralysis, and/or incoordination of the speech musculature. **Developmental anarthria** refers to a complete lack of speech as a result of profound paralysis, weakness, and/or incoordination of the speech musculature. The diagnosis usually implies that useful speech will not develop because of the severity of the oral motor involvement. **Developmental apraxia of speech** is an impaired ability to execute the appropriate movements of speech voluntarily in the absence of paralysis, weakness, and incoordination of the speech muscles.

The term childhood dysarthria implies a neurologic or neurogenic speech deficit caused by a dysfunction of the motor control centers of the developing central and/or peripheral nervous systems. Disturbances are in the areas of strength, speed, steadiness, coordination, precision, tone, and range of motion or movement in the speech muscles. Apraxia is considered a motor planning disorder of speech, whereas dysarthria is associated with a partial disturbance of the speech mechanism involving motor movements. Anarthria usually is associated with a total lack of speech as a result of severe to profound motor disturbances.[6]

Certain types of developmental dysarthria have been well studied; other types have received less attention in the speech pathology literature. The developmental dysarthrias found in the various forms of cerebral palsy, for instance, have been extensively studied for many years, whereas research on the dysarthrias of childhood muscular dystrophy is much less common. The speech signs commonly observed in the developmental dysarthrias are seen in Table 9-1.

Table 9-2 shows the major differences between dysarthria and apraxia from the point of muscle movements and range of motion as seen in many childhood motor disturbances such as cerebral palsy.

TABLE 9-1
Major Developmental Motor Speech Disorders

DISORDER	SPEECH SIGNS
Developmental apraxia of speech	Disorder in selection and sequencing of articulatory movements, with oral apraxia sometimes present; comprehension intact; expression poor; occasional nonfocal neurologic signs
Developmental Dysarthrias of Cerebral Palsy	
Spastic dysarthria	Bilateral corticobulbar involvement; dysphagia; articulation disorder; hypernasality; slowed rate; and loudness, pitch, and vocal quality disturbances; slow, stiff, and abrupt movements; increased muscle tone; muscle rigidity
Dyskinetic dysarthria	Athetosis (usually); dysphagia; hypernasality; articulation disorders; prevocalizations; loudness, pitch, and vocal quality disturbances; involuntary and often uncontrolled movements; often slow and writhing movements
Ataxic dysarthria	Articulation and prosodic disorders; unequal stress, loudness, and pitch; speech has an explosive, scanning quality
Mixed dysarthria	Often a combination of spastic and dyskinetic dysarthrias

TABLE 9-2
Differences between Apraxia and Dysarthria

APRAXIA	DYSARTHRIA
Sound substitutions not on the target sound	Sound distortions usually related to the target sound
Inconsistent errors; motor planning	Inconsistent speech sound substitutions from coordination problems
Often vocal or nonvocal groping behaviors	Groping for sound production precision is not noted verbally or nonverbally
Motor planning and execution difficulties	Motor disturbances causing distortions and not planning difficulties

CEREBRAL PALSY

Developmental dysarthria is most commonly seen in children diagnosed as having cerebral palsy. **Cerebral palsy** is a neurologic condition caused by injury to the immature brain; it is characterized by a nonprogressive disturbance of the motor system. Many associated problems often are seen, such as mental retardation, hearing and visual impairments, and perceptual problems produced by the infantile cerebral injury. Cerebral palsy is considered a major developmental disability.

Cerebral palsy has been variously classified, but most experts currently accept three major categories of clinical motor disorders: spasticity, dyskinesia, and ataxia. By far the most common type of dyskinesia is athetosis (see Chapter 6).

Table 9-3 presents a classification of the forms of cerebral palsy. As in adult disorders, spasticity implies a lesion in the pyramidal system, dyskinesia implies a

TABLE 9-3
Classification of Cerebral Palsy

LESION AREA	FUNCTION	SUBDIVISIONS	CLINICAL SIGNS	LIMB INVOLVEMENT
Pyramidal tract	Skilled movements of limbs and digits Innervation of motor neurons for flexor movements of the limbs	Corticospinal tract (see Fig. 9-1) Corticobulbar tract (see Fig. 9-1).	Interrupts motor information of the brainstem and spinal cord Weakness or paralysis of various muscles Upper motor neuron lesions	Paraplegia (lower extremities versus upper extremities), diplegia (lower extremities more than upper extremities) Quadriplegia (lower and upper extremities); hemiparesis (left or right side of body) or monoplegia (only one lower extremity)
Extrapyramidal tract or basal ganglia	Refer to Table 2-1 for the basal ganglia system Related to motor speech functioning Automatic execution of learned motor movements	Preferred term is basal ganglia; related pathways and subcortical nuclei	Either akinesia or lack of movements or dyskinesia or involuntary excessive movements; breathiness, roughness, hoarseness, tremor; exaggerated jaw movements; lip retrusion	Dyskinetic dysarthria (athetosis); choreoathetosis; dystonia; tremor, rigidity; upper extremity, lower extremity, neck, and trunk involvement
Cerebellum	Coordination of movements of the upper and lower extremities as well as at all stages of speech production; sensory input from larynx and articulators and speech processing	Inferior peduncle Middle peduncle Superior peduncle	Ataxia Sometimes diplegia	Upper extremities Lower extremities Trunk

lesion in the extrapyramidal system, and ataxia denotes a lesion in the cerebellar system. However, syndromes are often not as clear cut in the child as they are in the adult. Many children with cerebral palsy show a mixed picture. For instance, a child whose clinical picture is primarily athetoid, with typical slow, writhing movements of the limbs, grimaces of the face, and involuntary movements of the tongue and muscles of respiration, may also display hypertonic muscles and the upturning toes of the classic Babinski sign. The structural closeness of the pathways of the pyramidal and extrapyramidal tracts in the relatively small infant brain no doubt produces such mixed clinical pictures (Fig. 9-1).

Children with cerebral palsy may also be classified according to **topologic involvement**. Common topologic pictures are hemiplegia, diplegia, and quadriplegia (see Table 9-3). **Monoplegia**, **triplegia**, and paraplegia occasionally are seen. Children may also be classified by etiology. Common causes are **prematurity**, **anoxia**, kernicterus, birth trauma, and infection. Approximately 1 to 2 out of every 1000 schoolchildren have some form of cerebral palsy. Of the three major types, spasticity is the

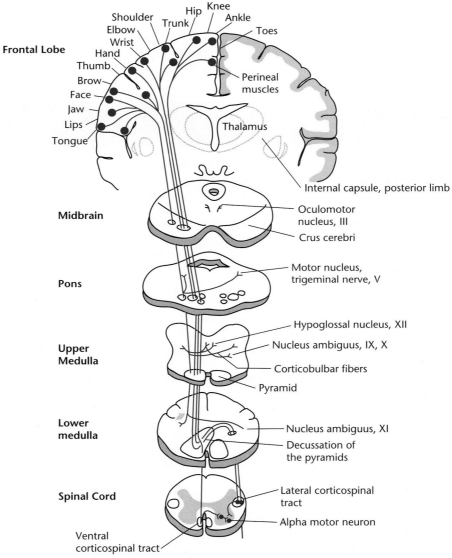

FIGURE **9-1**
Corticospinal and corticobulbar tracts of the central nervous system (pyramidal system). (Reprinted from Love, R. J. [1999]. *Childhood motor speech disability* [2nd ed.]. Boston: Allyn and Bacon.)

most prevalent, athetosis is next, and ataxia is the least common. Box 9-1 displays a summation of the major causes of cerebral palsy in children.

Developmental dysarthria is a major problem in the population with cerebral palsy, with 75% to 85% of the children showing obvious speech problems. Dysarthria may be complicated in some children by mental retardation, hearing loss, and perceptual disorders. Despite complicating factors, the two major dysarthrias—spastic dysarthria and dyskinetic dysarthria of athetosis—in cerebral palsy can be differentiated. Spasticity and athetosis cannot be identified by articulatory errors alone; however, when vocal and prosodic features are incorporated into perceptual judgments of speech, the two clinical types become distinct, just as spastic and hyperkinetic types are distinct among adult dysarthrias.[9,18]

Spastic Cerebral Palsy

Spastic cerebral palsy is characterized by hypertonic reflexes. With this type of reflex, when a muscle contracts the opposing muscle stretches abnormally,

---

BOX 9-1

Causes of Cerebral Palsy

Prenatal brain damage may result from:
- Impaired migration of new brain cells with the following risk factors:
  - Maternal infection, e.g., cytomegalovirus (CMV), HIV, meningitis, toxoplasmosis, rubella
  - Toxins
  - Drugs
  - Radiation exposure
- Prematurity and low birth weight with the following risk factors:
  - Low grade infection of mother's urinary-genital tract
  - Alcohol and drug abuse, cigarette smoking
  - Poor maternal nutrition
  - Multiple fetuses
- Trauma to mother

Perinatal brain damage may result from:
- Increased pressure on brain during delivery
- Impaired circulation to the fetal brain
- Poor respiration
- Low birth weight

Postnatal brain damage may result from:
- Physical trauma
- Infection
- Respiratory distress
- Cerebrovascular disorders

---

thus excessively increasing muscle tone.[13] This muscle group becomes rigid; movement therefore becomes extremely difficult. According to Owens et al,[13] these muscle movements can be described as laborious, jerky, and unusually slow. These children often exhibit infantile patterns of the rooting reflex that involve the tongue, lips, and mandible. The movement is toward the site of the stimulation. These reflexes usually become absent after the child reaches the age of 2 to 4 months.

Spastic Hemiplegia

According to Love,[6] children born with upper and lower extremity involvement on one side (hemi) exhibit signs of clasp-knife spastic paresis. Spastic hemiplegia usually is caused by damage to the corticospinal tract, with the possibility of corticobulbar involvement. Cranial nerve XII, the hypoglossal nerve, usually is also involved, with the tongue showing contralateral deviation from the affected side upon protrusion. Both dysarthric speech and dysphagia typically resolve after a brief period.

Phonologic development often is delayed in these children and is accompanied by a language delay and cognitive disturbances. Love[6] indicated that children with right hemiplegia display a shift of language centers from the left to the right hemisphere. Therefore visual spatial development, usually from the right hemisphere, is often expected to be compromised.

Spastic Paraplegia and Diplegia

Spastic paraplegia, which affects the lower extremities without involvement of the upper extremities, is uncommon in children. When it does occur, speech production usually is within normal limits without significant cognitive impairments.

Spastic diplegia usually involves all four extremities but the lower extremities display more involvement than the upper extremities, differentiating it from quadriplegia. Children with diplegia often display mild dysarthria with articulatory involvement only, but others with more severe dysarthric signs often display respiratory, laryngeal, palatal, and pharyngeal impairments in addition to articulation problems. Some dysphagia and drooling may also be present. Not all children with this diagnosis have cognitive difficulties.

Love[6] stated that flexion and adduction of the hips in diplegia also include "scissoring or crossing of the legs during walking, producing a 'scissors gait,' a widely known clinical sign of child spasticity" (p. 45). These children sometimes also display toe walking because of hamstring and Achilles tendon involvement.

Spastic Quadriplegia

Spastic quadriplegia usually displays equal involvement of both upper and lower extremities. In this condition both the corticospinal and corticobulbar tracts are affected. These children also display major problems with respiration, articulation, and laryngeal movements as well as compromised palatal and pharyngeal musculature. Language impairment is noticeable, as are cognitive difficulties and general speech and language delays. This type of spastic cerebral palsy usually has the highest incidence of mental retardation or developmental delay.

Table 9-4 summarizes the speech performance parameters found in children with spastic and athetoid cerebral palsy.

Athetoid Cerebral Palsy

The most common of the dyskinetic syndromes of cerebral palsy is **athetoid cerebral palsy**. It is much less common than spastic cerebral palsy. Love[6] reported that only approximately 5% of the total cerebral palsy population of children would be considered "pure" athetoid, whereas 10% would be diagnosed as dystonic athetosis.

Slower motor development and hypotonia are the first signs of motor difficulties in athetoid children. Sitting balance is either delayed or not developed at all. One of the most prevalent signs is the absence of the Moro and the tonic neck reflexes. Figures 9-2, 9-3, and 9-4 illustrate these reflexes, which are discussed later in this chapter.

In certain cases hypertonic athetosis progresses to a mixed type, usually spastic athetoid. In general, all four limbs are involved; a different presentation is rare. Speech problems usually are present along with swallowing difficulties and drooling. Severely affected motor movements of the upper and lower extremities usually correlate to the severity of the speech disorder present (see Table 9-4).

TABLE 9-4

Speech Performance in Spastic and Athetoid Cerebral Palsy

RESPIRATION	PHONATION	RESONANCE	ARTICULATION	PROSODY
Rapid rate	Poor pitch control	Hypernasality	Spastic slightly superior to athetoid	Reduced variations in intensity, frequency, and timing
Abdominal breathing	Poor loudness control	Nasal emission	Articulation development systematic but delayed	Voice commonly monotone through utterance
Reverse or paradoxic breathing in athetoid cerebral palsy	Monotone	Poor intraoral breath pressure	Motor complex sounds more difficult	Slowed rate
Limited upper thorax expansion	Breathiness	Varying types of velopharyngeal inadequacy	Athetoid cerebral palsy incorporates wide range of movement of articulators	No formal studies of prosody
Flared lower ribs	Poor adduction/ abduction of vocal folds	Inconsistency of velopharyngeal closure	Also uses jaw as major articulator	
Poor tidal air control	Varying tension of vocal folds	Incoordination of velar musculature	Adults show oral motion rates 50% slower than normal	
Increased subglottal pressure	Generalized laryngeal immobility Poor timing of voice and respiration		Athetoid cerebral palsy shows some out-of-class substitution; spastic cerebral palsy does not	

Reprinted from Love, R. G. (1999). *Childhood motor speech disability* (2nd ed.). Boston: Allyn and Bacon.

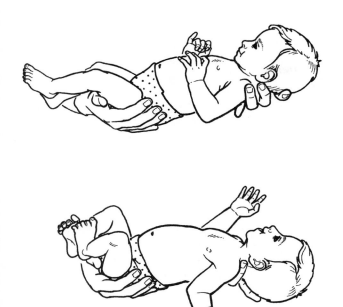

FIGURE **9-2**
The Moro reflex is elicited by dropping the head. The reflex is pathologic in the presence of a persistent symmetric abduction and upward movement of the arms with fingers splayed, followed by flexion of the arms in clasp manner as the child's back arches.

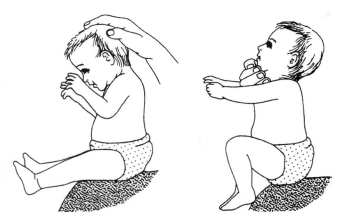

FIGURE **9-3**
Symmetric tonic reflex. The symmetric tonic neck reflex is elicited by passively extending and flexing the neck five times. The reflex is pathologic in the presence of obligatory arm extension or leg flexion with neck extension for more than 60 seconds. (Modified from Capute, A.J., Accardo, P.I., Vining, E.P.G., & Rubenstein, J.E. [1978]. *Primitive reflex profile*. Baltimore: University Park Press.)

Ataxic Cerebral Palsy

Love[6] reported that **ataxic cerebral palsy** is the most uncommon of the palsy syndromes. Dyssynergia that translates into incoordination of the upper and lower extremities typically is present. The most identifying sign is, as Fenichel[3] stated, a staggering, somewhat lurching, wide gait pattern. Disturbed balance usually is another sign of ataxic cerebral palsy. The child with ataxic cerebral palsy is often looked on as clumsy and awkward. Muscles are hypotonic and gait does not seem to have directional control. Ataxic cerebral palsy usually involves damage to the cerebellum. The cerebellum controls and monitors balance and proprioceptive information from muscles, including rate of movement, force of movement, and directional control of movement. Ataxia feedback from the cerebellar peduncles is lacking, thereby causing an incoordination, hence a difficulty in walking.

Table 9-5 summarizes the major differences among spastic, athetoid, and ataxic cerebral palsy, including characteristics and areas of damage to the brain.

CHILDHOOD SUPRABULBAR PARESIS

An isolated paresis or weakness of the oral musculature is sometimes seen in children without major motor signs in the trunk or extremities. This condition results in a form of developmental dysarthria and associated problems. Described by the neurologist Worster-Drought,[19] this condition usually affects the corticobulbar fibers that innervate cranial nerves X (vagus) and XII (hypoglossus). The etiology has been attributed to agenesis or hypogenesis of the corticobulbar fibers, but this theory has not been verified. The muscles of the lips, pharynx, palate, and tongue are involved to varying degrees. The dysarthria is marked by misarticulations and hypernasality. The individual may have a history of dysphagia and occasional laryngeal involvement and drooling.

This condition is called **congenital childhood suprabulbar palsy** because involvement generally is confined to the muscles innervated by the corticobulbar fibers. Paresis of the trunk and limbs is not present as in the child with obvious cerebral palsy. The condition is brought to the attention of the speech-language pathologist or neurologist because of an isolated dysphagia or dysarthria. Muscles of the oral mechanism are involved, but no other obvious neurologic signs are present in the motor system. Box 9-2 lists neurologic signs seen in the dysarthric syndromes of congenital and acquired suprabulbar paresis of childhood.

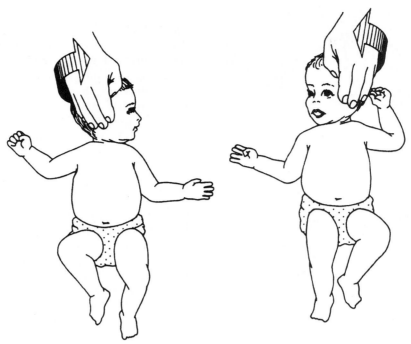

FIGURE **9-4**
The asymmetrical tonic neck reflex (ATNR) is elicited by turning the head to each side for 5 seconds. This movement is repeated five times to each side. The reflex is pathologic in the presence of obligatory extension and flexion of limbs for more than 60 seconds. (Modified from Capute, A.J., Accardo, P.I., Vining, E.P.G., & Rubenstein, J.E. [1978]. *Primitive reflex profile.* Baltimore: University Park Press.)

MUSCULAR DYSTROPHY

Next to cerebral palsy, **muscular dystrophy** is the childhood neurologic disorder most likely to present a developmental dysarthria. The most common type of muscular dystrophy is the pseudohypertrophic type, also called Duchenne dystrophy. **Duchenne dystrophy** is associated with a sex-linked recessive gene, occurs primarily in males, and usually is manifest by the third year of life. The disorder is marked by a characteristic progression of muscle weakness starting in the pelvis and trunk and eventually involving all the striated muscles, including those of the speech mechanism. The visceral muscles usually are spared. Enlargement of the calf muscles and occasionally other muscle groups accounts for the term **pseudohypertrophic**. Infiltration of fat and connective tissue produces the pseudohypertrophic effect.

In the later stages of the disease a flaccid dysarthria may appear, marked by articulation disorder and voice quality disturbances. Often the articulation disorder is mild, with only one or two phonemes in error. Dystrophic patients show reduced oral breath pressure and vocal intensity. They do not sustain phonation as

well as healthy children do, and they show serious involvement of the muscles of speech. Rate of tongue movement and strength of the tongue are poor. Retracting and pursing the lips as well as pointing and narrowing the tongue are noticeably disordered actions, and phonemes requiring tongue and lip elevation often are in error. A broadening and flattening of the tongue is sometimes seen in advanced cases. Respiratory and laryngeal muscles are also weakened, affecting respiratory and phonatory performance. Despite weakness, labial phonemes generally are produced more accurately than are tongue-tip consonants. Box 9-3 presents the speech and physical signs in the developmental dysarthria of pseudohypertrophic muscular dystrophy. Several uncommon childhood dysarthrias associated with lower motor neuron disorders are surveyed by Love.[6]

The speech-language pathologist, especially those in public schools or centers primarily working with a young child population, must understand the primitive reflex profile to discern whether dysarthria, primitive reflexes, or other speech, language, or cognitive problems exist in a child. An understanding of the Moro reflex and the symmetric and asymmetric reflexes

TABLE 9-5

Differences among Spastic, Athetoid, and Ataxic Cerebral Palsy

TYPE	CHARACTERISTICS	DAMAGE AREA(S)
Spastic	Spasticity: hypertonic Rigidity Stretch reflex Slow movements; laborious Presence of infantile reflexes	Pyramidal tract
Athetoid	Involuntary writhing movements Uncoordinated volitional movements	Extrapyramidal tract Basal ganglia tracts
Ataxic	Poor balance Poor direction control in gait Rate dysfunction in gait	Cerebellum

Adapted from Owens, R. E., Metz, D. E., & Haas, A. (2003). *Introduction to communication disorders: A lifespan perspective* (2nd ed). Boston: Allyn and Bacon.

(see Figs. 9-2, 9-3, and 9-4) as well as the other primitive reflex patterns of infants helps the speech-language pathologist understand the development of these reflexes into more permanent movement patterns. Furthermore, the speech-language pathologist also learns how primitive communication patterns such as

BOX 9-2

Dysarthria in Suprabulbar Paresis Syndrome of Childhood

Congenital Signs

Articulation disorder
Hypernasality
Lip, tongue, palate, and pharynx paresis
Isolated paresis (in some cases)
Possible agenesis of corticobulbar fibers
Drooling

Acquired Signs

Articulation disorder
Hypernasality
Lip, tongue, palate, and pharynx paresis
Some facial rigidity
Encephalitis
Traumatic head injury

BOX 9-3

Developmental Dysarthria in Pseudohypertrophic Muscular Dystrophy

Speech Signs (Flaccid Dysarthria)

Articulation disorder
Reduced vocal intensity
Respiratory weakness
Articulator weakness
Broad, flattened tongue

Physical Signs

Onset: 3 to 4 years
Proximal weakness
Pseudohypertrophic calf muscles
Proximal atrophy
Hyporeflexia, except ankles
Mental retardation (one third of cases)

cooing (as related to the emergence of reflex patterns and then more advanced movement patterns) and random sound productions of the newborn infant lead to speech sound development.

Diagnosis of Neurologic Disorder with Primitive Reflex

The neurologic examination of the newborn with suspected cerebral damage has in recent years relied heavily on the concept of a primitive reflex profile. Primitive and postural reflexes follow an orderly sequence of appearance and disappearance, beginning in the fetal period and extending through the first years of life. The reflexes are mediated at a subcortical level. First described by Rudolph Magnus (1873-1927), who received a Nobel Prize for his efforts, these reflexes can help determine degrees of prematurity or suggest neurologic dysfunction. If a normal reflex pattern does not appear on schedule, or if a reflex pattern persists beyond the age at which it normally disappears, the newborn or infant is considered at risk for cerebral injury or other neurologic involvement. Some pediatric neurologists assert that neurologic abnormalities at birth predict a diagnosis of minimal cerebral dysfunction at later ages, but others have found a limited association between neonatal abnormalities and neurologic signs, particularly at 1 year and beyond.

Despite questions about the reliability of prediction for a diagnosis of minimal neurologic abnormality, the careful evaluation of early primitive reflexes and later-evolving postural reflexes provides a basis for diagnosis and therapy of disturbed motor function. Examination can usually provide a locomotor prognosis, indicating when and how a child with cerebral palsy will walk. Table 9-6 summarizes the primitive and postural reflexes of the first year. Although the speech-language pathologist may be more interested in the neurologic status of oral and pharyngeal reflexes, an understanding of the primitive and postural reflexes is essential in the assessment of the neurologic maturity of a child suspected of cerebral injury.

A notable lack of consensus exists on the definition of the stimulus and response in the widely tested primitive reflexes. In addition, no agreement has been reached on how the responses change with time and growth. Seven reflexes are reviewed in this chapter. They are commonly assessed by neurologists and pediatricians and are typical of the first year of life, with the peak development at approximately 6 months. Testing during this peak time avoids assessing the

transitory neurologic signs of the newborn but is sufficiently early to allow a neurologic diagnosis before 1 year of age. These seven reflexes also appear to be predictive of later motor function in the child. Of the many infantile reflexes described by neurologists in the literature, these are the most studied.

ASYMMETRIC TONIC NECK REFLEX

The **asymmetric tonic neck reflex (ATNR)** probably is the most widely known of the early body reflexes. The reflex was shown to be universally present in the healthy infant by the outstanding child development specialist Arnold Gesell (1880-1961). When the healthy child is **supine**, he or she may lie with the head turned to one side. The extremities on that side (the chin side) are extended, with a corresponding flexion of the contralateral extremities on the opposite (occiput) side. This position is described as the fencer's position.

To test for the presence of the reflex, the child is placed in a supine position. Observations are made of active head turning and subsequent movement of the extremities. The head is then passively turned through an arc of 180 degrees to each side for 5 seconds. This maneuver is repeated five times on each side. Consistent changes in muscle tone in the extremities generally define the presence of the reflex. A clearly positive response is visible extension of extremities on the chin side and flexion on the occiput side when the head is passively turned. If extension of the extremities on the chin side and flexion on the occiput side last more than 30 seconds, the response may be called **obligatory**.

If the response is found beyond the eighth or ninth month, it is indicative of possible cerebral damage and poor motor development and suggests that the cortical control of upper motor neurons is not on schedule and that motor behavior is still controlled at subcortical levels. Obligatory tonic neck reflexes persisting into the second year and beyond usually are incompatible with independent standing and walking; they may disappear later, however, and the child may learn to walk alone. The ATNR may be seen in various types of cerebral palsy, predicting brain injury, but it is not useful for distinguishing between spastic and dyskinetic types. This reflex suggests brain injury only and is in no way completely diagnostic for cerebral palsy or its subtypes. The ATNR can reemerge after a catastrophe such as cardiac arrest and also may be present in progressive disease. It has little or no effect on the development of speech and shows little relation to the oral and pharyngeal reflexes. Elicitation procedures for the ATNR are illustrated in Figure 9-4.

TABLE 9-6

Primitive and Postural Infantile Reflexes of the First Year

REFLEX	RESPONSE
Asymmetric tonic neck reflex	Infant extends limbs on chin and flexes on occiput side when turning head
Symmetric tonic neck reflex	Infant extends arms and flexes legs with head extension
Positive support reflex	Infant bears weight when balls of feet are stimulated
Tonic labyrinthine reflex	Infant may retract shoulder and extend neck and trunk with neck flexion; tongue thrust reflex may occur
Segmental rolling reflex	Infant may roll trunk and pelvis segmentally with rotation of head or legs
Galant reflex	Infant arches body when skin of back is stimulated near vertebral column
Moro reflex	Infant may adduce arm and move it upward, followed by arm flexion and leg extension and flexion

SYMMETRIC TONIC NECK REFLEX

The **symmetric tonic neck reflex** is analogous to the ATNR, but the head is manipulated in flexion and extension in midline rather than turned laterally. The resulting responses are differences between upper and lower extremities rather than right-left differences in extremities. The normal reflex is an extension of the arms and flexion of the legs if the head is extended in midline. Flexion of the head has the opposite effect; the arms flex and the legs extend.

The technique of eliciting the reflex is to first ask the child to flex and extend his or her neck. The neck is then passively extended and flexed. This is repeated five times each for extension and flexion. If the reflex sign is absent at 5 to 6 months or persists into the second year, it is a symptom of motor abnormality. The symmetric tonic neck reflex does not appear to elicit any associated oral or pharyngeal reflexes (see Fig. 9-3).

POSITIVE SUPPORT REFLEX

Magnus saw the **positive support reflex** as necessary for support of erect posture. When the balls of the feet are stimulated, opposing muscle groups contract to fix the joints of the lower extremities so that they bear weight. To test the reflex, the infant is suspended around the trunk, below the armpits, with the head in midline and slightly flexed. The child is bounced on the balls of the feet five times. The feet are then placed in contact with the floor, and the degree to which the infant can support his or her weight is assessed. The positive support reflex is seen in fetal life and is considered abnormal if it persists beyond 4 months. A persistent strong response has been associated with spastic quadriparesis. The positive support reflex does not appear to elicit associated oral or pharyngeal reflexes (Fig. 9-5).

TONIC LABYRINTHINE REFLEX

The **tonic labyrinthine reflex (TLR)** is associated with the changes in tone related to different postures. The position of the extremities changes with respect to the position of the head in space because of the orientation of the labyrinth of the inner ear. The TLR is tested in both supine and **prone** positions.

To test in the prone position, the child is held in prone suspension. The head is extended approximately 45 degrees below the horizontal plane. Changes of posture and tone in the extremities are evaluated, with special attention to the shoulder area. When the head is flexed, a normal response involves protraction of the shoulders or flexion of the lower extremities. Consistent tone changes should be present in at least one upper and lower extremity for the reflex to be considered present (Fig. 9-6).

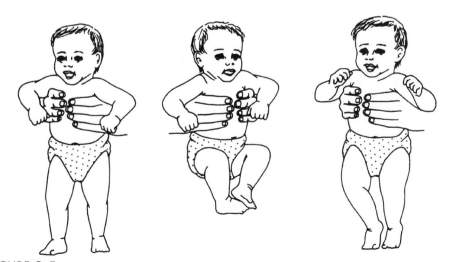

FIGURE **9-5**
The positive support reflex is elicited by suspending the child so that the balls of the feet can be bounced on a flat surface. The reflex is pathologic if the child remains on his or her toes and cannot move out of the position for 60 seconds or more. (Modified from Capute, A.J., Accardo, P.I., Vining, E.P.G., & Rubenstein, J.E. [1978]. *Primitive reflex profile.* Baltimore: University Park Press.)

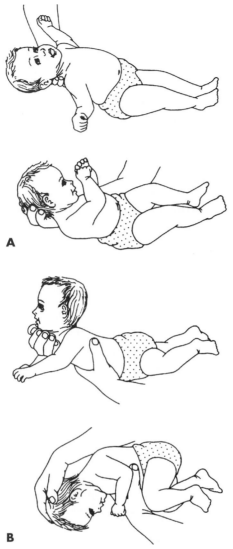

FIGURE 9-6
A, The TLR is elicited by placing support between the shoulders to extend the head 45 degrees. The head is flexed 45 degrees. The reflex is pathologic if severe extensor thrust or opisthotonos occurs. **B,** Extension and flexion. (Modified from Capute, A.J., Accardo, P.I., Vining, E.P.G., & Rubenstein, J.E. [1978]. *Primitive reflex profile*. Baltimore: University Park Press.)

In testing the TLR in the supine position, support is placed between the shoulders so that the head is extended at 45 degrees. Position and tone of the shoulders are assessed. Active neck flexion and grasp in midline are elicited. If the flexion and grasp responses are not noted, the head is flexed with the back supported and the midline grasp is sought again (see Fig. 9-6).

The normal response is shoulder retraction if the head is in extension. Trunk and leg extension accompanies shoulder retraction. Neck flexion results in shoulder protraction in 5 seconds and the disappearance of an extension posture.

An abnormal TLR may be accompanied by extensor hypertonia, and a persistent abnormal response may prevent the infant from rolling over normally. A pathologic response may make the legs so rigid that when the child is pulled to a sitting position, he or she will stand instead. The TLR is sometimes present in healthy children, but it is more common in children with pathologic conditions. Of the reflexes reviewed, it is the only one that may be routinely associated with oral reflexes. With the head extended 45 degrees, a reflex or tongue thrust may occur in the child with cerebral palsy.

SEGMENTAL ROLLING REFLEX

The healthy newborn shows a log-rolling response reflex associated with the activity of turning over. It is primarily a neck-righting reflex action. This early rolling response develops into a **segmental rolling reflex** in which turning of the head produces a reaction in which the infant attempts to undo the applied rotation by twisting the body at the waist, allowing one segment of the body to turn at a time. This corkscrew reaction allows the infant to roll over with a minimum of effort because only one segment of the body moves at a time. Abnormal responses are indicated by perseveration of a simple log-rolling response in which head rotation produces the simultaneous turning of the upper and lower extremities with no segmental control. The response is seen in motor-handicapped children with cerebral palsy.

To test the segmental rolling response, the child is placed in the supine position. The response is tested in two maneuvers. First, the child is rotated from the head; second, the child is rotated from the legs. For head rotation, the child's head is first flexed to approximately 45 degrees and then slowly rotated so that the shoulders are turned. The rotation is observed. The child's head is usually rotated with one hand on the side of the face near the chin and the other hand on the occiput of the head. When the child is rolled to the right, the examiner's left hand is the face hand and the right is the occiput hand. When the child is rolled to the left, the position of the examiner's hands is reversed (Fig. 9-7).

To test the leg response, one leg of the child is flexed at the hip and knee. The examiner holds the flexed leg below the knee, and the child is rotated to turn the pelvis toward midline. Rotation patterns are then observed (Fig. 9-8). Rotation responses have not been associated with oral or pharyngeal reflexes.

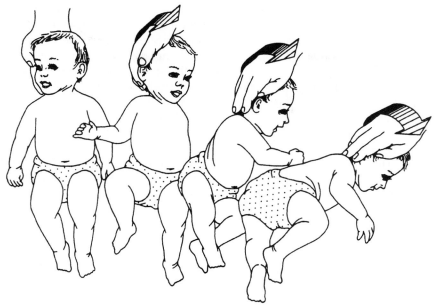

FIGURE **9-7**
The segmental rolling reflex (with rotation of the head) is elicited by rotating the head to turn the shoulders and by rotating the legs (see Fig. 9-8) to turn the pelvis. The reflex is pathologic if the child is obliged to roll in a log-rolling manner and cannot inhibit the reflex. (Modified from Capute, A.J., Accardo, P.I., Vining, E.P.G., & Rubenstein, J.E. [1978]. *Primitive reflex profile*. Baltimore: University Park Press.)

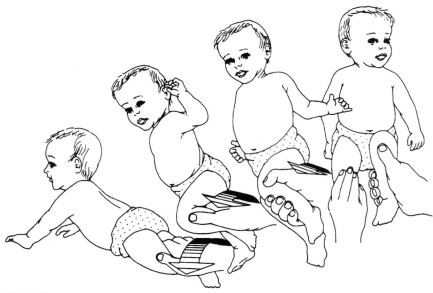

FIGURE **9-8**
Segmental rolling reflex: rotation of the legs. (Modified from Capute, A.J., Accardo, P.I., Vining, E.P.G., & Rubenstein, J.E. [1978]. *Primitive reflex profile*. Baltimore: University Park Press.)

GALANT REFLEX

The **Galant reflex** is an arching of the infant's body when the skin of the back near the vertebral column is stroked. The arching is usually forward, toward the stimulation. Arching in the other direction indicates the child is attempting to evade the stimulus. The responses may vary from total absence of response to an exaggerated hip flexion. In the majority of newborns the response is present bilaterally; unilateral responses have been reported in athetoid cerebral palsy. The response normally disappears by 2 months of age but persists in athetosis beyond that time. The Galant reflex is thought to be associated with delay of trunk stabilization and head control in athetoid cerebral palsy. Persistence of the response beyond 6 months is assumed to interfere with sitting balance. No association with oral or pharyngeal reflexes has been reported (Fig. 9-9).

MORO REFLEX

The **Moro reflex**, along with the ATNR, is one of the best-known and best-studied reflexes of child neurology. It is present in almost all newborns except for small premature babies. With sudden head lowering, a rapid and symmetric abduction and upward movement

of the arms occurs. The hands open, and gradual adduction and flexion of the arms occur. The lower limbs also show extension and then flexion.

Some debate has taken place about whether the Moro response and the startle response are continuous patterns. Both responses appear in the newborn, so they are thought to be discontinuous. The Moro usually reaches a peak at 2 months and diminishes by 4 months. A persistent reflex has been associated with cerebral palsy and mental retardation.

To test for the Moro reflex, the child is held in the examiner's arms, well supported at the head, trunk, and legs. The examiner suddenly lowers the child's head and body in a dropping motion (see Fig. 9-2).

The most significant aspect of the stimulus is the quality of suddenness. Primitive and postural reflexes sometimes reinforce more circumscribed reflexes, but no evidence exists that the primitive Moro reflex tends to reinforce oral and pharyngeal reflexes in children with cerebral palsy. The persisting Moro reflex is much less valuable to the neurologist as a sign of cerebral injury than is the ATNR.

In summary, persisting infantile primitive and postural reflexes have been a classic sign of central nervous system dysfunction. In particular, they have been extremely useful in the early diagnosis of cerebral palsy. Infantile reflex behavior also has been incorporated in motor treatment programs for children with

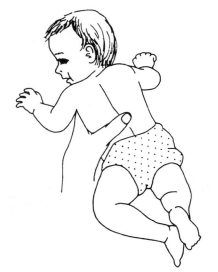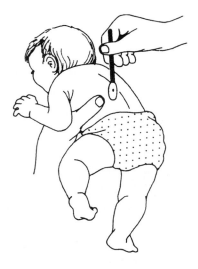

FIGURE **9-9**
The Galant reflex is elicited by stroking the back in the lumbar region with a blunt object. The reflex is pathologic in the presence of persistent curvature of the back and elevation of the hips. (Modified from Capute, A.J., Accardo, P.I., Vining, E.P.G., & Rubenstein, J.E [1978]. *Primitive reflex profile.* Baltimore: University Park Press.)

cerebral palsy. An important fact for the speech-language pathologist is that the primitive and postural body reflexes, with some exceptions, appear to have limited influence on oral and pharyngeal reflexes. Although these neonatal and early reflexes are important in assessing delayed development of motor function before age 12 to 18 months, they are of only limited use in the pediatric neurologic examination for the older child. The more conventional neurologic signs of altered muscle tone and abnormal muscle stretch and superficial reflexes, as well as the results of objective neurodiagnostic tests, are of equal value in making a diagnosis for the examining pediatric neurologist.

Oral and Pharyngeal Reflexes

Over the past half century, study of the normal infant reflexes and their relation to brain disease has promoted speech-language pathologists and others interested in the management of cerebral palsy to consider another set of reflexes—the oral and pharyngeal reflexes. Table 9-7 summarizes the major oral reflexes. Some speech specialists have assumed that abnormal oral and pharyngeal reflexes play a significant role in the speech development of the child with cerebral palsy who is dysarthric or is likely to develop dysarthria with the onset of speech. Absent or persisting reflexes, they argue, are predictive of dysarthria. Neurologists are more likely to argue that when the oral and pharyngeal reflexes are integrated into a spontaneous feeding pattern, they become more diagnostically and prognostically significant in neurologic disease. Similarly, speech-language pathologists are beginning to question whether the isolated artificially elicited reflexes of the first few months of life have as much diagnostic and prognostic importance in speech performance as do the dysphagic symptoms commonly seen in many children with cerebral palsy.

The type, number, and reliability of abnormal oral and pharyngeal reflexes found in those with cerebral palsy vary from study to study. Research strongly suggests that little or no correlation exists between the presence and number of abnormal oral and pharyngeal reflexes and the severity of dysarthria in cerebral palsy, as defined by a measure of articulation proficiency.[7] In fact, the dysphagic symptoms—disordered biting, sucking, swallowing, and chewing—are slightly better predictors of articulation proficiency than is an elicited set of neonatal oral and pharyngeal automatisms. The correlation, however, between speech impairment and dysphagic symptoms is not particularly strong. This limited relation between speech and dysphagia strongly implies that motor control for speech and the feeding reflexes may be mediated at different levels in the nervous system. Evidence indicates that the feeding reflexes are mediated at the brainstem level and that voluntary speech is controlled at the cortical, subcortical, and cerebellar levels, with the prime voluntary pathways for speech being the corticobulbar fibers. Brainstem reflex pathways apparently subserve only vegetative and reflex functions and are inactive during the execution of normal speech. Therefore early motor speech gestures probably are not directly related to the development of motor reactions in feeding during infancy and childhood, even though some of the motor coordinations and refinements in speech acquisition are analogous to some of the biting and chewing gestures in feeding.

Even though early oral motor behavior in feeding may only have a limited resemblance to actual motor patterns for speech, management programs to improve muscle function and coordination in eating have been initiated as a possible prophylactic measure for future dysarthria. The assumption of these programs is that any improvement in motor activity of the oral musculature gained through feeding therapy might conceivably result in improvement in speech performance because the parallel activities of speech and feeding have

TABLE 9-7
Infantile Oral Reflexes

REFLEX	STIMULUS	AGE OF APPEARANCE	AGE OF DISAPPEARANCE
Rooting	Perioral face region is touched	Birth	3-6 months
Suckling	Nipple in mouth	Birth	6-12 months
Swallowing	Bolus of food in pharynx	Birth	Persists
Tongue	Tongue or lips being touched	Birth	12-18 months
Bite	Pressure on gums	Birth	9-12 months
Gag	Tongue or pharynx being touched	Birth	Persists

muscles in common. At the very least, feeding therapy is likely to make eating faster and easier. This, of course, is an important consideration in the total management of the child with cerebral palsy, one that should not be overlooked by speech-language pathologists and neurologists. In fact, dysphagia may be just as disturbing as dysarthria in the young person with cerebral palsy. Direct motor training of the muscles during speech, rather than feeding training, appears to be the most effective method for improving the dysarthria because cortically mediated speech activities drive the muscles at a more rapid and coordinated rate than do brainstem-mediated feeding activities.

The feeding reflexes have sometimes been used diagnostically by speech-language pathologists in planning management programs in children with cerebral palsy. Persistent abnormal oral reflexes have also been factors considered in the decision to elect an augmentative communicative system with a nonspeaking motor-handicapped child. One pair of experts has asserted that "of all factors investigated, obligatory persistence of oral reflexes can in isolation lead to a decision to elect an augmentative communication system."[14] Their assumption is that retained oral reflexes indicate a poor prognosis for oral speech development. This claim may need to be reevaluated in the light of the aforementioned findings concerning the poor correlation between articulatory proficiency and the number of retained oral reflexes in a population with cerebral palsy.[7]

Despite the controversy about oral reflexes and speech in diagnosis, management, and prognosis, a description of six commonly tested oral pharyngeal reflexes is offered for the speech-language pathologist who wants to consider this aspect of disturbed oral motor functions in the cerebrally injured infant or child. In the typical infantile oral motor evaluation, eliciting each of these infantile automatisms artificially one by one is best to determine whether they are absent or abnormally persisting. Next, the spontaneous functions of mastication and deglutition in the feeding act should be assessed to determine how these neonatal reflex behaviors have become integrated into a more complex and voluntary oral-pharyngeal pattern of feeding. Infantile mastication and deglutition use the six cranial nerves (V, VII, IX, X, XI, XII) important for future speech, so evaluation of early feeding allows cranial nerve assessment for the child who is too immature to cooperate in standard cranial nerve testing.

ROOTING REFLEXES

If the perioral facial region is touched, two responses in combination make up the **rooting reflex**. The side-to-side

head-turning reflex usually is elicited by gently tapping on the corners of the mouth or cheek. The response is the head alternately turning toward and away from the stimulus, ending with the lips brushing the stimulus. Occasionally the response occurs without the stimulus when the infant is hungry.

This activity usually precedes any actual suckling. The side-to-side head-turning response is present in the term baby and premature infant. The reflex usually disappears by 1 month of age and is replaced by the direct head-turning response, a simple movement of the head toward the source of stimulation. The source is grasped with the lips and sucked. In the direct head-turning response, if the stimulus is applied to the corners of the mouth, the bottom lip usually lowers and the head and tongue orient toward the stimulus. The direct head-turning response is established at 1 month and disappears by the end of the sixth month of life. Persistence beyond a year may suggest cerebral injury, and asymmetry of response indicates damage to one side of the brain or facial injury. The cranial nerves involved in the reflex are V, VII, XI, and XII. The reflex is mediated by the pons, medulla, and cervical spinal cord (Fig. 9-10).

SUCKLING REFLEX

If a finger or nipple is placed in the infant's mouth, bursts of suckling behavior occur interspersed with periods of rest. The **suckling reflex** is integrated at birth, but within 2 or 3 months the action develops more purpose, and jaw activity is incorporated into the pattern. Involuntary suckling may disappear between 6 months and 1 year. Persistent suckling beyond 1 year suggests brain injury. The reverse, the inability to suckle, may also be an early sign of cerebral injury. The cranial nerves involved in suckling are V, VII, IX, and XII. The reflex is mediated at the pons and medulla (Fig. 9-11).

SWALLOWING REFLEX

The **swallowing reflex** develops after the suckling reflex is integrated into a total feeding pattern. Suckling activities produce saliva, which accumulates in the reflexogenic area of the pharynx. The swallowing reflex is triggered, and swallowing may be observed by visible upward movement of the hyoid bone and thyroid cartilage of the larynx. The upward movement of the thyroid cartilage of the larynx may also be palpated during the swallow. Separating suckling and swallowing is sometimes difficult because a swallow

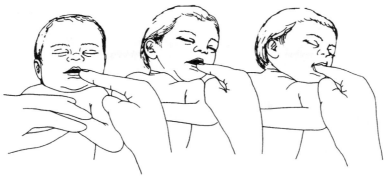

FIGURE **9-10**
The rooting reflex is elicited by stimulating the cheek lateral to the mouth. From birth, the infant normally turns the head toward the stimulus and then grasps the stimulus in the mouth. The reflex is pathologic if it is absent in infants from any cause or if it persists beyond the fourth month.

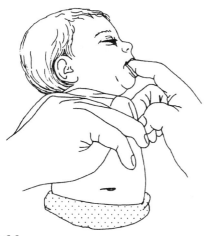

FIGURE **9-11**
The suckling reflex is elicited by putting the index finger 3 to 4 cm into the mouth of the infant. From birth, the infant normally engages in rhythmic sucking of the finger. The reflex is pathologic if it is absent or exaggerated or if it persists beyond the fourth month.

may precede a suck or follow a first or second swallow. The act of deglutition involves muscles of the mouth, tongue, palate, and pharynx and depends on a highly coordinated movement pattern. Cranial nerves V, VII, IX, X, and XII are involved in the act of swallowing. An immature swallow with tongue thrusting is sometimes seen until approximately 18 months of age. A mature swallow is present afterward. The reflex is mediated at the level of the brainstem in the medullary reticular formation. Disturbances in swallowing are frequent manifestations of neurologic deficits in the

infant and child, and they comprise the most important sign of neurologic disorder among the feeding reflexes.

TONGUE REFLEX

This reflex may be considered part of a suckle-swallow reaction in which the tongue thrusts between the lips. If lips or tongue are touched, cranial nerve XII predominates. Excessive thrusts beyond 18 months are abnormal. The **tongue reflex** is mediated at the medulla.

BITE REFLEX

Moderate pressure on the gums elicits jaw closure and a bite response. The **bite reflex** is present at birth; in the normal infant it disappears by 9 to 12 months, when it is replaced by a more mature chewing pattern. The reflex may be exaggerated in the brain-injured child and may interfere with feeding and dental care. Its persistence inhibits the lateral jaw movements of chewing seen in the spontaneous mastication pattern. A weak response is seen with brainstem lesions, and corticobulbar lesions exaggerate the response. Cranial nerve V innervates the reflex, which is mediated at the low midbrain and pons.

GAG REFLEX

A stimulus applied to the posterior half of the infant tongue or on the posterior wall of the pharynx causes rapid velopharyngeal closure. This primary action is

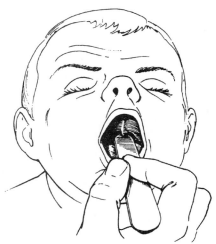

FIGURE 9-12
The gag reflex is elicited by stimulating the posterior half of the infant's tongue with a tongue blade or stimulating the posterior pharyngeal wall. The reflex is present from birth and is pathologic when absent or exaggerated.

accompanied by mouth opening, head extension, and depression of the floor of the mouth with elevation of the larynx and diaphragm. This **gag reflex** is present at birth and continues throughout life. The gag serves as a protective mechanism for the esophagus. Brain-damaged children often show a hyperactive gag. In the severely motor-involved child, the gag may be difficult to elicit. In the ataxic child, the gag is sometimes hypoactive. Cranial nerves IX and X innervate the gag, and the reflex is mediated at the level of the pons and medulla (Fig. 9-12).

Relation of Reflexes, Brain Development, and Speech Development

The development and progression of the reflexes presented in this chapter help the speech-language pathologist understand the way early speech and language development occurs in progression after reflexes are in place and as they mature. Once many of the reflexes are extinguished as the child's brain develops, pleasure sounds, cooing, babbling, and eventually phonemic development occurs, as previously discussed. Neurolinguistic theory postulates that the developing brain ontogenetically allows the child to form the eventual sounds that comprise that individual's phonemic system. This is attributable to brainstem development and other relevant neurologic systems (central nervous system and peripheral nervous system).

Reflexes develop first, and a delayed or persistent reflex should trigger a red flag to the speech-language pathologist that the development of phonemes may be interrupted and subsequently the morphemic and perhaps pragmatic systems for that child.

ASSESSING MASTICATION AND DEGLUTITION

In the infant or child at risk for neurologic injury, the clinical evaluation of neural control of the oral and pharyngeal activities involved in chewing and swallowing allows the speech-language pathologist to estimate the motor potential of those muscles, which ultimately fall under the control of higher nervous centers devoted to the production of speech. The fact that speech and feeding are mediated at different levels within the nervous system implies that evaluation of chewing and swallowing predicts future muscle activity in speech in only a limited manner. Only gross estimates of muscle potential for speech can likely be derived from any nonspeech examination because of the semiautonomous control of the muscles for the dual function.

In addition to gross estimation of muscle function in mastication and deglutition, the infantile oral motor examination of the cranial nerves for speech permits the speech-language pathologist and neurologist to observe signs of possible neurologic disorder that may not be readily apparent in other motor behaviors. **Mastication** and **deglutition**, as relatively complex motor behaviors in the repertoire of infant motor activity, are highly sensitive to neurologic dysfunction. Dysphagia may be an early and even sometimes isolated sign of brain injury.

Modified Feeding
Examination of chewing and swallowing is best accomplished through the technique of **modified feeding.** In the preverbal child, this technique can replace the more traditional procedures of the adult speech cranial nerve test, which requires a level of maturity not yet developed in the infant and very young child. By selectively placing small morsels of solid food in different locations in the oral cavity of the child, an examiner can judge the integrity of the bulbar muscles and the brainstem neural pathways innervating these muscles. Healthy children from birth to 36 months respond well to the technique, which may also be used with motor-handicapped children with oral motor involvement well beyond 3 years of age. In the healthy child, spontaneous feeding emerges from the neonatal oral and pharyngeal reflexes and reaches its full

maturity at approximately age 3 years. Experiences with solid foods provide a gradual refinement and integration of movements of the lips, tongue, palate, and pharynx for chewing and swallowing.

When testing the infant or motor-handicapped child without sitting balance, the child should be placed in a chair in which the body and head can be well supported (e.g., a tumble-form chair) or in the primary caregiver's or clinician's lap in a well-supported position. In the child with some sitting balance, placement in a relaxed sitting position with adequate head support is preferred. See Chapter 7 for a summary of the cranial nerves.

Cranial Nerve VII

Placement of a small food bolus on the lower lip in midline and observation of the child's oral reaction to it provide evidence of the ability to use the muscles of the lip and lower face purposefully. Pursing the lips during rooting and sucking indicates intact facial movement. Lack of a smiling response may suggest severe bilateral facial muscle involvement. The healthy baby smiles to a human face at 2 to 4 months of age. A sober expression and sluggish grin must be carefully evaluated as possible neurologic signs of a bilateral corticobulbar system involvement ultimately affecting the paired nerves of cranial nerve VII. An asymmetric smile with a unilateral flattening of the nasal fold on one side of the face may be associated with unilateral paresis. This sign is not as obvious in the infant and young child as it is in the adult. Lack of lip tonicity may be present, and lip seal may not be maintained. In the brain-damaged child, drooling may result from the poor lip seal.

Cranial Nerve XII

The child with cerebral injury often is unable to shape, point, and protrude the tongue in retrieving food from the lower lip by licking. The lack of tongue protrusion is common in both spastic and athetoid children. In the brain-injured infant, the tongue often will not cup, even during crying. Neither will the tongue thin, nor will the tip elevate with precision. This inability to produce any fine tongue movements suggests motor involvement of both the intrinsic and the extrinsic tongue musculature.

Unilateral or bilateral atrophy of the tongue may be seen in young children, and this loss of muscle bulk suggests lower motor neuron disease. However, fasciculations are rarely seen in the tongue muscles of infants.

Excessive tongue thrust, sometimes called the tongue reflex, is common in children with severe brain damage. It is particularly common in athetosis, and it may be associated with orthodontic problems and excessive drooling. In addition, occasional wavelike involuntary movements are seen in the body of the tongue, mimicking the involuntary movements of limb and trunk in extrapyramidal athetosis.

Cranial Nerve V

When confronted with a small food bolus on the lips or tongue, the young child begins the total act of deglutition by initiating voluntary mastication. The aim of the evaluation at this point is to determine whether the bolus of food can be pulverized and whether the particles of food can be selectively manipulated to be transported to the back of the oral cavity. With a large food bolus, the tongue is usually elevated, so the bolus is placed between the tongue surface and the anterior hard palate and crushed. Smaller boluses of food are crushed between the hard palate and tongue, and the tongue directly begins a wavelike, peristaltic movement, carrying the food to the pharynx. If the food bolus is large, the tongue often acts in a whiplike fashion to propel the food laterally between the molars for grinding and pulverization. Observation of the vigorous tongue actions confirms the integrity of the neural control of the tongue. Disorders involving neurologic integrity of the tongue and jaw innervation often limit cerebrally damaged children to eating only diced or liquefied food.

Adequate biting and vigorous anterior-posterior movements of the mandible plus lateral grinding action of the jaws assure the speech-language pathologist that cranial nerve V innervation is intact and that muscles innervated from the pons are functional. On the other hand, an exaggerated and too-powerful bite may be a manifestation of an abnormal jaw reflex, suggesting an upper motor neuron lesion above the level of the pons. In older children with brain damage, a firm tap on the lower jaw may elicit a clonus, suggesting a hyperactive jaw reflex. If the lower jaw deviates to one side on opening or during mastication, pterygoid muscle weakness may be present on the side of deviation. In athetosis the jaw may become a major articulator, producing the motor power for elevating a poorly controlled tongue in achieving tongue tip–alveolar ridge contact and other tongue-elevation gestures.

Integration of Cranial Nerves V, VII, IX, X, and XII

When the food bolus is well masticated, the final involuntary stage of deglutition is initiated. The nasopharynx is closed by the muscles of the soft palate and the pharyngeal constrictors. Cranial nerves IX and X produce this closure. Saliva or the food bolus is pushed through the palatal fauces, into the pharynx, and onto the esophagus in a peristaltic wave. Muscles of the soft palate, the pharyngeal constrictors, and muscles of the tongue and larynx work in intricate coordination to propel the food bolus to the esophagus. In one sense, swallowing becomes the ultimate integration of the nervous mechanisms to be used later in motor expression of speech.

Speech, however, requires more intricate coordination of muscles than do chewing and swallowing. This fine coordination is accomplished through increasing cortical and cerebellar control of the pontine and bulbar muscles. Certain other complex motor adjustments are seen in speech that are not seen in chewing or swallowing. As an example, the grooved fricative /s/ requires finer motor control than is seen in mastication. To produce an adequate /s/, a central groove in the tip and blade of the tongue must be formed, with the sides of the tongue firmly anchored between the lateral dentition. This specific tongue configuration, common to speech, is not seen in brainstem-mediated functions. Intricate coordination of intrinsic and extrinsic tongue muscles is needed for the grooved fricatives. These fine motor configurations are not present in feeding. Thus assessment of mastication and deglutition in a preverbal child suspected of neurologic impairment is most appropriate, but when speech emerges the evaluation should be based on the motor control for phonemes, syllables, words, and sentences assessed in the traditional articulation test format and on the results of a standard oral examination that includes assessment of the speech cranial nerves (see Chapter 7).

The actions of the cranial nerves for speech and the corticobulbar system, which activate the cranial nerve nuclei, can be assessed in infancy through observation of chewing and swallowing. All the nervous action of the bulbar muscles is integrated into the single act of feeding in infancy.

Childhood Apraxia of Speech (Developmental Verbal Dyspraxia)

Childhood apraxia of speech is a childhood condition reportedly similar to apraxia of speech (acquired) seen in the adult. The disordered movements of the articulators frequently appear to contribute to a serious phonologic problem in the school-aged child. If an apraxic disorder of the oral muscles is present in the preschool years, it may well delay the development of speech and language, and the language developmental milestones of one-word utterances, two-word combinations, and three-word sentences may be disrupted. A clear-cut syndrome has not yet emerged despite considerable clinical research on the topic. The prime sign of the disorder is awkward movement of the speech muscles that cannot be attributed to developmental dysarthria. This single sign appears to be the only clearly reliable and consistent feature for diagnosis of the disorder. Some question exists whether the articulation errors of children diagnosed as having speech apraxias can reliably and validly be separated from the articulation errors of children with severe functional developmental phonologic disorders.

Acceptance of the disorder in a true apraxic context is also difficult. Apraxia of adulthood has been unequivocally associated with verified brain lesions; in children, however, this has not been the case. In some instances no brain lesion has been demonstrated at all; in other instances inconsistent soft signs have been found. Doubt has arisen in these cases about the actuality of cerebral dysfunction because no demonstrable structural lesion or evidence of dysfunction has been found.

Childhood apraxia of speech associated as a motor speech disorder may be summarized with the following speech and nonspeech symptoms recognized in the literature as characteristic of these children. Box 9-4 refers to these characteristics.

BOX 9-4

Speech and Nonspeech Characteristics of Childhood Apraxia of Speech

Speech Symptoms

Errors are inconsistent
Cannot imitate particular speech sounds
Distortion of vowels
Omission, distortion, and addition errors
Voicing errors
Prolongations and repetition of sounds
Consonant clusters are in error
Errors in fricative and affricative productions
Articulatory groping behavior
As length and complexity of utterance increase, more errors are noted
Some prosody incongruencies

Nonspeech Symptoms

Oral apraxia
Alternating movement rate disturbance
Oral motor deficits
Language disorder may be present

(Modified with permission from Lass, N. J., McReynolds, L. V., Northern, J. L., & Yoder, D. E. (eds), [1988]. *Handbook of speech-language pathology and audiology.* Toronto: BC Decker.)

In summary, childhood apraxia of speech is still controversial. Many researchers do not agree on symptomatology, causes, assessment, or treatment procedures. Further study into this disorder is needed, and agreement among speech-language clinicians is not expected regarding how to serve this population.

INTRODUCTION TO NEUROLINGUISTICS

As children mature and develop from the basic oral reflex stage to more sound or articulatory development, some simply become delayed in phonologic and/or articulatory development without a neurologic motor speech component. Articulation disorders have their roots in the phonetic (sound) development that children progress through as their oral motor skills mature. These children currently are referred to as having phonologic processing disorders. Phonologic disorders have their basis in the study of phonology from a linguistic point of view. These children, now served in clinics, do not necessarily have a motor speech component that must be addressed either linguistically or neurolinguistically.

Salient differences exist between children with an articulation disorder and those with a phonologic disorder. Much is distinguished by phonetic versus phonemic errors. Phonetically, this child struggles with speech sound form and development, but phonemically the child displays problems with language-based functions of phonemes.[2] This becomes a matter of sound formation (articulation disorder) versus phonemic function (phonologic disorder). Because motor speech delay or impairment is not present, children with articulation disorders display disturbances in the neurologic processes of sound development, and children with phonologic disorders represent an impairment of the phonemic system within the language. Articulation disorders are phonetic in nature, whereas phonologic disorders are phonemic.[2]

NEUROLINGUISTICS DEFINED

Neurolinguistics is the science concerned with the biologic basis of language development. For human study, the processes of interest include comprehension, production, and abstract knowledge of language, including phonology, morphology, syntax, semantics, and pragmatics, whether in spoken, signed, or written communication. According to Ahlsén,[1] "neurolinguistics studies the relation of language and communication to different aspects of brain function...it tries to explore how the brain understands and produces language and communication" (p. 3). Neurolinguistics has its roots in the field of aphasia and aphasiology.

The speech-language pathologist knows that as a child matures and develops, the brain increases in weight and functional abilities. This primarily occurs from increased myelination of the child's brain tissue. For the most part, motor and sensory pathways are formed before the higher cortical functions are developed. Genetics usually plays an important factor in the brain's "wiring" that eventually forms the mature central nervous system. This is how neural pathways are formed, especially in the first month or two of life. Speech-language pathologists are trained to understand that the central and peripheral nervous system tracts devoted to speech and language are not fully matured, at least until the late toddler stage of development.[10,12] Owens[11] postulated that while this is happening in brain development the infant begins vocalizations as the brainstem and pons develop. An increase in babbling may be related to development of the motor cortex and maturation of the larynx and face. Stark[16] and Owens[10] discussed that the arcuate fasciculus and other auditory association areas link auditory areas with corresponding cortical motor areas as the child's brain develops. This usually occurs by the time the child is turning 2 years of age and is essential for the child's ability to imitate sounds and intonation patterns of the people with whom the child comes in contact on a daily basis

Locke,[5] of the University of Sheffield in England, offers a theory of neurolinguistic development to explain how an infant develops from simply recognizing faces and voices to learning his or her parent or caregiver's vocal characteristics. Locke explains that "the first phase is indexical and affective" (p. 265), in which the infant is strongly oriented to a person's face and voice. The infant's second phase is "primarily affective and social...whereby its function is to collect utterances for social purposes" (p. 266) regulated by the right hemisphere. The third phase facilitates discovery and is ultimately responsible for the child's development of speech and language rule usage. The fourth and last phase is integrative in nature.[5] This underlies Locke's idea that "children who are delayed in the second phase have too little stored utterance material to activate their analytic mechanism at the optimum biological [neurolinguistic] moment and when sufficient words are learned, the capability has already begun to decline" (p. 266).[5] This could explain, from a neurolinguistic viewpoint, the delay in speech development in infants and young children. Finally, Locke suggested that "the resulting neurolinguistic resources, not being specialized for phonological operations, are minimally adequate but not optimal for development of spoken language" (p. 266).[5]

TABLE 9-8

Phases and Processing Systems and Neurolinguistic Correlates

AGE OF ONSET	DEVELOPMENTAL PHASES AND SYSTEMS	NEUROLINGUISTIC AND NEUROCOGNITIVE MECHANISMS	LINGUISTIC DOMAIN
0-3 months	Vocal learning	Specializing in social understanding	Prosody and sound segment development
5-7 months	Utterance acquisition	Specializing in social understanding	Stereotypic utterances
20-37 months	Analysis and computational	Grammatical analysis skills	Phonology, morphology, and syntax
3+ years	Integration and elaboration	Social understanding and grammatical analysis	Automatic operations and expanded lexicon and sound development

Modified from Locke, J. (1997). A theory of neurolinguistic development. *Brain and Language, 58,* 265-326.

Table 9-8 outlines Locke's system, including the neurolinguistic components of speech development and language capacity.

A delay in or the absence of neurolinguistic development can lead to speech delays, phonologic disorders, and motor speech problems. Children develop through periodic phases, as described in Table 9-8, and if an interruption (e.g., cerebral palsy, muscular dystrophy) or delay (e.g., mental retardation, Rhett's syndrome) occurs, speech development would either be absent or significantly altered.

Wingate[17] introduced an interesting concept of how to define **fluent** speech, or fluency. He spoke of it as a *continuity* in speech but not in words. He postulated that "fluency is not equivalent to words in uninterrupted sequence" (p. 201). Sequencing of speech involves the words that are uttered as well as the complicated motor speech movements executed when saying those words. Relatively speaking, it involves many prosodic elements often assumed to be the rhythm of speech. These other suprasegmental elements of speech fluency often are filtered out or even go unnoticed by the listener. Many times when the listener has to pay close attention to the way someone speaks (prosody, etc.), the comprehension of the actual message is interrupted. Listening for hesitations, prolongations, and sound repetitions often hinders communication. After all, as Wingate[17] pointed out, "listening for hesitation...is quite a demanding task" (p. 201). These hesitations, whether a simple "uh" or "you know," are an intrusion into the fluency of a conversation. Understanding this intrusion may be comprehended through an understanding of the relation of neurolinguistics to fluency disorders.

NEUROLINGUISTICS AND FLUENCY DISORDERS

According to Wingate,[17] studying and understanding **fluency disorders** may be enhanced by looking at the field of neurolinguistics. As children develop their neuronal capacities, dysfluent behaviors may be noticed at the age of 2 or 3 years. The brain is genetically wired, and capacity is developed as the person ages, starting at infancy. What matters is that even though the human brain is wired for speech production, sometimes the cognitive and emotional aspects of speech output can be altered through neural development. Neurolinguistic programming is the ability to re-wire cortical structures on the basis of behaviors and emotions. According to Wingate, the thalamus is substantially involved in both the production of speech and the disorderliness of speech production.

There are numerous subcortical neuronal structures that affect speech production. Wingate stated that the thalamic nuclei are especially significant. Because the thalamus is the center where all sensory information is processed (other than the sense of olfaction), it acts as a relay station to control information coming in and going out from a variety of cortical areas. This gating function of the thalamus will be further elaborated in Chapter 10. Wingate suggests that this could explain how, neurolinguistically speaking, the brain may be mis-wired and thereby cause some sensory information to manifest itself as disordered speech production in the form of dysfluency.

Silverman[15] referred to Kent,[4] who proposed that "...stuttering results (at least in part) from a central nervous system disturbance, the nature of which is a reduced ability to generate temporal patterns whether for sensory or motor purposes, but especially the latter" (p. 156). Based on this hypothesis, those who stutter would not have the same abilities as those who do not to sequence motor movements for fluent speech. This reduction in temporal ability would result in dysfluent speech patterns and therefore require neurolinguistic programming to effect change. Thus, by empowering an individual to reprogram the brain to think in terms of fluency, the neurolinguistic aspects (or programming) of the brain may be altered. That is why, according to Mackesey,[8] "by optimizing the environment through education and empowerment [neurolinguistic programming] we can increase the reinforcement of fluency and a healthy self-esteem and in turn limit negative reinforcement, teasing, and the like."

Synopsis of Clinical Information and Applications for the Speech-Language Pathologist

- Early cerebral injury of the speech mechanisms in the infant brain result in motor speech disorders.
- These include developmental dysarthria, anarthria, and apraxia of speech.
- Developmental dysarthria is characterized by weakness, paralysis, and incoordination of the speech musculature.
- Developmental anarthria is characterized by a lack of speech as a result of profound paralysis, weakness, or incoordination of the speech muscles.
- Dysarthria is characterized by a disturbance in the motor control centers of the developing brain.
- Disturbances include strength, speech, steadiness, coordination, precision, tone, and range of motion.
- Apraxia is a motor planning disorder characterized by a disturbance in selecting and sequencing movements.
- Dysarthrias can be categorized as spastic, dyskinetic, ataxic, or mixed.
- Spastic dysarthria is characterized by bilateral corticobulbar involvement, increased muscle tone, slowed rate, and loudness.
- Dyskinetic dysarthria is characterized by athetosis, dysphagia, hypernasality, articulation disorder, and vocal quality disturbance.
- Ataxic dysarthria is characterized by unequal stress, articulation and prosodic disorder, disturbance of balance, and an awkward gait.
- Cerebral palsy can be subdivided into three major categories: spasticity, dyskinesia, and ataxia.
- Approximately 75% to 85% of children with cerebral palsy have dysarthria to some extent.
- Other complications of cerebral palsy include mental retardation and hearing loss.
- Spastic cerebral palsy is characterized by hemiplegia, paraplegia, diplegia, and quadriplegia of upper and lower extremities.
- Athetoid cerebral palsy is the most common of the dyskinesias of cerebral palsy and is characterized by hypotonia and the absence of the Moro and tonic neck reflexes.
- Ataxic cerebral palsy is the most uncommon of all cerebral palsy syndromes and is characterized by disturbed balance, lurching gait, hypotonic muscles, and damage to the cerebellum.
- Next to cerebral palsy, muscular dystrophy is the most likely condition to display dysarthria. Flaccid dysarthria may appear with an articulation problem, reduced vocal intensity, respiratory weakness, and a broad and flattened tongue; one third of the cases include mental retardation.
- Major infantile reflexes in the developing child are the asymmetric tonic neck reflex, symmetric tonic neck reflex, positive support reflex, TLR, segmental rolling reflex, Galant reflex, and the Moro reflex.
- Oral reflexes in the developing child that appear at birth include rooting, suckling, swallowing, tongue, bite, and gag; the gag reflex persists throughout life, but the others usually disappear by 6 to 18 months of age.
- Swallowing is controlled by the integration of functions of central nerves V, VII, IX, X, and XII; it requires coordination but not in a form as intricate as speech.
- Developmental apraxia is controversial; in the developing child, apraxic speech disorders may delay speech and language development, including the milestones of first word utterances, two-word combinations, and three-word sentences.
- Neurolinguistics is concerned with the underlying process of communication, including phonology, morphology, syntax, semantics, and pragmatics in regard to various aspects of brain function.
- The human brain is wired genetically; neurolinguistic programming enables "re-wiring" cortical structures on the basis of behaviors and emotions. Dysfluency has a neurologic component.
- Stuttering results from a central nervous system disturbance, according to Kent.
- The ability to sequence motor movements for fluent speech is impaired in those who stutter; stuttering is a reduction of temporal abilities and results in dysfluent speech patterns.

CASE**STUDY**

H. T., a 10-year-old boy, was brought to the emergency department by his parents. H. T. was home alone with his younger sister after his parents went out with friends. After putting his sister to bed, H. T. found liquor bottles in the wet bar of the family room and some beer in the refrigerator. He consumed a fifth of vodka and two bottles of beer within 5 hours. His parents came home and found him passed out on the kitchen floor. They called 911 and H. T. was rushed to the hospital. His blood alcohol level was four times the legal limit set for an adult. The medical team revived him and he was admitted to the hospital. A few hours later H. T. began to have several severe grand mal seizures. Seizure activity was intermittent for almost 6 hours. Magnetic resonance imaging (MRI) was completed at this time. Several areas of diffuse damage appeared on the image, but the radiologist could not determine if any particular parts of the central nervous system were affected. Imaging was ordered to be repeated. On wakening in the morning, the house neurologist on call and physical and speech therapists were summoned for an evaluation. H. T. was disoriented ×3 and had to be prompted to answer questions. Speech was slurred, with intermittent loudness and softness in voice output, reminding the staff of the drunken state he was in when brought to the emergency department. Physical therapy provided minimal assistance to have H. T. walk across the room. Gait was wide and unsteady. Both fine and gross motor skills were tremulous and unbalanced. Alternating motion rates were slow and deliberate, and H. T. often stopped and started again several times. Many phonemic errors were noted. Social Services was consulted, and history indicated that this has happened several times before but this was the first time that H. T. passed out and had seizures, according to the parents.

QUESTIONS FOR CONSIDERATION:

1. The speech symptoms, gait, and other behaviors appear to be reminiscent of which type of dysarthria?
   a. Flaccid
   b. Ataxic
   c. Spastic
   d. Mixed
2. What primary area of the central nervous system do you think was affected in this child?
3. Will this damage resolve as in the past, or will it be more permanent this time?

REFERENCES

1. Ahlsén, E. (2006). *Introduction to neurolinguistics.* Philadelphia: John Benjamins Publishing Co.
2. Bauman-Waengler, J. (2004). *Articulatory and phonological impairments: A clinical focus.* Boston: Allyn and Bacon.
3. Fenichel, G. M. (1997). *Clinical pediatric neurology: A signs and symptoms approach,* (3rd ed.). Philadelphia, W. B. Saunders.
4. Kent, R. D. (1983). Facts about stuttering: Neurologic perspectives. *Journal of Speech and Hearing Disorders, 48,* 249-255.
5. Locke, J. (1997). A theory of neurolinguistic development. *Brain and Language, 58,* 265-326.
6. Love, R. J. (2000). *Childhood motor speech disability* (2nd ed.). Boston: Allyn and Bacon.
7. Love, R. J., Hagerman, E. L., & Tiami, E. G. (1980). Speech performance, dysphagia and oral reflexes in cerebral palsy. *Journal of Speech and Hearing Disorders, 45,* 59-75.
8. Mackesey, T. (2007). *Logical levels of stuttering,* www.stuttering-specialist.com/development.html. Retrieved January 21, 2007.
9. Meyer, L. A. (1982). A study of vocal, prosodic and articulatory parameters of the speech of spastic and athetotic cerebral palsied individuals [doctoral dissertation], Nashville, TN: Vanderbilt University.
10. Owens, R. E. Jr. (2001). *Language development: An introduction* (5th ed.). Needham Heights, MA: Allyn and Bacon.
11. Owens, R. E. Jr. (2004). *Language disorders: A functional approach to assessment and intervention* (4th ed.). Boston: Pearson.
12. Owens, R. E. Jr. (2005). *Language development: An introduction* (6th ed). Needham Heights, MA: Allyn and Bacon.
13. Owens R. E., Metz D. E., & Haas, A. (2003). *Introduction to communication disorders: A lifespan perspective* (2nd ed.). Boston: Allyn and Bacon.
14. Shane, H. C., & Bashir, A. S. (1980). Election criteria for adoption of an augmentative communication system: Preliminary considerations. *Journal of Speech and Hearing Disorders, 45,* 408-414.
15. Silverman, F. H. (2004). *Stuttering and other fluency disorders,* (3rd ed.). Long Grove, IL: Waveland Press, Inc.
16. Stark, R. (1986). Prespeech segmental feature development. In Fletcher, P., & Garman, M. (Eds.), *Language acquisition* (2nd ed.). New York: Cambridge University Press.
17. Wingate, M. E. (2002). *Foundations of stuttering.* San Diego: Academic Press.
18. Workinger, M. S., & Kent, R. D. (1991). Perceptual analysis of the dysarthrias in children with athetoid and spastic cerebral palsy. In Moore, C. A., Yorkston, K. M., & Beukelman, D. R. (Eds.). *Dysarthria and apraxia of speech: Perspectives on management.* Baltimore: Paul H. Brookes.
19. Worster-Drought, C. (1974). Suprabulbar paresis. *Developmental Medicine and Child Neurology, 16* (suppl 30), 1-30.

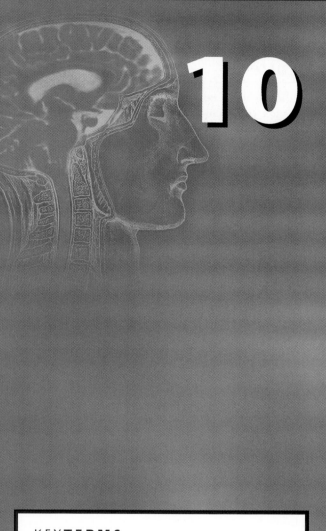

10

Central Language Mechanism and Learning

It was Wernicke's paper which made the first searching attempt to link the facts of anatomy with the facts of behavior in a way that permitted prediction of syndromes and the organized test of hypothesis. Like Meynert he gave the brain life.
—Norman Geschwind, *Cortex*, 1967

CHAPTER**OUTLINE**

KEY**TERMS**

autoassociator network
cognition
constraint-induced
  therapy (CIT)
declarative memory
executive functions
graceful degradation
input fibers
intrinsic neurons
  (interneurons)
long-term memory
metacognition
neocortex (archicortex)
neurogenesis
neuroplasticity
pattern associator
  network

perisylvian cortex
phoneme
presynaptic inhibition
procedural memory
projection neurons
reasoning
selective engagement
short-term memory
spatial summation
summation
supramarginal gyrus
synapses
temporal summation
thalamic reticular
  nucleus
transcranial magnetic
  stimulation (TMS)

Earlier chapters in this text have primarily concentrated on the anatomy and physiology associated with the input to the cortex from sensory mechanisms and the output of the cortical neurons in terms of motor responses. Chapter 2 reviewed the structure of neurons, the lobes of the cortex, and the primary and association areas of the cortex. This information should be reviewed and re-digested before studying this chapter., We now take a simplified, but expanded, look at the cortical mechanisms underlying the extraordinary capacity of human beings to use and understand language and to learn and create new ideas. These abilities begin to form a foundation from birth and, barring injury or disease, continue throughout life. This chapter introduces current thinking regarding how neurons work together to accomplish this task. Also highlighted are the anatomic structures involved in language processing, as well as some of the historically popular models of language underlying explanations of language disorders acquired from brain damage. The more common acquired adult language disorders and cognitive-linguistic disorders are discussed in Chapter 11.

Language and learning disorders of children are covered in Chapter 12.

Neocortex

The highest level of cortex in terms of cytoarchitecture is **neocortex** (or **archicortex**), covering approximately 90% of the brain. The total area of cortex is approximately 2500 cm^2, with a range of 2 to 4 mm in thickness; sensory cortex is thinner than motor and association areas. The thickness is determined by the aggregation of neuronal cell bodies. The cortex contains approximately 50 billion neurons, 500 billion neuroglial cells, and an extensive capillary network. This chapter primarily is concerned with the work of the neurons.

LAMINAR ORGANIZATION

The neocortex is composed of six layers. Table 10-1 summarizes the name and composition of each layer.

TABLE 10-1
Summary Description of the Laminar Organization of the Neocortex

LAYER NUMBER	LAYER NAME	DESCRIPTION	SPECIAL FEATURES
I	Molecular	Contains mostly horizontal axons and a few neuronal bodies	
II	Outer granular	Contains a mixture of small neurons (granule cells) and slightly larger neurons (pyramidal cells); apical dendrites extend up to layer I and axons descend into and through deeper layers	
III	Outer pyramidal	Contains primarily medium and large pyramidal cells; apical dendrites extend up to layer I and axons descend into and through deeper layers	
IV	Inner granule	Contains stellate (starlike) neurons, smooth and spiny; no pyramidal cells	Primary target layer for ascending sensory information from the thalamus
V	Inner pyramidal	Contains medium and large pyramidal cells; apical dendrites of medium size extend up one or two layers; large cells project to layer I	Large pyramidal = major source of cortical efferent fibers that send axons to corpus striatum, brainstem, and spinal cord; some corticocortical connections
VI	Multiform	Contains an assortment of neuron types	Axons project to subcortical structures such as thalamus; also make corticocortical connections

SYNAPTIC ORGANIZATION

For these cortical neurons to transmit and process neural information, connections must be made through **synapses**. Synaptic organization is concerned with the way neurons form circuits that mediate the function of different regions of the brain. These different centers or regions have pathways that run between them, with connections being made within the centers (locally) as well as outside the particular region, perhaps a relatively long distance away. Essentially three types of neural elements make the connections possible. **Input fibers** synapse onto the cell body and/or dendrites or dendritic spines found on the dendrites. **Projection neurons** (also called principal or relay neurons) send out a long axon fiber that carries information signals to other regions. The third type are cells concerned only with local processing within a certain region, the **intrinsic neurons**, or **interneurons**. Sometimes a projection neuron takes action locally and behaves as an interneuron; the distinction between the two is not rigid. The relations among these three elements of synaptic organization vary in the different regions of the brain and determine the function of that region.

There are approximately 10 billion cells in the human cortex and probably 60 trillion synapses. Given the density of tissue in the cortex, as many as 1 billion synapses may be present per cubic millimeter of cortical tissue.[45] These connections form circuits, though they are not of a simple input and output nature. The nervous system is organized in a complex hierarchical manner from the molecular level to complex behavioral systems. **Microcircuits**, formed from small bunches of synapses,

give way to local circuits, then interregional circuits that result in systems of behavior. Figure 10-1 breaks this organization down further. Microcircuits form dendritic connections and subunits within the connections between dendrites of individual neurons. These neurons with their connections interact, forming local circuits and performing the operations of a particular region of the brain. These regions are organized with interregional pathways, columns, and laminae. Neural impulses traveling by the interregional connections between these multiple local circuits account for behaviors. The assembly of synapses and the connectivity of these assemblies, especially during development, produce the behaviors of interest in the study of neurology.

The neural microcircuits are the most localized synaptic patterns that can be studied. Chapter 4 presented two basic patterns of connectivity—divergence and convergence. These are important to remember when thinking about how information processing occurs within these circuits. Microcircuits are built of three types of elements: divergence, convergence, and a variation of convergence called presynaptic control.

To summarize, synaptic divergence means that an action potential can trigger multiple excitatory postsynaptic potentials simultaneously, affecting many dendritic terminals at once. This amplifies the activity of a single axon. This kind of divergent synaptic action is found, for example, in the cerebellum, which demonstrates great divergence, and in the sensory afferents of the thalamus. Another method of achieving divergence is also found in the nervous system. Axons branch into collaterals and give rise to multiple terminals, thus

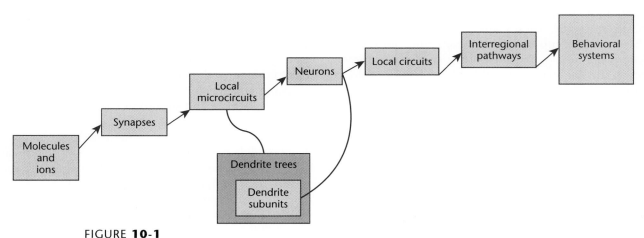

FIGURE **10-1**
Levels of hierarchical organization in the nervous system. *Arrows* should be read as "organize into." *Curved line connection* indicates that local microcircuits are grouped to form dendritic subunits within the dendritic trees, which are part of the individual neurons.

resulting in numerous synaptic contacts. This kind of divergence is common in the cortical cells.

Synaptic convergence, on the other hand, occurs when multiple synapses occur on one postsynaptic dendrite. When this occurs, two kinds of **summation**, or additive effects, may take place. **Temporal summation** may occur in which the effect of the neurotransmitters may be enhanced, for example, if all synapses are excitatory. The convergence may also summate with the excitatory and inhibitory potentials canceling each other out, resulting in the resting potential being maintained. The integration of the excitatory and inhibitory synapses usually function, however, to *modulate* the action; thus there is a change in potential but it is not as strong as it would have been without the convergence. Another kind of summation is **spatial summation**, in which the varied sites of synapse along the dendritic surface of the neuron cause responses to rise in the different parts of the neuron. This may increase the possibility of more local mechanisms during activation from the site on one dendritic tree to another.

A third type of action that is similar to convergence is **presynaptic inhibition**, in which two sequential axonic synapses occur. One axon terminates on another with inhibitory action. When this second axon then is presynaptic to a third axon, there is an inhibitory effect on the synapse that will occur on the postsynaptic membrane of the third axon. Box 10-1 summarizes the three kinds of connectivity patterns.

DENDRITES AND NEURONS

The complexity of neuronal processing is exemplified by the extensive variety of patterns of dendritic branching unique to different types of neurons. The different branching patterns are said to impose geometric constraints on activity. These patterns, combined with the different sites of input and the passive and active electronic properties of the membrane of the dendrites, account for the complex nature of the activity of dendrites and consequently the neurons. This text does not go in depth into this complex organization of the dendritic input to the neuron. However, the fact that the dendritic tree is responsible for the variety of actions the neuron may undertake is important to understand.

Of note, the smallest functional unit within the dendritic tree is the dendritic spine, which is, as it sounds, a thornlike protuberance on the dendrite. Being quite numerous in the nervous system, they account for most postsynaptic sites in the brain, especially within the cerebellum, basal ganglia, and cortex. Within the cortex most excitatory synapses are made onto spines, and approximately one third of the inhibitory synapses

---

BOX 10-1

Synaptic Connectivity Patterns

Synaptic Divergence
- Occurs when action potential triggers multiple excitatory postsynaptic potentials, affecting many dendrites; can also occur when axons branch into collaterals, creating multiple terminals and synaptic contacts
- Acts to increase amplification of a single axon
- Commonly found in the cerebellum, the sensory afferents of the thalamus, and in cortical cells

Synaptic Convergence
- Occurs when multiple synapses fire on one postsynaptic dendrite, adding activity from multiple axons to one dendrite
- Two kinds of summation can occur at a synaptic convergence:
  - Temporal summation—effect of neurotransmitter may be enhanced if all synapses are excited or if resulting excitatory and inhibitory potentials create a resting potential
  - Spatial summation—various sites along synapse cause responses in different parts of neuron

Presynaptic Inhibition
- Occurs when two axonic synapses are in sequence and an inhibitory effect occurs on the postsynaptic membrane of the third of three axons

---

occur there. Approximately 15% of all dendritic spines carry potential for both kinds. Aside from the obvious function of increasing the surface area available for connective integration, spines are theorized to have significance for rapid signal processing.[45] Long-term potentiation is a long-lasting change in synaptic efficiency of cortical neurons thought to be related to learning and memory. This processing utility may also involve chemical and structural changes at the level of the dendritic spines.

The foundational study of neuronal functioning in Chapter 4 discussed the basics of impulse initiation and synaptic connection, with the impulse being generated at the axon hillock and traveling down the axon to synapse with another neuron. Also discussed was the graded potential set up in the cell itself. To take this further, evidence exists that to various degrees electronic backspread of this propagated current occurs back into the soma and the dendrites. This may be sufficient to activate dendrite to dendrite (dendrodendritic) synapses, further facilitating or inhibiting action within that neuron's local circuit.

Basic Circuits

The basic cortical neuron (usually a pyramidal cell type) is structured well for the integrative actions beginning to emerge. The typical cortical neuron has dendritic trees that are divided into apical and basal parts, with dendritic spines on both parts and different excitatory and inhibitory synapses occurring at different levels of the parts of the dendritic tree.[45] It also, of course, has an axon that gives off collateral axons that synapse within the local circuit as well as at sites some distance from that region.

In the neocortex, the best-studied neural connections are those of the visual system. Basic circuitry began to be studied with the visual system. Two basic models were proposed. A feed-forward model is one in which processing is strictly serial. In this model input arrives at the cortex, is fed forward through a short chain of neurons within the local area, and then is transmitted to other areas by the output neurons. Another model, called the recurrent model, theorizes that the rich connections between the cortical layers form a cortical circuit that is more unitary, with input, association, and output layers being difficult to distinguish. In this model impulses circulate in recurrent circuits with association fibers modifying the action so that the effect of the input depends on what is happening within the circuit at that point in time.

When these models were being discussed by scientists in the early literature of neural processing, they agreed that processing was local and vertical, moving only up or down through the different laminae. Early cortical maps displayed an essentially vertical organization. This was the way it appeared through research with the microscope. When newer methods of study became available, however, functional maps of processing (such as visual maps) could be drawn up for the lateral dimension. The cortical maps of areas such as the visual cortex or the auditory cortex then appeared more as slabs or pinwheels. Thus both vertical and lateral connections could be traced within these local circuits.

NEURAL NETWORKS

The concept of processing neural information within local circuits and interregional circuits has changed the way many neuroscientists have begun to think about the brain in the last few decades. In the 1970s, Barlow[3] proposed the "neuron doctrine," championing localized encoding for perceptual processes. This theory invoked the power and specificity of individual cortical neurons in building a hierarchical organization of processing by single cortical areas, resulting in an output neuron specific to a certain percept (for instance, in vision, a "chair" cell). This is being gradually replaced by neural network processing explanations.

Neural network theories usually involve comparison and simulation done with computer processing. The scientific discipline of parallel distributed processing (PDP), or connectionism, has grown up around this work. PDP asserts that circuits of neurons in regions of the brain work through joint interactive behavior involving possibly millions of neurons in these neural networks. Two kinds of networks are used in simulations of behavior: autoassociator networks and pattern associator networks. An **autoassociator network** simply implies that every unit in the network is connected to every other unit with associations stored within a layer of neurons. The associations between neural activities in a given pattern are stored in the connection weights. Because of the connections among the units, these networks can support any number of different patterns of activity. A pattern of activity in a network establishes a representation. A **pattern associator network** allows transformation of a pattern of activity across its input units into a pattern of activity across its output units. The pattern associator stores associations between a pattern of neural activations in an input layer and a pattern of activations in an output layer. Once stored in the connection weights between these layers, a pattern of output activity can be recalled by presentation of the input pattern.

All the primary and association cortices in the brain are thought to be essentially collections of pattern associator networks, many of them working in parallel. For example, when auditory phonologic representations are transformed into articulatory phonologic representations, a pattern associator network is in action.

PDP, or neural network theory, proposes that the efficiency and effectiveness of processing information in the brain occur through the activation of the connections between the neurons in the circuits. The information processed is thought to be stored in the multitude of connections rather than in the neurons themselves. The strength of the connection in terms of excitatory versus inhibitory synaptic action and the likelihood of neural firing provide constraint on the flow of activation in a particular circuit. A steady state can be obtained and a representation (percept or concept) results the instant that particular pattern of activity occurs. The strength of the connections in a network, occurring within and across association cortices, defines the capability of the network for generating a particular representation at any point in time.

The units or components of the "grand representation" appear to be distributed across the association areas. This helps explain why a breakdown in processing rarely results in a total loss of a percept or concept. The loss of one component of this distributed processing network results in a reduced level of performance, but not a complete inability to process. For example, in word retrieval failures, patients often know something about the word or object they are trying to think of. They have not completely lost all information about it. This reduction in performance of the system is called **graceful degradation** in engineering terms and has been a useful concept in neural processing. Speech-language pathologists often use it to great advantage in treatment.

Graceful degradation also is responsible for the ability to deal successfully (sometimes) with ambiguous input into the system. For example, in a place where so much noise is present that a person can only hear part of what his or her conversational partner is saying, the brain can often fill in because patterns of activation occur for possible representations of what would make sense. At times the wrong guess is made, but what was thought to be said is not nonsensical because that would be eliminated from possibilities through further processing of probable versus improbable. Again, in engineering terms, graceful degradation allows human beings to tolerate "noisy" input from the sensory systems and organize it to make sense, if possible. The human brain is an excellent processor of fragmentary information because of the distribution of representations across it.

The brain is the ultimate information processor. No computer built to date can process information, learn new information, and create from imagination with the efficiency and productivity of the human brain. Because of (1) the properties of the neurons and their links across association cortices; (2) the input from sensory mechanisms, limbic structures, basal ganglia, cerebellum, and so forth; and (3) output back to some of these areas, processing in this ultimate PDP network is a two-way function. Processing is both from the bottom up and from the top down. From peripheral sensory input comes a forward press of converging neural information, traveling through the intermediate subcortical pathways to early sensory association cortical processing areas (unimodal and polymodal association cortex) to higher and higher cortical association areas (supramodal or heteromodal cortex). At each local circuit station are also backprojections occurring at the synapses onto the neuron, with this output from the circuits occurring in a mostly divergent rather than convergent manner.

This convergent/divergent action within neuronal circuits enhances or changes the strength of connections within the circuit and thus output to other regions. This allows changes in behavior. These neuronal operations allow translation of what is thought into what is said, written, or signed; in other words, to communicate thoughts.

Neuroanatomy of Language

The contribution of Pierre Paul Broca's study of the brain of two patients with language loss was acknowledged earlier in this text. Broca's discovery of a specific speech-language area in the left hemisphere of the brain had dramatic consequences for neurology. It prompted European neurologists to formulate numerous hypothetical models of the central language mechanism. Several of these models were highly speculative and based on limited evidence of the correlation between behavioral deficits and brain lesions. Even today the central mechanism for language is not completely understood, and it remains risky to attempt to formulate a model for normal and abnormal communication. However the model formulated by Carl Wernicke is generally conceded to be the most valid and powerful model of the central language mechanism.[6] The model presented here is based on Wernicke's conception and its modern variations, primarily elaborated by Dr. Norman Geschwind (1926-1984).[17] The Geschwind model is a connectionist conception of the higher mental functions of speech and language and as such it gives importance to the classic language and speech centers and highlights the significance of the interconnection of the association fibers between major centers. The model has been of significant use to the clinical neurologist because it allows a high degree of predictability of symptoms associated with specific lesion sites. In addition, the model also predicts possible aphasic syndromes not yet described. It does this by postulating possible lesion sites for these syndromes. In general the model has been confirmed by clinical studies. The classic language centers have been established through computerized tomography and other current objective neurodiagnostic procedures.

Geschwind,[17] however, pointed out that some conditions exist under which the model has not always fulfilled its promise. First, certain features of aphasic syndromes are not readily explained by the model. Second, aphasic cases occasionally occur whose existence is not predicted by the model. Third, in a few cases the expected symptoms do not appear when an adequate lesion exists Despite these limitations, the model has been extremely useful for neurologists, linguists, and speech-language pathologists.

In recent years research in acquired communication disorders has felt the impact of the field of cognitive neuropsychology as experimental psychologists test and develop their information-processing models of cognition in individuals with aphasia or other types of brain damage. Much of the initial work was done in the United Kingdom, mainly with investigations of reading.[10] These models are testimony to the belief in cognitive neuropsychology that investigations of individual patients from a particular theoretical stance are preferable to comparisons of groups of patients categorized by the classic syndrome models.[8]

Many cognitivists believe that attempting to map brain structure to cognitive function is not a useful task at this time because current definitions of what constitutes a function, such as naming or reading, are too broad. For example, Rothi and Moss[41] have demonstrated that failure to read a word aloud correctly may result from a breakdown in any number of processes involved in the task. Thus information-processing models require that a task be fractionated into its different components. Individuals are then studied in such a manner as to identify where during the process the breakdown may occur, resulting in inaccurate or inefficient performance.

These models usually represented the brain as a specialized computer that has domain-specific modules associated with defined neural structures, with input and output routes mapped as the model becomes more specific to function. The modules were usually represented as boxes with the input and output routes as arrows.[9,25,39] These models appealed to clinicians because techniques for assessment and treatment can be adapted from them.

The development and use of such models are well established in both speech-language pathology and neuropsychology. Their acceptance is variable, however, because much controversy exists regarding the independence of language from other psychologic operations. Also argued is that no model, as of yet, can deal with the complexity of human language. Marin[24] points out that the organism strives mainly to understand or express meaning in all communication and that a model is needed where meaning is the primary emphasis. Science is not there yet, even with the advances made in neural networks and PDP theories and simulations. However, knowledge is rapidly advancing. The use of positron emission computed tomographic studies and functional magnetic resonance imaging have advanced knowledge of how all areas of the brain work together and how other cognitive processes interact with language.

Despite the existence of the newer models and the criticism of the Wernicke/Geschwind model, emphasis will continue to be placed on learning the structures and the function of the traditional language areas. We do not have to limit this study to a simple connectionist approach. Knowledge has advanced beyond that, as evidenced by the discussion leading into this chapter. The regional anatomy serves to localize where the action is but primarily may be thought of as representing local processing networks, as just discussed. Interconnections between these networks exist, as do interconnections with subcortical structures. But what are distributed between these areas appear to be patterns of neural activity that are transformed into all the things studied in communication, such as sounds, words, sentences, and thoughts. These may be represented as output through several different modalities. Although science has made tremendous progress, none of these processes or regions is definitively mapped or understood. However, the proposed regional specialization for language that develops over time, and in most human beings develops in the left hemisphere, has stood the test of time. Advanced studies of language processing in normal subjects rather than patients with lesions may alter the view somewhat but so far has not radically changed opinion about which cortical structures are primarily involved in language production and comprehension.

A Model for Language and Its Disorders

PERISYLVIAN ZONE

The major neurologic components of language are situated in the area of the dominant hemisphere known as the **perisylvian cortex**. Table 10-2 summarizes the components of the language model. This zone contains Broca's area, Wernicke's area, the supramarginal gyrus, and the angular gyrus as well as the major long association tracts that connect the many language centers. These areas are composed of primarily supramodal association cortex. Figure 10-2 shows the central language mechanism of the dominant hemisphere.

Before describing the basic function of each of these areas, determining how the processing within these areas may occur may be helpful. Nadeau et al[32] provide a simplified description of the processing in these areas that should facilitate understanding. As previously mentioned, the smallest unit of language is the **phoneme**, many of which can be written as letters and all of which a speech-language pathologist can write in phonetic symbols. It is thought that the cortex of the perisylvian area contains a distributed representation of phonemes and that this representation is in all the various forms

TABLE 10-2

Major Components of the Central Language Mechanism Model

STRUCTURE	FUNCTION
Broca's area	Motor programming for articulation
Motor strip	Activation of muscles for articulation
Arcuate fasciculus	Transmission of linguistic information to anterior areas from posterior areas
Wernicke's area	Comprehension of oral language
Angular gyrus	Integrates visual, auditory, and tactile information and carries out symbolic integration for reading
Supramarginal gyrus	Symbolic integration for writing
Corpus callosum	Transmission of information between hemispheres

in which they are used. There are motor, auditory, visual, and tactile representations. Depending on the communication system (e.g., verbal vs. signing), the representation of one type may be stronger than others because of the strengthening of the connections through use. These representations are supported by their links or connections with appropriate cortical processing areas within the perisylvian cortex. These links allow abstract representations of phonemes to be translated into reality. The translation allows a sound to be spoken, a letter representation to be written or signed, and a spoken representation of that phoneme to be correctly understood as that particular phoneme as opposed to other ones.

Another functional aspect of the perisylvian cortex is to sequence these individual phonemes into combinations found in a particular language, the phoneme blends, syllables, and words that make up a language. This is the first step, but without a consequent linking to a particular neural pattern that corresponds to meaning, these combinations would have no value. Science believes and research is supporting that "meaning corresponds to the particular pattern of neural activity distributed across association cortices throughout the brain that actually represents a particular concept" (p. 544).[32] This is the fundamental concept underlying the neural association and function of the areas now discussed.

BROCA'S AND WERNICKE'S AREAS

The location and limits of Broca's area in the frontal lobe are well defined by research from several sources (see Chapter 2). Considerable documentation shows that the area primarily functions as a center for the motor programming of speech articulation movement. That is, Broca's area is the link in the system for the motor representation of the phonemes. Here the motor patterns are sequenced into the movements underlying the production of the phonemes and their combinations. Recent research with transcranial magnetic stimulation has validated a function division in this area.[19] These experiments found that the anterior (pars triangularis) and ventral (pars orbitalis) parts seemed to be involved in semantic processing, whereas the posterior portion (pars opercularis) was engaged with syntactic and phonologic processing as well as motor control of speech.

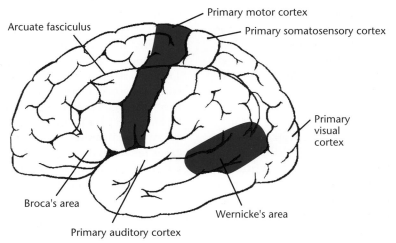

FIGURE **10-2**
Important perisylvian cortical regions of the central language mechanism. (From Brookshire R. [2007]. *Introduction to neurogenic communication disorders* [7th ed.]. St. Louis: Mosby.)

Wernicke's area, found in the temporal lobe, rivals Broca's area as a major component in a model of neurologic language functioning. The function of the center is well agreed upon, although its borders are sometimes disputed. In contrast to Broca's area, which serves the expressive aspects of motor speech, Wernicke's area is devoted to another major aspect of language–reception of speech. Neural structures in Wernicke's area are assumed to allow for comprehension of oral language and, in some as-yet-undefined manner, underlie the formulation of internal linguistic concepts. During speaking these concepts are transmitted anteriorly in the brain, traveling forward to Broca's area for the motor programming and expression of language. Little is actually known about the neural correlates of this internal aspect of language. However, links with patterns of neural activity are believed to be involved in many association areas. Links to auditory association cortices are certainly present. The formulation of these internal linguistic concepts may require links to neural circuit patterns present in limbic, somatosensory, and visual cortices as well as other supramodal association areas. Which areas are linked will depend on the prior association and knowledge, the way the particular knowledge was learned or is to be learned, and the complexity. There is much research still to be done to explain this processing.

ARCUATE FASCICULUS

Wernicke[53] must be given credit for developing a language model that highlights the connective association pathways between the frontal and temporal speech-language areas. The major fiber connections between Broca's area and Wernicke's area are now generally agreed on to be the arcuate fasciculus. The fibers, as described in Chapter 2, leave the auditory association area in the temporal lobe, arch around and under the supramarginal gyrus, and pass through the parietal operculum. They travel forward as part of the long association tract known as the superior longitudinal fasciculus, finally ending in Broca's area.

ANGULAR GYRUS

Included as a significant component of the language model is the angular gyrus in the left parietal lobe. Joseph J. Dejerine (1849-1917) suggested that this area was one of two sites associated with the reading disorder alexia. Alexia can also be associated with a lesion of the left occipital lobe accompanied by a lesion of the splenium of the corpus callosum. The left occipital lobe lesion produces a right hemianopsia. The lesion in the splenium prevents the right occipital cortex from transmitting information to the left angular gyrus. The hemianopsia, compounded by this disconnection syndrome, produces severe alexia.[12,13]

SUPRAMARGINAL GYRUS

Anterior to the angular gyrus is the **supramarginal gyrus**, curving around the posterior end of the sylvian fissure. Together with the angular gyrus, it is known as the inferior parietal lobule. Sensory information is analyzed and integrated in this area, which is thought to play an important role in perception. Lesions of the supramarginal gyrus in the dominant hemisphere are associated with agraphia, or writing disorders.

UNDERSTANDING SUBCORTICAL LANGUAGE MECHANISMS

The strictly cortical model of language mechanisms displayed in Figure 10-2 has been questioned numerous times because patients with what appeared to be only subcortical lesions were found to have language problems. Wilder G. Penfield and Lamar Roberts were among the first investigators to present evidence for possible subcortical mechanisms for language and speech.[37] They suggested that the pulvinar and ventrolateral nuclei of the thalamus serve as relay stations between Broca's and Wernicke's areas. They demonstrated massive fiber tracts to and from the thalamus and the major cortical speech and language areas. In addition, direct electrical stimulation of the left pulvinar and ventrolateral nuclei has produced naming problems.

Subcortical aphasias have been reported since the nineteenth century, but their existence has remained controversial. Although the language disturbance observed after thalamic infarct or damage to other subcortical mechanisms (caudate, globus pallidus, internal capsule) was originally believed to be a direct result of damage to a structure that must be somehow responsible for language, better imaging capability has shown that to be incorrect. New explanations have recently been put forth that describe the complicated nature of subcortical-cortical connections and their influence on language processing and production when those connections are interrupted by damage to certain subcortical structures.

THALAMIC LESIONS

Wallesch and Papagno[51] suggested that subcortical structures involved in a cortical-subcortical loop serve to monitor and select lexical input, which is then sent forward to the anterior language cortex in a modular fashion. The lexical alternatives from which the loop selects information originate in the posterior language cortex of the left hemisphere. In 1992 Crosson[11] proposed that cortical-striatal-pallidal-thalamic-cortical loops are involved in language. He suggested that the loop triggers the release of language segments at the appropriate time after semantic monitoring, thus serving more of a regulatory than an information-processing function. Crosson also theorized that the thalamus arouses the anterior language cortex and transmits semantic segments from the anterior to the posterior cortex for monitoring. These theories were early indictments of the assumption that the language deficits found in patients with thalamic stroke or hemorrhage were directly related to the damage to the thalamus itself. This premise of language disorder being caused directly by dysfunction of the thalamus alone has been shown to be essentially incorrect. Rather, the language disorder (aphasia) appears to result from the disruption of *cortical* function caused by the thalamic damage. It is an indirect cause resulting in a neural system disruption. Nadeau and Crosson[31] present an extensive analysis and discussion of the mechanisms summarized here.

Chapters 2 and 5 discuss the primary relay functions of the thalamic nuclei. A vast number of relays are synapsing in the thalamus, going from peripheral sensory nerve organs to the cortex. Also mentioned are extensive relays from the cortex to the thalamus. Most of the connections of thalamic nuclei and cortical areas are two-way, with numerous projections back to the thalamus from the cortex, as well as the more typically discussed projections from the thalamus to the cortex. In relation to language function, the two most interesting thalamocortical loops relay from the dorsomedial nucleus and the pulvinar-lateral posterior nucleus of the thalamus. The dorsomedial nucleus relays information originating from prefrontal cortex areas involved in executive functioning as well as some subcortical areas. This neural information originates from these areas and is relayed back to them after processing in the thalamus. For the pulvinar-lateral posterior nucleus, projections are from the frontal, temporal, and parietal cortices and back.

The specific function of the thalamus in language and cognition is now thought to be not a simple relay mechanism in the neural pathway, but a regulated or gated relay mechanism. A cogent and lengthy discussion of these mechanisms, their purported function, and relevance to treatment can be found in Nadeau and Rothi.[33] To summarize their points, deeper discussion of the structure of the thalamus is required. PDP, as discussed at the beginning of this chapter, also plays an important role.

Most of the thalamus has a layer of cells enveloping it that forms what is called the **thalamic reticular nucleus**. These cells do not send their axons out, but rather send them back into the thalamus and synapse on either relay neurons or on inhibitory interneurons. The reticular neurons themselves employ gamma-aminobutyric acid (GABA) and are inhibitory. Thus the action of these neurons can be to facilitate transmission to the cortex (through inhibition of the inhibitory action of the interneurons) or block transmission to the cortex (by inhibiting the relay neurons).

These reticular neurons are under the control of (or regulated by) a number of different brain systems, with two important ones being the reticular formation of the midbrain and projections from the cerebral cortex. Global and nonselective are said to describe the impact of the midbrain on thalamic transmission. With high levels of arousal comes a strong excitation of the thalamic cells, causing inhibition of the interneurons and consequently allowing ready transmission through the thalamus in an unregulated fashion. During low arousal (with sleep and coma being the most common examples) little can quell the action of the inhibitory interneurons, and most transmission through the thalamus is blocked. Compared with the global and nonselective effect of the midbrain is the impact of the cortical-thalamic-cortical projections, which are thought to be local and selective. Thalamic transmissions from specific nuclei are believed to be selectively gated to the cortex. Nadeau and Rothi,[31] acknowledging that errors do occur in localization of stroke damage, indicate that lesion data support that patients found to have aphasia after thalamic lesions show primary involvement of structures related to this gating mechanism of the thalamus. Thus it is proposed that rather than damage to the thalamus per se causing the dysfunction, the deleterious effect on cortical language mechanisms results in the symptoms seen in these patients with thalamic lesions.

In the proposal developed by Nadeau and Rothi,[31] the thalamus is involved in normal language functioning by regulating the engagement of certain neural networks in different association cortices to participate in lexical semantic access. They theorize that the cortical-thalamic disruption that occurs in the presence of damage to certain parts of the thalamus impairs the cortical network that supports declarative memory (knowledge of facts and events). The language function most dependent on declarative knowledge and memory is naming, which is, in neurolinguistic terms, lexical-semantic access. The patients with subcortical damage affecting the thalamus show the most difficulty with naming, whereas most of the other aspects (grammar, comprehension, articulation, and repetition) are maintained.

NONTHALAMIC SUBCORTICAL LESIONS

In addition to thalamic lesions causing aphasia, lesions in the internal capsule, striatum, and globus pallidus also have been documented as seeming to give rise to language disturbances. These descriptions are discussed in Chapter 11. Again, the language disturbance documented in these patients is most likely caused by cortical dysfunction that is an indirect result of the subcortical damage. Metter et al[28,29] found that a subcortical lesion is accompanied by remote hypometabolism, indirectly affecting the left perisylvian area. This was found to be related to language functioning in the patients studied. In their study of patients with striato-capsular lesions (head of the caudate nucleus, anterior half of the putamen, and anterior limb of the internal capsule in these cases), Nadeau and Crosson[31] found that the infarct was caused by the spread of the thrombus or the movement of the embolus into the portion of the middle cerebral artery that serves the lenticulostriate arteries, which perfuse these structures, naturally resulting in their cellular death. However, beyond this effect, a reduced flow of blood to the middle cerebral artery branches serving the overlying cortex was also discovered. If the collateral circulation mechanisms through the anterior cerebral and posterior cerebral arteries are vital, the cortex will be minimally affected in function. If poor collateral structure and operation are present, however, a much larger stroke will occur. Despite this, the damage to the cortical region that takes place through the secondary mechanism of infarct initially is not visible on imaging studies, though cortical atrophy can be imaged later.[52] Because the mechanism of damage to cortical areas is much the same as in direct cortical damage, the resulting language disorders will predictably be of many different types depending on the site of cortical hypoperfusion.

RIGHT HEMISPHERE

The role of the right hemisphere in communication had been trivialized until relatively recently. It had been referred to as the silent, or minor, hemisphere while much of the research on the central language mechanism in the left hemisphere was being done through studies of aphasia. The right hemisphere was acknowledged as having a major role in visual perception and as having a special (perhaps minor) role in visuospatial processing. In the 1960s the technique of commissurotomy (disconnecting the two hemispheres by severing part of the corpus callosum) was found to be successful in controlling seizures if the corpus callosum was almost completely severed and the two hemispheres

almost completely disconnected. This resulted in the research on split-brain patients (see Chapter 2) and heralded a new interest in right brain function. Evidence from hemispherectomies and callosal sections suggests that the right hemisphere can assume some language function, although the extent of recovery may be limited. In adult patients with hemispherectomy with no cortical tissue remaining, language behavior is similar to that in a person with extensive infarction of the perisylvian area and a global aphasia. What language remains appears to be completely the product of the right hemisphere.

Research began later on right hemisphere function in non–brain-damaged patients. These studies have indicated that the right hemisphere differs from the left in discrete functions and in its role in communication and cognition. Myers[30] reports that research began to show that the right hemisphere was important in visual processing as well as holistic, nonlinear, and parallel processing. Important to information synthesis, the right hemisphere seemed to be superior in seeing the "big picture" or the gestalt and in incorporating and dealing with novel stimuli. The current concept of right hemisphere functions shows it to be superior for the following:

- Visuospatial processing and visual perception
- Integration of different types of incoming stimuli
- Comprehending and producing emotion in the face and voice
- Maintaining a normal state of arousal and alertness
- Attending to the left side of space
- Attention in general, selecting what to attend to and maintaining attention or shifting attention

At approximately the same time that this interest in right hemisphere processes was burgeoning, the concept of communication began to change and expand beyond the traditional informational processing input-output model. Communication style, nonverbal aspects of communication, as well as language use or the pragmatic aspects of language, were now of interest to clinicians and researchers. Speech-language pathologists, linguists, and neuropsychologists began to look at discourse versus just words, phrases, and sentences and to put much more emphasis on meaning (both literal and implied). As in research with patients with left hemisphere damage, the communication abilities of patients with right hemisphere damage were studied and analyzed. As Myers discusses throughout her book, when studying patients with right hemisphere damage who have trouble communicating normally (not all patients have difficulty), the problems clearly are not language based in the traditional sense; the patients have problems with communication in the broader context. The problems may be complex and are just beginning to be understood. Communication problems of the patient with right hemisphere damage are discussed in Chapter 11.

The right hemisphere is known to become more active in language processing after left hemisphere damage to language areas. Some treatment methods, such as melodic intonation therapy, have tried to capitalize on this neural effort by homologous areas in the nondominant hemisphere. Some evidence from **transcranial magnetic stimulation (TMS)** studies shows that this activity in the right hemisphere can be actually interfering with language recovery in the left hemisphere.[34] Improvement in naming in a person with chronic, global aphasia was noted and maintained over time after TMS treatment was targeted to inhibit function of the pars triangularis area in the right hemisphere. A negative effect occurred, however, when the inhibitory stimulation was applied to the posterior portion (pars opercularis) of the homologous Broca's area in the right hemisphere. Stimulation to other areas in the right hemisphere did not improve speech or language performance. TMS was hypothesized to suppress overactivity in the right hemisphere area of the pars triangularis and consequently improved interhemispheric modulation of semantic processing for naming pictures. Much interesting research remains to be done on the role of the right hemisphere in normal communication and recovery of language after brain insult.

ROLE OF COGNITION IN COMMUNICATION

As Chapey[7] notes in her discussion of cognitive intervention in aphasia, the definition of cognition varies greatly across the speech-language literature as well as that of other professions. An acceptable generic definition often used is that **cognition** is any process whereby an organism becomes aware of or obtains knowledge of an object.[15] Examining cognition at work is examining "functional mental events" that take place during behavior.[40] These events are such things as perception, recognition, reasoning, judgment, concept formation, and problem solving. In laying the groundwork for cognitive communicative evaluation and intervention with traumatic brain-injured patients, Gillis[18] discusses four key aspects of cognition as critical for the clinician to understand: (1) attention and information processing, (2) memory, (3) reasoning and problem solving, and (4) metacognition and executive functions. The following sections briefly describe these functions and their neurologic bases.

Attention and Information Processing

The word *attention* has many definitions. This text uses that of Solberg and Mateer,[46] who define it as "the capacity to focus on particular stimuli over time and to manipulate flexibly the information." This definition implies that an active response occurs rather than simply reflexive behavior. For attention to occur as a process, the organism must be in a general physiologic state of readiness, called arousal. Arousal, or as some have termed it, alertness, is the initial stage of attention. Arousal is mediated by the reticular activating system and is subject to internal and external influences. For attention to take place, perception must also occur. Perception is the recognition of sensory input. Gillis points out that it is often difficult to separate and distinguish perception from other aspects of cognition.

When studying attention, the organism's attentional capacity or information processing capacity and the capability for attentional control must be considered. Attentional capacity is the amount of information that can be attended to at any one time. Attentional control is the process of guiding or directing this attentional capacity where it is needed. This control may be automatic in process, such as when overlearned tasks are performed, or it may be controlled processing, which is used for novel or complex stimuli. The latter is conscious processing.

Some simply characterize attention as either intentional or reactive. However, some researchers and clinicians divide attention into different subcomponents because attentional mechanisms are seemingly not damaged in an all-or-none manner in brain injury. Solberg and Mateer[46] break attention down into five component areas: focused attention, sustained attention, selective attention, alternating attention, and divided attention.

Nadeau et al[32] present attention as a part of the more general neural process they call **selective engagement**. They describe this process in engineering terms as bringing certain neural networks (depending on the task) "online" while taking others "offline" because they are not needed for that task. This is part of the self-organizing system of the brain. Two systems are said to be critical for many of the higher level tasks that require selective engagement. These are corticocortical systems and corticothalamocortical systems. The latter was previously discussed in the section on subcortical language mechanisms. This gated relay function of the thalamus is thought to be part of the mechanism that allows the cortex to engage one neural network selectively over another.

The corticocortical system actively participating in selective engagement (a large part of which is manifest in attention) is thought to reside in the dorsolateral prefrontal cortex. This part of the cortex is the supramodal cortex involved in planning and other executive functions. It also is critical to the orienting response, allowing movement of the eyes, head, and perhaps whole body to attend to something. The neural basis of attention is strongly related to the neural basis of the orienting response. This area of the cortex seems to process the significance of neural activity communicated from posterior association areas. Studies of lesioned monkeys also indicate that this prefrontal area allows the engagement to be maintained neurally and thus process information in working memory. The next chapter discusses the attention and memory problems of patients with closed-head injury. These patients have frequently had damage impairing function of the prefrontal cortex.

Memory

Duhai[14] defines learning as an experience-dependent (including changes related to maturation, injury, and fatigue) generation of enduring internal representations or modification in these representations. Memory is the retention of these experience-dependent changes over time.[4] Separating memory from attention or from the other aspects of cognition is difficult. Memory is not a unitary construct. Varying temporal domains exist, such as short-term and long-term memory, and different stages of information processing are necessary before a memory is constructed. The first step in information processing leading to memory is a sensory store, with visual and auditory information storage being the most familiar. Some refer to the sensory storage as a sensory register because it is extremely brief in duration. Some perceptual analysis may take place at this stage, or it may simply be a brief holding tank for information that will need attention.

Sensory registration or storage initially occurs in the process of encoding or information processing for memory. Some level of meaning is extracted during encoding. A person's associations, experiences, and perceptions influence this extraction. These are unique to each individual, although everyone shares some associations. During encoding the information is organized, and the level of analysis and organization is important to its storage and later retrieval. Two main types of storage exist in many theories of memory processing: short-term memory and long-term memory. **Short-term memory** is temporary in nature, and the brain has limited capacity for this storage. Information in short-term memory must be continually acted upon (rehearsed, imaged, etc.) or the memory will decay in a brief time. The decay time posed by the research literature varies from 30 seconds to a few minutes.[18] Short-term memory and working memory are considered synonymous terms by some; others consider short-term memory as the storage site and working memory as the active processing to hold the information.[36] **Long-term**

memory is the permanent storage of information with unlimited capacity. The two primary types of knowledge store in memory are referred to as **procedural memory** (also known as implicit memory) and **declarative memory** (also known as explicit memory or propositional memory). Information thought to be stored in procedural memory is an integral part of rule-based skills and behaviors, and this type of memory can be accessed only through performance of learned behaviors. This primarily involves motor behaviors, but acquisition of some mental behaviors also is included. Nadeau and Rothi[33] proposed the concept that grammatical function depends on procedural rather than declarative memory and therefore may require a different approach in treatment than other deficits, such as semantic access problems. Declarative memory is directly accessible through recognition and recall tasks. These memories may be brought to mind verbally or visually. Semantic and episodic memory are two subdivisions of declarative memory.

Rahmann and Rahmann[38] point out that information processing and storage are immensely complex processes and that many factors still stand in the way of research aimed at localizing memory. Some of the factors listed are (1) the exceedingly complex organization of the brain with its several hundred trillion synapses, (2) the total length of all neuronal fibers in the brain (similar in length to the distance from the earth to the moon and back), and (3) the enormous number of neurons activated during each memory event. According to these authors, "memory is ultimately stored in the form of molecular changes in the synapses of the neuronal structures involved in perception, analysis, and further processing of acquired (learned) information" (p. 264). This storage is in the brain and spinal cord, not in the sensory or neuronal pathways. Research on the visual system has suggested that memory storage events may occur through reciprocal feedback mechanisms between neuronal representations in the cortex and neuronal assemblies in subcortical regions. The formation of a memory is likely caused by an alteration in the strength of neural connection. The connections are enhanced when the neurons are simultaneously active.

The two subcortical regions that participate in memory formation are thought to be the hippocampus and the amygdala. A system in the basal forebrain depends on acetylcholine transmission (a cholinergic system) to assign a certain value to the pattern of neural activity being accessed. This is a crucial task of the limbic system and the hippocampus in particular. The limbic system "judges" the neural activity regarding import and communicates this to the rostral cholinergic system that, in turn, supplies cholinergic input to the targeted cortical area. The message to the cortical area from the limbic system is that this information is important and worth learning. Chemical changes can then be facilitated in the targeted cortical area and the hippocampus that produce permanent changes in neural connectivity and establish that representation in memory. The amygdala may partially be responsible for feelings or emotions that accompany the processing of certain sensory input or certain memories.

Reasoning and Problem Solving

Reasoning is the process of evaluating information to come to a conclusion.[18] Two different types of reasoning are discussed and evaluated clinically. In deductive reasoning, a number of premises, facts, and opinions are considered and a conclusion is made about one thing (person, fact, circumstance, etc.). In inductive reasoning generalization from one fact or instance is turned into a broad interpretation. In most cases problem solving and reasoning are simultaneous mental activities performed while trying to reach a conclusion needed to solve a problem. Guilford and Hoepfner[20] think of problem solving as having five steps: preparation, analysis, production, verification, and reapplication. These steps obviously point to problem solving (and reasoning) as being a multifaceted process. Impairments in problem solving and reasoning are often associated with lesions in prefrontal regions of the brain, though subcortical damage also can cause difficulties.[49] A recent study using rats with lesioned orbitofrontal cortex demonstrated that this area appears to be important for decision making.[43] When faced with a problem to solve when a previously learned strategy did not work and a new way was needed, the neural firing rate in the orbitofrontal cortex of the lesioned animals was slow and sluggish. Consequently, they were not able to change behavior efficiently to accomplish a task under new demands. The researchers hypothesized that the orbitofrontal cortex seems to process visual and other informational cues that help make decisions in the presence of new information. Damage to this area of the brain may cause persons to have difficulty adapting their behavior to new situations despite being able to learn new information in a fairly normal way.

Metacognition and Executive Functions

Metacognition and executive functioning were not routinely discussed by speech-language pathologists until recently, when work with patients with cognitive communicative disorders became more widespread. **Metacognition** is knowledge about all cognitive processes and involves the monitoring of these processes.[18] Metacognition, then, refers to the seemingly subconscious ability to know how and when to attend, remember, and organize information and recognize and solve certain problems with certain strategies.

Executive functions refer to the skills human beings use to carry out nonroutine processes.[18] The executive functions are thought to be mediated by the prefrontal cortex in the frontal lobes. These functions include anticipation, goal direction, planning, monitoring of internal and external events, and interpretation and use of feedback. The fact that most nonroutine processes are carried out in a deliberate, coordinated manner and that human beings are typically self-regulating and able to inhibit inappropriate behaviors are testament to the executive system of the frontal lobes. Mesulam[27] notes that the prefrontal cortex of the frontal lobes is composed of a heteromodal cortex that integrates information from both unimodal and other heteromodal areas. The frontal lobes have multiple direct and indirect connections to all other areas of the brain. They are well positioned and equipped to perform this important central executive officer job. Box 10-2 summarizes the four key concepts that the clinician should consider when performing a cognitive assessment.

Changing the Brain

Any neurology text that is written is behind in its acknowledgment and explanations of new discoveries and research the day it is surrendered for publication. In the past 2 decades the research findings and the technology enabling this science to proceed has exploded. Although still slow, the transmission of these findings to others is much more rapid than once was possible. Many more journals are being published, some online, and many more conferences and other interactions are taking place. This engages other scientists and advances even more discovery.

A text such as this, with the task of teaching students the names, locations, primary purpose and physiologic mechanisms of parts of the brain most important to a certain function (in this case, communication), is of necessity simplistic in nature. It tends to present the brain as developing over time into an essentially hard-wired structure. This is not the impression that students should leave with. The brain, as implied by some studies much earlier and confirmed more and more by recent research, is an extremely flexible organ, capable of much more change and development than has previously been generally accepted by scientists and medical practitioners.

NEUROGENESIS AND NEUROPLASTICITY

Through studies duplicating earlier findings in animals, scientists seem to be accepting that new neurons are being born (**neurogenesis**) in the adult brain, at

BOX 10-2

Cognitive Factors in Communication

Attention and Information Processing

- Attention requires a certain level of arousal (alertness) as well as perception of sensory input
- Attentional capacity refers to the amount of information one can hold; it is directed by attentional control mechanisms
- Concept of attention can be considered as reactive in nature or as part of general neural processes described as selective engagement
- Thought to reside in dorsolateral prefrontal cortex, which also is involved in planning and other executive functions, the orienting response, and additional executive functioning

Memory

- Retention and recall of internal representations of experience-dependent changes over time
- Visual and auditory sensory storage that can be broken into two types of information processing:
  - Short-term memory—temporary storage that begins to decay in 30 seconds to a few minutes
  - Long-term memory—permanent storage of unlimited capacity
- Two kinds of information stored in memory:
  - Procedural (implicit) memory—recalled from performance of repetitive, learned motor behaviors over time
  - Declarative (explicit) memory—recalled through verbal or visual sensory recognition and recall cues

Reasoning and Problem Solving

- Two types of reasoning:
  - Deductive reasoning—evaluation based on a number of facts to create a conclusion about one thing (person, fact, event, etc.)
  - Inductive reasoning—evaluation based on generalization of one fact to create a broad interpretation and conclusion
- Problem solving involves evaluation based on reasoning and application to produce a conclusion
- Lesions to the prefrontal and subcortical areas have been shown to impair both reasoning and problem-solving processes

Metacognition and Executive Functioning

- Metacognition refers to the ability to recognize how and when to use reasoning and problem-solving skills to solve specific problems with the most effective cognitive strategies
- Executive functions include anticipation, goal direction, planning, monitoring of internal and external events, and feedback interpretation
- Frontal lobes carry out metacognitive and executive functioning processes

least in the hippocampus.[16,44,50] The neurons are able to generate because the brain has a reserve of neural stem cells that can differentiate themselves into neurons or other cells of the nervous system. These new neurons can make new connections and establish themselves into functional circuits that already exist, enhancing the structure as well as the function. Thus even the adult brain is now believed to demonstrate neuroplasticity, though certainly not to as great an extent as that of a young child.

Just how much **neuroplasticity** the brain is capable of demonstrating has been surprising. Studies of congenitally blind persons who use Braille have demonstrated that the visual cortex, along with the somatosensory cortex, is activated when Braille is being read.[42] An early study[35] showed the same kind of reorganization in the brains of adults deaf since birth or early childhood when evoked potentials were measured in response to a flash of light. The response of persons who were deaf to the flash was stronger than that of normal hearing subjects and was registered from the auditory cortex rather than the visual cortex. This indicated that the brain's auditory region, denied of its normal input, had somehow begun picking up signals from the retinas. Visual cortex activity has been found in blind adult subjects when verbal processing tasks also are studied.[2] When the visual cortex was inhibited in these subjects, performance deteriorated, confirming the primary participation of the visual cortex.[1] This may help explain why blind children often are found to be delayed in language development.

The findings of many studies of neuroplasticity in different regions of the brain support the concept that the brain does organize and, in many cases, reorganize itself according to what it experiences.[5] Studies in language development of children deprived of auditory stimulation certainly support this. Animal studies of "enriched environments" and the consequent effect on learning as well as neural development also strongly support this.

Many studies wait to be done based on the belief and increasingly documented evidence that brain development can be enhanced through structured experiences. Ways to be more effective in the educational system, train new skills in adults, and maintain optimal cognitive function into advanced age must be found. Further research in neuroscience will pave the way for this progress.

RECOVERY IN THE DAMAGED BRAIN

Speech-language pathologists must believe that the brain can change and reorganize. If they did not, no one would show up to work every day to treat clients attempting to improve their communication skills. Research in neuroscience supports the belief that a permanent change in behavior does involve a change in brain organization. This does not mean change only in the strength of connections in the neural networks involved in the behavior, as takes place when memories are formed. It also may mean a change in where in the brain these connections are made or in which pathways are used—a type of "rezoning" or reassignment of the duties of cells in a certain part of the brain. With better technology and more elegant research design, we will one day perhaps be able to know exactly what changes are taking place in the brain during successful (or in some cases, unsuccessful) treatment for a communication disorder.

One new treatment method that has resulted from the curiosity of a neuroscientist about brain reorganization and its usefulness in rehabilitation is **constraint-induced therapy (CIT)**, introduced by Taub et al[47] for improving the use of the paralyzed arm after a stroke. In CIT the functional arm is restrained in a sling, with the hand covered to prevent use. In the initial study, the patients who were 1 year or more poststroke received intensive treatment for 10 days and performed all tasks for most of their waking hours with the paralyzed limb as best they could. At the end of the 10-day period, clients had regained considerable functional use of the formerly paralyzed limb, whereas control subjects who did not receive treatment showed no change. Taub hypothesized a "use-dependent cortical reorganization." Investigation using TMS to map the cortical activity before and after CIT proved Taub's hypothesis.[21] Treatment resulted in improved motor functioning and caused the area of the motor cortex controlling the hand to enlarge with recruitment of more neurons in the motor cortex, particularly those adjacent to the area that originally controlled the arm. With more extensive damage to the motor cortex, neurons in the premotor cortex or even in the opposite hemisphere are hypothesized to participate in the network supporting the improved function.

The strong evidence for success with CIT for paralyzed limbs of stroke patients[48] led to interest in CIT for improvement of communication in persons with aphasia. Several studies were initially performed in Europe showing that constraint-induced aphasia therapy involving the principles of prevention of compensatory communication and massed practice produced significant and stable improvement. Changes in performance on standardized testing as well as in communication as measured by patient and family report and communicative effectiveness ratings were all significantly greater than for patients who participated in the same amount of therapy with more traditional treatment methods allowing compensatory communication use.[26] A pilot study from the Houston Veterans Administration Hospital also demonstrated more consistent improvement of patients receiving constraint-induced language therapy when compared with more traditional treatment, though both groups had positive outcomes.[23] The conclusion is that use-dependent learning may be a viable tool for improving communication after stroke. Evidence is being amassed and studies of the changes in brain organization ideally will follow.

Students interested in more in-depth study of the brain's capacity for change are encouraged to begin by reading a recently published book by the science columnist for the *Wall Street Journal*, Sharon Begley.[5] The book, titled *Train Your Mind, Change Your Brain*, seems at first glance at the title like one of the pseudo-science self-help texts that are stacked high in bookstores. However, the book documents the collaboration between leading scientists, many of whom are referenced in this text, and the Dali Lama, which resulted in a landmark study at the University of Wisconsin on brain reorganization and differences in monks who are highly advanced in meditation.[22] It also provides a highly readable summary of the history of neuroscientific study of brain-behavior relations and how the brain is transformed by the environment, experience, and thought.

This chapter ends on a positive note for the clinician because of the work of neuroscientists to prove that the brain can be changed by chemical and surgical intervention as well as by behavioral treatments that replace or supplement other treatments. Chapter 11 describes some of the acquired disorders of communication that adults may experience when damage occurs to language processing areas of the brain. It is hoped that clinicians will not only learn from the literature of neuroscience, but will continue to contribute findings that support enhancement of brain function even after the brain has been damaged.

Synopsis of Clinical Information and Applications for the Speech-Language Pathologist

- Six layers comprise the neocortex, consisting primarily of pyramidal cells with axons and dendrites ascending and descending from one layer to another.
- Synaptic organization is concerned with the way input neurons, projection neurons, and interneurons organize themselves and connect through synapses, becoming neural circuits.
- Dendritic connections and subunits within microcircuits form local circuits in regions of the brain. The connections between these regions and their circuits account for behaviors.
- The brain's vast circuitry is made possible by convergence and divergence of synapses in the nervous system.
- Most postsynaptic sites in the cerebellum, basal ganglia, and cortex are on dendritic spines, increasing the surface area and probably enabling rapid signal processing and long-term potentiation.
- The existence of neural networks involved in parallel distributed processing (PDP) has begun to explain how information is transferred in the brain.
- In autoassociator networks, each unit in the network is connected to every other unit, storing the associations within the layers and capable of storing many patterns within the connections.
- A pattern-associator network allows the input patterns to be transformed into output patterns (e.g., sequences of letters transformed into spoken words read aloud).
- All the primary association areas are thought to be collections of pattern-associator networks in which neural representations (percepts, concepts, etc.) are formed. Information for these representations is stored in the connections, and the connections are strengthened by practice, exposure, learning, and so forth.
- This pattern of connections strengthened into a representation is difficult to lose completely. Rather, some components of the representation may be activated though others are not, degrading the representation. This is called "graceful degradation." This often allows people to deal successfully with ambiguous or partial information.

- Geschwind's model of language, based in large part on the work of Wernicke, is a traditional localization or connectionism model but has held up over time and is not negated by neural network theory or by evidence from neuroimaging. However, other areas of the brain function fairly well in language production and comprehension in some circumstances.
- Geschwind's model emphasizes Broca's area, Wernicke's area, the arcuate fasciculus, and parietal areas of the angular and supramarginal gyrus. These areas comprise the perisylvian language zone.
- Language disorders appear to result from damage to subcortical structures, especially the thalamus and parts of the basal ganglia. However, research into the etiology of the language difficulty has demonstrated that the language disorders result from the indirect effects on cortical language areas. A thalamic gating mechanism is theorized to exist that assists in engagement of different association cortices in declarative memory tasks for lexical-semantic access. Patients with thalamic damage primarily have difficulty with naming.
- Hypoperfusion of the cortex follows basal ganglia and capsular damage because of reduced flow through the lenticulostriate arteries. The language symptoms depend on what area of the perisylvian zone is affected.
- The right hemisphere is dominant for visuospatial processing, integration of different kinds of stimuli, attention, intention, and holistic processing. Right hemisphere damage affects communication in a broader sense with discourse and communication style as well as processing of more intangible input (e.g., humor, sarcasm).
- Cognition is the process by which an organism obtains knowledge of an object. It is the examination of mental events, such as perception, reasoning, problem solving, and concept formation.
- Four key aspects of cognition important to the treatment of patients with cognitive-linguistic disorders are (1) attention and information processing,

Continued

Synopsis of Clinical Information and Applications for the Speech-Language Pathologist—cont'd

(2) memory, (3) reasoning and problem solving, and (4) metacognition and executive functioning. The study of these cognitive functions involves the dorsolateral cortex, the hippocampus and amygdala, orbitofrontal cortex, and the greater association area in the frontal lobes.

- New neuroimaging techniques and interest in neurogenesis (the birth of new neurons) and neuroplasticity of the brain have spawned exciting research into enhanced learning and recovery after brain damage.
- New treatment methods such as CIT are being developed on the basis of this research and knowledge.

CASE**STUDY**

A 64-year-old former van driver experienced sudden onset of confusion, slurred speech, and left-sided paralysis of the arm and leg. He was admitted to the hospital stroke unit and begun on blood thinners after computed tomography ruled out hemorrhage. He was admitted to the acute rehabilitation unit in 2 days. Testing showed mild unilateral upper motor neuron dysarthria with fair intelligibility, poor pragmatics (poor eye contact, inattention to speaker if on his left, poor topic maintenance, apathy during communication), mild to moderate neglect of left side of space, mild anomia on confrontation naming and questioning, and constructional deficits in drawing and copying. After a 3-week stay, he was ambulatory with a leg brace, had little functional use of his left upper extremity, had improved intelligibility, and was learning to compensate for his left side neglect.

QUESTIONS FOR CONSIDERATION:
1. What part(s) of the brain were affected by this stroke?
2. Why is neglect more prominent with this location of damage to the brain?
3. What could be the cause of the perception of apathy in the patient's communication interactions?

REFERENCES

1. Amedi, A., Floel, A., Knecht, S., Zohary, E., & Cohen, L. G. (2004). Transcranial magnetic stimulation of the occipital pole interferes with verbal processing in blind subjects. *Nature Neuroscience, 7*, 1266-1270.
2. Amedi, A., Raz, N., Pianka, R., Malach, R., & Zohary, E. (2003). Early visual cortex activation correlates with superior verbal memory performance in the blind. *Nature Neuroscience, 6*, 758-766.
3. Barlow, H. B. (1972). Single units and sensation: a neuron doctrine for perceptual psychology. *Perception, 1*, 371-394.
4. Baxter, H. F., & Baxter, D. A. (1999). Neural mechanisms of learning and memory. In Cohen, H. (Ed.), *Neuroscience for rehabilitation*. Philadelphia: Lippincott Williams & Wilkins.
5. Begley, S. (2007). *Train your mind, change your brain*. New York: Ballantine Books.
6. Buckingham, H. W., Jr. (1982). Neuropsychological models of language. In Lass, N., McReynolds, L., Northern, J., & Yoder, D. (Eds.), *Speech, language, and hearing (vol. 1)*. Philadelphia: W. B. Saunders.
7. Chapey, R. (2001). Cognitive intervention: Stimulation of cognition, memory, convergent thinking, divergent thinking and evaluative thinking. In Chapey, R. (Ed.), *Language intervention strategies in adult aphasia* (4th ed.). Baltimore: Williams & Wilkins.
8. Code, C. (Ed.) (1990). *The characteristics of aphasia*. New York: Taylor and Francis.
9. Coltheart, M. (1987). Functional architecture of the language processing system. In Coltheart, M., Samtori, G., & Fob, R. (Eds.), *The cognitive neuropsychology of language*. London: Lawrence Erlbaum and Associates.
10. Coltheart, M., Patterson, K., & Marshall, J. C. (Eds.) (1980). *Deep dyslexia*. London: Routledge and Kegan Paul.
11. Crosson, B. (1992). *Subcortical functions in language and memory*. New York: Guilford Press.
12. Dejerine, J. (1891). Sur un cas de cecite verbal avec agraphie, suivi d'autopsie. Mémoires de la Société de Biologie *3*, 197-201.
13. Dejerine, J. (1892). Contributions à l'étude anatomo-pathologique et clinique des différentes variétés de cécité. Mémoires de la Société de Biologie, *4*, 61-90.
14. Dudai, Y. (1989). *The neurobiology of memory: concepts, findings, trends*. New York: Oxford University Press.
15. English, H. B., & English, A. C. (1958). *A comprehensive dictionary of psychological and psychoanalytic terms*. New York: McKay.
16. Eriksson, P. S., Perfilieva, E., Bjork-Eriksson, T., Alborn, A. M., Nordborg, C., Peterson, D. A., & Gage, F. H. (1998). Neurogenesis in the adult human hippocampus. *Nature Medicine, 4*, 1313-1317.

17. Geschwind, N. (1969). Problems in the anatomical understanding of aphasia. In Benton, A. L. (Ed.), *Contributions to clinical neuropsychology*. Chicago: Aldine.

18. Gillis, R. J. (1996). *Traumatic brain injury: rehabilitation for speech-language pathologists*. Boston: Butterworth-Heinemann.

19. Gough, P. M., Nobre, A. C., & Devlin, J. T. (2005). Dissociating linguistic processes in the left inferior frontal cortex with transcranial magnetic stimulation. *Journal of Neuroscience, 25*, 8010-8016.

20. Guilford, J. P., & Hoepfner, R. V. (1971). *The analysis of intelligence*. New York: McGraw-Hill.

21. Liepert, J., Bauder, H., Wolfgang, H. R., Miltner, W. H., Taub, E., & Weiller, C. (2000). Treatment-induced cortical reorganization after stroke in humans. *Stroke, 6*, 1210-1216.

22. Lutz, A., Greischar, L. L., Rawlings, N. B., Richard, M., & Davidson, R. J. (2004). Long-term meditators self-induce high-amplitude gamma synchrony during mental practice. *Proceedings of the National Academy of Sciences, 101*, 16369-16273.

23. Maher, L. M., Kendall, D., Swearengin, J. A., Rodriguez, A., Leon, S. A., Pingel, K., Holland, A., & Rothi, L. J. (2006). A pilot study of use-dependent learning in the context of constraint-induced language therapy. *Journal of the International Neuropsychological Society, 12*, 843-852.

24. Marin, O. S. M. (1982). Brain and language: the rules of the game. In Arbib, M. A., Caplan, D., & Marshall, J. C. (Eds.), *Neural models of language processes*. London: Academic Press.

25. Marshall, J. C. (1985). On some relationships between acquired and developmental dyslexias. In Duffy, F. H., & Geschwind, N. (Eds.), *Dyslexia: a neuroscientific approach to clinical evaluation*. Boston: Little, Brown and Company.

26. Meinzer, M., Djundja, D., Barthel, G., Elbert, T., & Rockstroh, B. (2005). Long-term stability of improved language functions in chronic aphasia after constraint-induced aphasia therapy. *Stroke, 36*, 1462-1466.

27. Mesulam, M. M. (1985). *Principles of behavioral neurology*. Boston: F. A. Davis.

28. Metter, E. I., Riege, W. H., Hanson, W. R., Jackson, C. A., Kempler, D., & van Lancker, D. (1988). Subcortical structures in aphasia: an analysis based on (F-18)-fluorodeoxyglucose, positron emission tomography, and computed tomography. *Archives of Neurology, 45*, 1229-1234.

29. Metter, E. J., Riege, W. H., Hanson, W. R., Kuhl, D. E., Phelps, M. E., Squire, L. R., Wasterlain, C. G., & Benson, D. F. (1983). Comparison of metabolic rates, language, and memory in subcortical aphasias. *Brain and Language, 19*, 33-47.

30. Myers, P. S. (1994) Communication disorders associated with right-hemisphere brain damage. In Chapey, R. (Ed.), *Language intervention strategies in adult aphasia* (3rd ed.). Baltimore: Williams & Wilkins.

31. Nadeau, S. E., & Crosson, B. (1997). Subcortical aphasia. *Brain and Language, 58*, 355-402, 436-458.

32. Nadeau, S. E., Ferguson, T. S., Valenstein, E., Vierck, C. J., Petruska, J. C., Streit, W. J., & Ritz, L. A. (2004). *Medical neuroscience*. St. Louis: Saunders Elsevier.

33. Nadeau, S., & Rothi, L. G. (2001). Rehabilitation of subcortical aphasia. In Chapey, R. (Ed.), *Language intervention strategies in adult aphasia* (4th ed.). Baltimore: Williams & Wilkins.

34. Naeser, M. E., Martin, P. I., Nichols, M., Baker, E. H., Seekins, H., Helm-Estabrooks, N., Cayer-Meade, C., Kobayaski., M, Theoret, H., Fregni, F., Tormos, J. M., Kuran, J., Doran, K., and Pascual-Leone, A. (2005). Improved naming after TMS treatments in a chronic, global aphasia patient—case report. *Neurocase, 11*, 182-193.

35. Neville, H. J., Schmidt, A., & Kutas, M. (1983). Altered visual-evoked potentials in congenitally deaf adults. *Brain Research, 266*, 127-132.

36. Parenté, R., & DiCesare, A. (1991). Retraining memory: theory, evaluation, and applications. In Kreutzer, J., & Wehman, P. (Eds.), *Cognitive rehabilitation for persons with traumatic brain injury*. Baltimore: Paul H. Brookes.

37. Penfield, W. G., & Roberts, L. (1959). *Speech and brain mechanisms*. Princeton, NJ: Princeton University Press.

38. Rahmann, H., & Rahmann, M. (1992). *The neurobiological basis of memory and behavior*. New York: Springer-Verlag.

39. Roeltgen, D. P., & Heilman, K. M. (1985). Review of agraphia and a proposal for an anatomically-based neuropsychological model of writing. *Applied Psycholinguistics, 6*, 205-230.

40. Rosenthal, T., & Zimmerman, B. (1978). *Social learning and cognition*. New York: Academic Press.

41. Rothi, L. G., & Moss, S. E. (1985). *Alexia/agraphia in brain-damaged adults*. Presented at the American Speech-Language-Hearing Association Convention, Washington, D. C.

42. Sadato, N. (1996). Activation of the primary visual cortex by Braille reading in blind subjects. *Nature, 380*, 526-528.

43. Saddoris, M. P., Gallagher, M., & Schoenbaum, G. (2005). Rapid associative encoding in basolateral amygdala depends on connections with orbitofrontal cortex. *Neuron, 46*, 321-331.

44. Santarelli, I., Saxe, M., Gross, A., Surget, A., Battaglia, F., Dulawa, S., & Weisstaub, N. (2003). Requirement for hippocampal neurogenesis for behavioral effects of antidepressants. *Science, 301*, 805-809.

45. Shepherd, G. M., & Koch, C. (1998). Introduction to synaptic circuits. In Shepherd, G. M. (Ed.), *The synaptic organization of the brain* (4th ed.). New York: Oxford University Press.

46. Solberg, M. M., & Mateer, C. A. (1987). Effectiveness of an attention-training program. *Journal of Clinical and Experimental Neuropsychology, 9*, 117-130.

47. Taub, E., Miller, N. E., Novack, T. A., Cook E.W., III, Fleming, W. C., Nepomuceno, J. S., & Crago, J. E. (1993). Technique to improve chronic motor deficit after stroke. *Archives of Physical Medicine and Rehabilitation, 74*, 347-354.

48. Taub, E., Uswatte, G., King, D. K., Morris, D., Crago, J. E., & Chatterjee, A. (2006). A placebo-controlled trial of constraint-induced movement therapy for upper extremity after stroke. *Stroke, 37,* 1045-1049.

49. Tompkins, C. A. (1995). *Right hemisphere communication disorders: theory and management.* San Diego: Singular Publishing Group, Inc.

50. Van Praag, H., Christie, B. R., Sejnowski, T. J., & Gage, F. H. (2002). Functional neurogenesis in the adult hippocampus. *Nature, 415,* 1030-1034.

51. Wallesch, C. W., & Papagno, C. (1988). Subcortical aphasia. In Rose, F. C., Whurr, R., & Wyke, M. A. (Eds.), *Aphasia.* London: Whurr.

52. Weiller, C., Willmes, K., Reiche, W., Thron, A., Insensee, C., Buell, U., & Ringelstein, E. B. (1993). The case of aphasia or neglect after striatocapsular infarction. *Brain, 116,* 1509-1525.

53. Wernicke, K. (1874). *Der aphasische symptomkomplex.* Breslau: Kohn and Neigert.

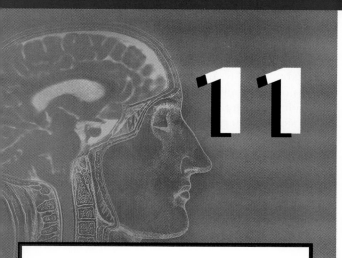

11

Adult Disorders of Language

Let the young know they will never find a more interesting,
more instructive book than the patient himself.

—Giorgio Baglivi

KEY TERMS

acceleration-
 deceleration injury
agraphia
alexia
alexia with agraphia
alexia without agraphia
Alzheimer's disease
amyloid plaques
aneurysm
anomic aphasia
aphasia
aphasic alexia
aprosodia
arteriosclerosis
arteriovenous
 malformation (AVM)
border zone
Broca's aphasia
capsular
central (parietal-
 temporal) alexia
cerebrovascular
 accident (CVA)
circumlocution
cognitive-
 communicative
 disorders
conduction aphasia
confabulation
confusional state
deep dyslexia
dementia
dementia of the
 Alzheimer's type (DAT)
diffuse axonal injury
 (DAI)

dyslexia
dysprosody
encephalopathy
extinction
focal lesions
frontal alexia
frontotemporal
 dementias (FTD)
glioma
global aphasia
ischemia
neoplasm
neologistic jargon
 aphasia
neurofibrillary
 tangles
paraphasia
phonologic alexia
Pick's disease
posterior (occipital)
 alexia
primary progressive
 aphasia (PPA)
prosopagnosia
subcortical aphasia
surface dyslexia
thrombus
transcortical
 aphasia
transient ischemic
 attack (TIA)
traumatic brain
 injury (TBI)
unilateral
 inattention
Wernicke's aphasia

CHAPTER OUTLINE

Aphasia
Etiology and Neuropathology of Aphasia
 Cerebrovascular Accident
  Occlusive mechanisms
  Hemorrhage
   Cerebral aneurysm
   Arteriovenous malformation
 Neoplasms in the Brain
Aphasia Classification
 Dichotomous Classification
 Classifications under the Boston System
  Broca's aphasia
  Wernicke's aphasia
  Conduction aphasia
  Global aphasia
  Transcortical aphasias
  Anomic aphasia
  Subcortical aphasia
Testing and Intervention for Aphasia
Role of the Speech-Language Pathologist
Pharmacology in Aphasia
Associated Central Disturbances
Alexia
 Alexia without Agraphia
 Alexia with Agraphia
 Aphasic Alexia
Psycholinguistic Classifications
Agraphia
Cognitive-Communicative Disorders
Communication Disorders Related to Right Hemisphere
 Damage
 Neglect, Inattention, and Denial
 Prosopagnosia
 Visual-Perceptual Deficits
 Spatial Organizational Deficits
 Language Disorders of Visual-Spatial Perception
 Prosodic Deficits

The speech-language pathologist (SLP) who chooses a career path working with adults quite often works with patients with acquired neurogenic language disorders. This chapter discusses language disorders that have focal brain damage as the etiology—aphasia, alexia, and agraphia—as well as disorders of communication referred to as cognitive-communicative (or cognitive-linguistic) disorders. Although communication disorders of patients with right hemisphere lesions and dementia are not treated as intensively by the SLP as are the aphasias and the problems resulting from traumatic brain injury, the SLP should understand the underlying pathology, the communication deficits, and the contribution the SLP can make to the quality of life for these patients.

Aphasia

Persons with brain damage that is focal in nature and affects the functioning of the cortical and/or subcortical language mechanisms of the dominant hemisphere (i.e., in most people, the left hemisphere) may experience some form of aphasia. **Aphasia** is defined by Rosenbek et al[39] as follows: "Aphasia is an impairment, due to acquired and recent damage of the central nervous system, of the ability to comprehend and formulate language. It is a multimodality disorder represented by a variety of impairments in auditory comprehension, reading, oral-expressive language, and writing. The disrupted language may be influenced by physiological inefficiency or impaired cognition, but it cannot be explained by dementia, sensory loss or motor dysfunction."

Etiology and Neuropathology of Aphasia

As stated previously, aphasia results from focal damage to areas of the brain that are primarily responsible for the understanding and production of language. A focal lesion is different from diffuse damage to several parts of the brain. **Focal lesions** are caused by interruption in the blood flow to the area of the brain supplied by the particular arterial distribution. The blood supply to the brain is discussed in Chapter 2 and should be reviewed to understand the discussion of etiology of aphasia. Figure 11-1 elaborates slightly on what is presented in Chapter 2, showing the branches of the middle cerebral artery, also known as the "artery of aphasia." It clearly demonstrates that the middle cerebral artery perfuses most of the perisylvian language areas.

Reduction of blood flow to an area is called **ischemia**. Blood carries oxygen to the brain, which is the biggest user of oxygen, consuming approximately 20% of the body's supply at any given time. Without an ongoing flow of oxygenated blood, the brain cannot function for long. If the brain is deprived of blood for approximately 10 to 12 seconds, the average person will lose consciousness; after 3 to 5 minutes irreparable brain damage or death may result. Exceptions exist, such as interruption to blood flow in the presence of hypothermia. The reduction in body temperature seems to have a protective effect on the brain, reducing the consequences of reduction of flow. When an area of the brain is damaged because of a lack of blood, cell death or infarction has occurred. If an area of the brain is infarcted, necrotic tissue then remains in that area. Eventually the infarcted area softens and liquefies, with this waste removed, probably by astroglial action (gliosis). This usually leaves a cavity that has the appearance of a crater in the brain with a rim of scar tissue around it formed by the astrocytes.

Several different medical conditions may interrupt the vital oxygenated blood supply to the brain. These include cerebrovascular accident, trauma, brain infections leading to focal abscess, vasculitis (or arteritis), and neoplasm. Trauma is discussed later in this chapter, though we will be emphasizing the diffuse damage that results in a cognitive-communicative disorder rather than the focal damage that can occur and result in an aphasia. Keep this in mind while studying the trauma section. The following discussion of common causes of interruption to blood flow concentrates on CVA and neoplasms.

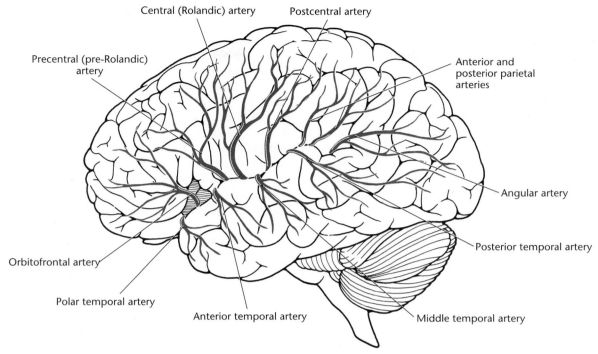

Figure **11-1**
Branches of the middle cerebral artery on the lateral surface of the hemisphere. Polar temporal and anterior arteries are branches of M_1; the remaining arteries represent branches of M_4. (Reprinted from Haines, D. [2006]. *Fundamental neuroscience* [3rd ed.]. Philadelphia: Churchill Livingstone.)

CEREBROVASCULAR ACCIDENT

The most frequent cause of interrupted blood flow is **cerebrovascular accident (CVA)**, also known as stroke (or "a brain attack"). Stroke, although decreasing in incidence in the United States, is the third leading cause of death in persons older than 55 years, and approximately 700,000 strokes occur per year according to the American Heart Association. CVA can result from two different mechanisms of interruption: occlusion or hemorrhage.

Occlusive Mechanisms

In a stroke of occlusive origin, the opening of an arterial vessel has been occluded, reducing or stopping the flow of blood through that artery. The most common cause of arterial occlusion is a disease process known as **arteriosclerosis**, which is characterized by a thickening or hardening of the arterial wall with consequent reduction of elasticity of the vessel. The diagnosis of atherosclerosis is frequently made before or after CVA and indicates a form of arteriosclerosis in which blood vessel walls thicken. This thickening is caused by

a proliferation of cells, particularly blood platelets, along the wall. Also found are abnormal fatty deposits in the artery with deterioration of the inner coating of the wall, again resulting in loss of elasticity, or fibrosis, of the vessel wall. The thickening plaques on the wall continue to enlarge and hinder diffusion of nutrients from blood to deeper tissue of the wall. This results in fraying and ulceration of the wall. Eventually a protrusion into the vessel begins to build up. If this accumulation is formed exclusively of blood platelets, it is known as a **thrombus**. As the deterioration of the wall begins to build in the vessel, the wall increases in rigidity, leading to a rise in hypertension (high blood pressure), which puts the person at an even higher risk for CVA.

Current thinking is that most CVAs are embolic in origin, meaning that this extraneous material in the vessel has occluded a cerebral vessel distal to the point of origin. This embolus has broken away from the vessel wall, traveled through the vessel and become lodged in some part of the brain, stopping or disrupting the flow through that vessel's distribution (Fig. 11-2). If a thrombus has built up on a vessel wall and completely occluded the vessel at that point, the CVA would be

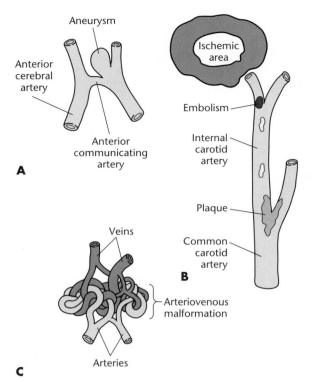

FIGURE 11-2
An aneurysm (**A**), an embolism (**B**), and an arteriovenous malformation (**C**). (From Haines, D. [2006]. *Fundamental neuroscience* [3rd ed.]. Philadelphia: Churchill Livingstone.)

considered thrombotic in origin, but that is often quite difficult to determine and the diagnosis may often be thromboembolic stroke. This kind of occlusion may take minutes or weeks to clog an artery fully. The resulting dysfunction arises suddenly and increases in severity over minutes, hours, or even days. When the symptoms seem to increase, it is referred to as "stroke in evolution" and it may proceed in a stepwise fashion. The maximal deficit is referred to as a completed stroke.

The most common source of emboli is the heart. Other extraneous material building up in the vessel may be tumor cells, a clump of bacteria, air, or plaque from the fatty deterioration. Emboli may also be a secondary effect of trauma. With an embolus that suddenly reaches a point at which it cannot continue flowing with the blood through the artery, the time for occlusion is quicker or more abrupt and the time to maximal deficit may be seconds or minutes.

Another term heard when working with patients with compromised vascular systems is **transient ischemic attack (TIA)**. A TIA is often referred to by the layperson as a "mini stroke," which is acceptable because the symptoms often mimic the effects of a completed stroke. However, with a TIA the disruption of

blood flow is temporary and the neurologic signs are transient, lasting usually less than 1 hour and completed within 24 hours. The occurrence of a TIA usually indicates that platelet formation is underway, generally in the internal carotid artery distribution. There is a 20% chance of suffering a stroke during the first year after the TIA and a 30% to 60% chance within 5 years. A TIA is a warning and should be taken seriously.

Hemorrhage

The rupture of a vessel in the brain causes a cerebral hemorrhage. Trauma to the brain often results in hemorrhage into the subarachnoid area and can cause hemorrhaging into other areas. The two most common causes of hemorrhage of a cerebral artery without trauma occurring are rupture of an aneurysm and arteriovenous malformation.

Cerebral Aneurysm

An **aneurysm** is a dilated blood vessel, usually an artery, that involves a stretching of all layers of the wall, weakening the vessel. Often the weak part of the wall can be seen extending from the vessel surface (see Fig. 11-2). Approximately 85% of aneurysms are found on branches of the internal carotid artery system, with 10% to 15% in the vertebrobasilar distribution.[18]

Points at which cerebral vessels branch off or make a sharp turn are the most vulnerable for aneurysm development. Many of the aneurysms are congenital in nature. Hemorrhage into the subarachnoid space is referred to as a subarachnoid hemorrhage and in the brain proper as an intracerebral hemorrhage. Small aneurysms may never rupture and remain silent throughout life. Large aneurysms may cause symptoms before rupture because they compress adjacent structures, such as cranial nerve roots.

Arteriovenous Malformation

Arteriovenous malformation (AVM) occurs when the capillary network between arteries and veins is absent and vessels are twisted and tangled (see Fig. 11-2). This is presumably a congenital condition and may not be detected until a seizure or a hemorrhage occurs. An aneurysm can grow and change in configuration and may damage adjacent structures. With deterioration of the walls in these abnormal vessels, a hemorrhage can occur into the subarachnoid space, brain tissue, ventricles, or brainstem, depending on where the AVM is located.

NEOPLASMS IN THE BRAIN

A **neoplasm** is an abnormal mass of tissue, better known as a tumor. Benign tumors do not spread and are not recurrent. Malignant tumors expand and are resistant to treatment, though new treatments are being developed daily. As a brain tumor spreads, it presses on adjacent structures and may invade and destroy the tissue, obstructing circulation. If the damage is directly to the language areas or indirectly affects normal function of the language mechanisms, an aphasia may result. With a slow-growing tumor, the surrounding tissue may accommodate it for a time with few symptoms noted.

Tumors are classified according to their origin, with the most common source in the brain being the neuroglia; the term **glioma** is the general name for a tumor arising from these supportive tissues of the brain. Of the gliomas, astrocytomas, ependymomas, oligodendrogliomas, and tumors with mixtures of two or more cell types (fibrillary astrocytomas) are the most common primary brain tumors in adults. In the medical workup the tumor is graded, indicating its tendency to spread. Tumors with distinct borders are classified as grade I because they usually are benign, do not grow, or grow slowly. Grade IV indicates a fast-growing, destructive tumor.

As previously stated, any condition or disease process that can damage a blood vessel carrying blood to the brain, and thus oxygen, can result in a focal lesion affecting function of the language areas of the brain.

Aphasia Classification

The aphasia literature is characterized by a proliferation of clinical classification schemes. The history of aphasia is peopled by students of the disorder who either communicated poorly to each other about the disorder or were in clear disagreement about the nature of the syndromes. Syndromes were often named or classified in terms of personal bias. This situation has resulted in a number of confusing classification systems. Similar names in two classification systems may be used to describe radically different language syndromes, each with strikingly different lesion sites.

SLPs who have devised classification systems have generally disregarded the site of lesion in their systems, basing their classifications on patterns of performance on standardized language tests. Tests that use classification systems based on performance alone, rather than extensive neurologic data, are Wepman and Jones' Language Modalities Test for Aphasia,[45] Schuell's Minnesota Test for Differential Diagnosis of Aphasia,[41] and the Porch Index of Communicative Ability.[35,36] The approach to classification based on language performance alone has further complicated the issue of classification.

DICHOTOMOUS CLASSIFICATION

Patients commonly are broadly classified into one of two categories on the basis of the general locus of the presumed lesion before specific syndromes are identified. The dichotomous classification of receptive and expressive aphasia, introduced in 1935 by the neurologist Theodore Weisenburg and the psychologist Katherine McBride, has been one of the most widely used modern divisions. Expressive aphasia generally is associated with anterior lesions and receptive aphasia with posterior lesions.

The motor and sensory division of aphasia introduced by Wernicke has been widely used. Motor aphasia usually implies an anterior cortical pathology, usually located in the frontal lobe. Sensory aphasia implies a posterior lesion in the temporal lobe. Some experts have done away with the classic terms "motor" and "sensory" and directly classify the aphasias as anterior and posterior, referring to lesion site.

A widely used dichotomy for spontaneous language in aphasia is fluent versus nonfluent. All persons with aphasia show some degree of expressive involvement in conversational language, and, for most, their expressive language can be appropriately described as fluent or nonfluent. In general, the person with a fluent aphasia has expressive output that is perceived by the listener (even a listener unfamiliar with the language) as smooth and effortless, though some speakers show a hyperfluency in which the output is constant and fairly unrelenting. A person with a nonfluent aphasia, on the other hand, is perceived by the listener as having difficulty with getting words out, with notable hesitancies, revisions, inappropriate silences, and perhaps even visible struggle. This dichotomy often is considered to be better than classification as expressive versus receptive because it recognizes that practically all persons with aphasia demonstrate some expressive difficulty.

Much of the supposed confusion in classification is artificial. In general, more agreement exists on the critical features that distinguish various aphasia syndromes than on the names applied to them. The syndromes of the language area, or perisylvian zone, are the most widely accepted of the aphasic syndromes. These include Broca's, Wernicke's, and global aphasia, generally considered the most common aphasic syndromes. Conduction aphasia is a less-common perisylvian syndrome. The transcortical aphasias and various alexic or agraphic syndromes have their lesion sites outside the perisylvian zone, and they are even less common. These syndromes became popular as the primary classification system for aphasias that could be grouped by pattern of performance. The research and development supporting two assessment instruments still in use today, the

Western Aphasia Battery[21] and the *Boston Diagnostic Aphasia Exam*[15] resulted in the widespread use of this classification system known as the Boston Classification System.

CLASSIFICATIONS UNDER THE BOSTON SYSTEM

Broca's Aphasia

Broca's aphasia is marked by nonfluent conversation, decreased verbal output, increased effort in speaking, shortened sentence length, **dysprosody**, and agrammatism (reduction of syntactic filler words with retention of nouns, verbs, and adjectives). Motor speech disorders often are present, such as apraxia of speech and dysarthria. Some neurologists believe that what are referred to as speech apraxic symptoms by SLPs are merely a form of transient nonfluent aphasia. Lesions limited to Broca's area alone produce speech apraxia or this form of transient aphasia. More widespread lesions produce a chronic and classic clinical picture.

Comprehension of spoken language is always qualitatively better in Broca's aphasia than is production of language. Language production varies widely from near normal to clearly abnormal. Persons with Broca's aphasia often have difficulty in understanding syntactic relations and show deficits in comprehending syntactical items they have difficulty expressing. Repetition is always abnormal, and confrontation naming (naming objects and pictures) is poor. Oral reading and reading comprehension usually are poor, although some patients do relatively well. Writing is poor, marked by misspellings and letter omission. In addition, the patient usually has a right hemiparesis and uses the left hand for writing. Some patients cannot write at all because of paresis. Figure 11-3 shows a computed tomographic scan of a patient with a left hemisphere CVA resulting in Broca's aphasia.

Wernicke's Aphasia

Wernicke's aphasia is a fluent aphasia characterized by difficulty in understanding language as well as difficulty in repetition of language. The speech is fluent but paraphasic. **Paraphasia** includes the omission of parts of words, incorrect use of correct words, use of neologisms ("new words"), and substitution of incorrect phonemes for correct ones. Verbal or semantic paraphasia is

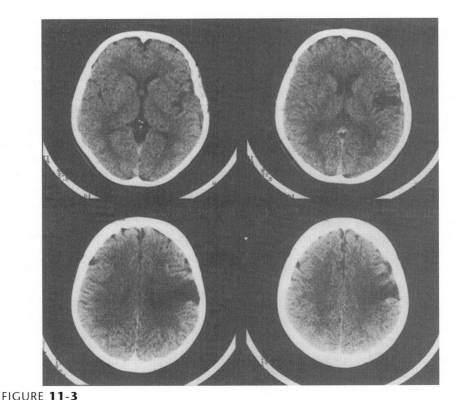

FIGURE **11-3**

Computed tomography scans of four horizontal slices from a patient with Broca's aphasia and a right hemiparesis. Note the darkened area in the left hemisphere, which defines the infarction. (Courtesy Howard S. Kirshner, MD, Department of Neurology, Vanderbilt University School of Medicine, Nashville, TN.)

the incorrect use of words; literal paraphasia is the substitution of incorrect phonemes for correct phonemes.

The fluent verbal output may be excessive, a condition called logorrhea. Phrase length is normal, and in most cases syntactic structure is acceptable. Articulation and prosody are usually not abnormal. The speech often lacks meaningful and substantive words and clinically is described as empty speech. Use of jargon is common. Sometimes neologistic jargon is documented, implying that meaning is incomprehensible because output primarily consists of excessive jargon and neologistic terms (neologistic jargon aphasia).

With Wernicke's aphasia, comprehension of language is poor, especially early after onset, and some patients appear to understand no spoken language at all. Others understand only some words, and certain patients have distinct problems in discriminating phonemes. Patients with Wernicke's aphasia characteristically demonstrate poor awareness of their comprehension or expression difficulty. Repetition of spoken language is poor, and failure and paraphasic errors characterize confrontation naming tasks. Reading is generally disturbed, often paralleling the disturbance in comprehension of spoken language.

The damage in Wernicke's aphasia is to the posterior portion of the superior temporal gyrus of the dominant hemisphere, the auditory association area, or to Wernicke's area in the sylvian fissure.[10] Extension into the area of the supramarginal gyrus and angular gyrus has also been found to be present in patients with persisting Wernicke's aphasia.[22] Because the damage is to posterior portions of the brain, the motor areas in the frontal lobe and those pathways usually are spared. Therefore the patient with Wernicke's aphasia will only infrequently show any motor weakness in the limbs or the face. A visual field deficit should be ruled out because of this posterior lesion site.

Conduction Aphasia

One form of fluent aphasia is characterized by intact comprehension and fluent, melodic speech. Despite the good comprehension, repetition is poor in contrast to the fluency in spontaneous speech. Phoneme substitutions are frequent because of the inability to match acoustic information with motor plans for the output of phonemes; word retrieval deficits are present. Wernicke postulated a disconnection theory, proposing the cause to be a lesion in the arcuate fasciculus, the connection between Broca's and Wernicke's areas. **Conduction aphasia** is less well accepted as a diagnosis than Broca's or Wernicke's aphasia because of questions about the site of lesion. The lesion is not always in the arcuate fasciculus as Wernicke postulated, and conduction aphasia is almost never seen in diseases that

interrupt white matter tracts and may involve the arcuate fasciculus (such as multiple sclerosis). However, the language syndrome has been repeatedly described and can be diagnosed from symptoms alone without neuropathologic evidence. Two distinct locations of pathology have been demonstrated in conduction aphasia. One involves the arcuate fasciculus in the dominant hemisphere, usually deep in the supramarginal gyrus. Some experts argue that the supramarginal cortex or the inferior parietal cortex rather than deep white matter is the critical site. The other major site is said to be in the left temporal lobe in the auditory association area.

Conversational speech is fluent and often paraphasic, but generally the speech quantity is reduced compared with that of Wernicke's aphasia. Reactive pauses and hesitations from awareness of incidents of word-finding difficulties are common, so the melodic line may be interrupted; however, the fluency is much better than in Broca's or global aphasia. Literal paraphasia is often present. Articulation is good. Comprehension of spoken language is also adequate in most cases. If comprehension is disturbed, the diagnosis of conduction aphasia should be questioned.

Repetition of language presents a serious problem to the person with conduction aphasia, and the dramatic difference between comprehension and repetition is a clue to correct diagnosis. Repetition is much poorer than the ability to produce words in conversational speech, and paraphasic substitutions of words often are present in repetition attempts. Errors also are present in confrontation naming. Reading comprehension usually is intact, but reading aloud often results in increased paraphasia. Writing disturbance or dysgraphia is present. Spelling is poor, with omissions, reversals, and substitutions of letters. Words in sentences may be reversed, omitted, or misplaced.

Associated characteristics vary. Some patients show a right hemiparesis and/or hemisensory loss. Patients may also show a visual field deficit. Some patients may also demonstrate an ideomotor apraxia.

Global Aphasia

Global aphasia is marked by severe impairment of both understanding and expression of language. The person usually is mute or uses repetitive vocalization. This aphasia is usually associated with a large lesion in the perisylvian area. The lesion does not serve as a localizing one for the neurologist except when in the left perisylvian area.

Expressive language always is limited, although true mutism rarely appears other than initially. The patient can often use inflected phonation and sometimes simple words, such as expletives, repetitively. Comprehension is often reported to be better than production with global aphasia; patients may also become adept at interpreting nonverbal communication through gestures and facial and body language. This nonverbal comprehension may be mistaken for comprehension of the spoken word.

The person with global aphasia does not repeat. If a patient who appears to have global aphasia repeats adequately, the SLP and neurologist should suspect that one of the transcortical aphasic syndromes, described below, is present instead of a true global aphasia. Confrontation naming is severely or completely impaired, and reading and writing are also severely or totally impaired. Many of the language dysfunctions are not reversible with treatment.

Transcortical Aphasias

These language disturbances are a set of aphasic syndromes whose lesions fall outside the perisylvian area. They have been given various names, but Lichtheim[26] identified them as **transcortical aphasias**, and they are probably identified most commonly by this name. Benson[5] called them **border zone** aphasic syndromes because the lesions usually are found in the association cortex in a vascular border zone (also known as a watershed area) between the field of the middle cerebral artery and the area supplied by the anterior or posterior cerebral arteries. A hallmark of the transcortical aphasias is the retention of the ability to repeat with good accuracy. In contrast, the aphasias of the perisylvian area all present a repetition defect.

Three transcortical aphasias are generally recognized: transcortical motor aphasia, transcortical sensory aphasia, and mixed transcortical aphasia. This last type also has been called a syndrome of isolation of the speech area.

Transcortical motor aphasia is a nonfluent aphasia marked by more dysfluency and effort in conversation than usually is seen in Broca's aphasia. Serial speech, repetition, and comprehension appear surprisingly adequate. The lesion is anterior or superior to Broca's area in the dominant hemisphere.

Transcortical sensory aphasia is fluent and marked by paraphasia with semantic and neologistic substitutions. Comprehension is poor, in sharp contrast to repetition, which is surprisingly good. Reading, writing, and naming are poor. The site of the lesion is controversial. It is usually found deep to and posterior to Wernicke's area in either the temporal or the parietal border zone, or it may be located in both of these sites.

Mixed transcortical aphasia is rare. The most striking feature is severely disordered language except in one area—repetition. Patients do not speak unless they are spoken to and answer only in repetition. The most striking feature is echolalia, the repetition of heard phrases.

Examples of echolalia may be incorporated into the patient's speech. The articulation of phonemes is good, but the expressive language as a whole is nonfluent. Comprehension is defective, with little or no demonstrable understanding of spoken language. Visual field defects and other neurologic signs are common. The pathology is mixed but generally appears to involve the vascular border zones of the left hemisphere.

Anomic Aphasia

Word-finding difficulty, known as anomia, is common in many types of aphasia as well as in nonaphasic medical conditions. In fact, many neurologists believe a diagnosis of aphasia should not be considered without evidence of some anomia. Further, anomia occurs in most types of dementia and is a clear diagnostic feature of Alzheimer's syndrome, a major dementia. Anomia often is the only major language residual after recovery from aphasia of any clinical type and may remain a long-lasting problem in the recovered aphasic.

Clearly anomia is not a good localizing symptom for the neurologist. Rather, it is a common symptom in what is called nonfocal brain disease. In those neurologic conditions in which the whole brain is generally affected, anomia is a common language symptom. It occurs in many brain conditions, including encephalitis, increased intracranial pressure, subarachnoid hemorrhage, concussion, and toxic-metabolic **encephalopathy**.

When anomia is the most prominent symptom in the aphasic syndrome, the condition is known as **anomic aphasia**. The clinical picture generally includes only limited receptive or expressive difficulty, but on occasion a disorder of confrontation naming may take an extreme form in these patients, and given patients may be unable to produce virtually any appropriate names. Spontaneous speech usually is fluent but interrupted by word-finding difficulties. Nonspecific words may be substituted for precise lexical items. These verbal paraphasias are usually semantic rather than phonemic errors. Usually the patient exhibits good expressive syntax except for pauses for word recall. **Circumlocution**, the utterance of circuitous and wordy descriptions for unrecalled words, is common in anomic aphasia. Comprehension is normal or near normal and repetition generally is intact. Reading and writing are more variable, and word-finding difficulties are obvious in written language.

Anomic aphasia may appear as an isolated syndrome or be the final stage of recovery from other syndromes, such as Wernicke's, conduction, and transcortical aphasias. Some controversy exists regarding whether a recovered aphasic who becomes anomic at the end point of recovery should be classified as an anomic aphasic or according to the primary syndrome at the onset of the aphasia.

Associated neurologic defects vary. The site of the lesion causing anomia also varies, but anomic symptoms in and of themselves are less variable than in other classic aphasic syndromes. In severe and isolated anomia, a possible focal lesion may be found in the left hemisphere. A prominent site for a lesion is in the left angular gyrus. Anomia is a common early sign in the syndrome called primary progressive aphasia.

Subcortical Aphasia

With the continued advancement of imaging technology, a new category of aphasia based on lesion site emerged and is known as **subcortical aphasia**. Although many aphasia experts have hypothesized the existence of subcortical speech and language disturbance over the years, not until the lesions were documented did the brain-behavior relation became an interest of study. The reports of several investigators suggested that basal ganglia and thalamic lesions are primarily responsible for subcortical aphasia. Subcortical aphasia associated with thalamic hemorrhage without involvement of the cerebral cortex established the disorder, and then the availability of better imaging techniques used in cases of ischemic infarction of the thalamus allowed more precise localization than had been attempted earlier. Bogousslavsky et al[6] looked at the presence of aphasia with infarction of four separate vascular territories. They found aphasia characterized by hypophonia, verbal paraphasia, impaired comprehension, and intact repetition to be present after infarction affecting the vascular supply to the anterior thalamus, including the ventral anterior and part of the ventral lateral nuclei.

Radanovic and Scaff[37] studied patients with left and right thalamic lesions. Their findings showed primarily deficits in naming and some difficulty in individual patients with auditory comprehension. These problems were thought to be possibly related to verbal memory and attention deficits rather than true language deficit. The aphasias reported after thalamic lesion do not match any of the classic cortical aphasia syndromes, and research indicates primary difficulty with naming in these patients, though some difficulty with comprehension is noted in the worst cases. As discussed in Chapter 10, the etiology of the lexical-semantic access deficits is most likely related to the indirect effect on cortical function that results from the thalamic gating mechanism damage. Nadeau and Rothi[33] propose that treatment be directed to remediation of the declarative memory deficits.

Subcortical aphasias associated with basal ganglia lesions have sometimes been classified by anatomic sites. Each site is said to be associated with a different cluster of speech and language symptoms. Several speech and language syndromes affecting the basal ganglia have been described. The syndromes vary widely, and no general clinical descriptions are associated with basal ganglia lesions. Kirshner[23] identified the head of the caudate nucleus, anterior limb of internal capsule, and anterior putamen as the most commonly reported lesion sites causing an aphasia (Fig. 11-4). These lesions result in the anterior subcortical aphasia syndrome, which is characterized by dysarthria and decreased fluency but has a longer phrase length than in Broca's aphasia. Paraphasia is also noted.

Alexander and Naeser[2] have suggested that four distinct syndromes affecting language and/or speech exist. Each is associated with a different subcortical anatomic site or combination of sites. These sites include (1) striatal lesions (basal ganglia alone), (2) internal capsule lesions, (3) striatal and internal **capsular** lesions, and (4) insular and capsule lesions. Figure 11-5 lists the signs and symptoms of each of the subcortical speech or language disorders that they identified. Other findings have been described in the literature as well. For example, disproportionate impairment of writing has been reported with subcortical lesion.[43]

A simplified localization scheme based on current knowledge for all major aphasia syndromes is provided in Box 11-1. As described in Chapter 10, the aphasic deficits seen with subcortical lesions are most likely related to the indirect effect on perfusion of cortical language and speech areas from the blockage of flow through lenticulostriate areas and poor collateral filling. These deficits probably should be treated as a cortical aphasia of the same nature.[33]

Testing and Intervention for Aphasia

Aphasia testing has had a long history in neurology and speech-language pathology. Broca reportedly tested his patients with conversational questions in addition to testing tongue movements, writing, and arithmetic. He also described their gestures. In 1926 the British neurologist Henry Head (1861-1940) published the first systematic aphasia examination in English. The test was not standardized and contained some items that were even difficult for healthy people to perform. Today clinical neurologists usually assess language and aphasia disturbances as part of the mental status examination of higher cerebral functions, which is part of the traditional neurologic examination. The mental status examination assesses major functions of the total nervous system and lateralizes and localizes dysfunction when it is present.

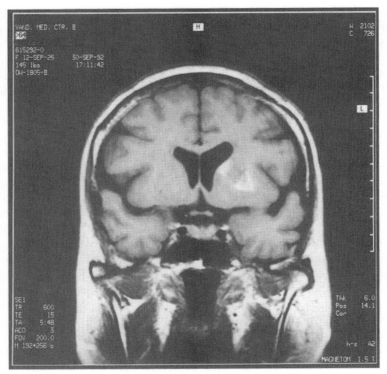

FIGURE **11-4**

MRI scan showing a lesion in the head of the caudate, anterior putamen, and anterior limb of the internal capsule resulting in a mild subcortical aphasia characterized by hesitant speech and anomia. The patient showed good recovery after a period of speech therapy. (Courtesy Howard S. Kirshner, MD, Department of Neurology, Vanderbilt University School of Medicine, Nashville, TN.)

Subcortical Aphasia

Striatal Lesions	**Striatal and Internal Capsule Lesions**
No aphasia Dysarthria possible Hypophonia	No definite aphasia Dysarthria possible

Internal Capsule Lesions	**Insular and External Capsule lesions**

No aphasia
Left dysarthria possible
Right affective dysprosody
	Fluent aphasia
	Anomia
	Paraphasias in
	  repetition
	  oral reading
	  spontaneous speech
	No dysarthria

FIGURE **11-5**

The signs and symptoms of language and speech disorders associated with subcortical lesions. (Modified from Alexander M., & Naeser, M. [1988]. Cortical-subcortical differences in aphasia. In Plum, F. [Ed.]. *Language, communication and the brain*, New York: Raven Press.)

BOX 11-1

Localization of the Aphasias in the Central Language Mechanism

Aphasias of the Perisylvian Zone

Broca's aphasia
Wernicke's aphasia
Global aphasia
Conduction aphasia

Transcortical Aphasias of the Border Zone

Transcortical motor aphasia
Transcortical sensory aphasia
Mixed transcortical aphasia

Aphasias of the Subcortical Areas

Thalamic aphasia
Striatal disorders
Internal capsule disorders
Striatal or capsular disorders
Insular or capsular disorders

Data from Alexander, M. P., & Naeser, M. A. (1988). Cortical-subcortical differences in aphasia. In Plum, F. (Eds). *Language, communication and the brain*. New York, Raven Press.

TABLE 11-1					
Language Functions of Major Classic Aphasias					
	SPONTANEOUS SPEECH	COMPREHENSION	REPETITION	READING	WRITING
Broca's	Nonfluent	+	−	±	−
Wernicke's	Fluent	−	−	−	Paragraphic
Conduction	Fluent	+	−	+	−
Global	Mute	−	−	−	−
Anomic	Disorder of word recall	+	+	+	+
Transcortical motor	Nonfluent	+	+	+	−
Transcortical sensory	Fluent	−	+	+	−
Mixed transcortical (isolation of speech area)	Nonfluent	−	+	−	Paragraphic

+, Relatively intact; −, impaired; −, variable.
Developed by Howard S. Kirshner, MD, Department of Neurology, Vanderbilt University School of Medicine, Nashville, TN.

The language functions tested by the neurologist are found in Table 11-1. An example of a bedside examination of speech and language designed for the clinical neurologist is found in Appendix C.

SLPs and psychologists have been more concerned about developing aphasia tests that precisely measure language behavior under standardized conditions than about providing tests that predict and confirm possible lesions or verify the validity of classic models of neurologic language mechanisms. Testing is performed to assist in discharge and treatment planning. Direct intervention for the language deficits may be provided on an individual or group basis, and literature is growing on treatment techniques.

Role of the Speech-Language Pathologist

The SLP is perhaps the most critical member of the rehabilitation team for the person with a significantly limiting aphasia. Numerous books, articles, websites, and treatment programs are devoted to language therapy with patients with aphasia. An attempt to describe treatment methods would not do justice to this vast amount of literature and is not the purpose of this text. At this writing, promising research studies and treatments involving constraint-induced aphasia therapy,[29] transcranial magnetic stimulation,[25] and group communication therapy were underway.[14] The SLP should be well versed and dedicated to evidence-based medical and behavioral treatments and, as a member of the rehabilitation team, know something about pharmacologic intervention as well.

Pharmacology in Aphasia

The use of medication to aid the language-impaired patient has been attempted for many years. The internationally known Russian neurologist Alexander Luria was one of the first to use a powerful anticholinesterase agent, galanthamine, to improve speech and gnostic and praxic functions in brain-injured individuals.[27] In recent years intensive study of the actions of neurotransmitter systems has increased the use of drugs in aphasia rehabilitation, though the number of studies reported in the literature remains limited. de Boissezon et al[12] recently reviewed the PubMed database for studies on the use of drugs to improve communication in persons with aphasia. This review found 24 studies published between 1970 and 2005. These included trials of bromocriptine (a dopaminergic agent), amphetamines, cholinergics, GABAergics, and serotoninergic agents. The review and summary indicated that two pharmacologic agents, piracetam (a gamma-aminobutyric acid derivative "cognitive enhancer") and amphetamines, showed limited efficiency in enhancing and maintaining the communication of persons with the type of aphasia studied for those reports. All studies that looked at it reported that drug therapy was more efficacious if it was combined with language therapy.[12]

In brief, biochemical intervention appears to be a useful adjunct to the more traditional methods of behavioral therapy used with persons with aphasia. Drug therapy certainly will not supersede traditional methods of therapy, but the future appears brighter for more effective drug therapies combined with other approaches for the rehabilitation of aphasia.[12]

Associated Central Disturbances

While testing the language system, the SLP or the neurologist often finds or suspects that other disturbances are present that are not a part of the aphasia but accompany the true aphasia. The examiner may also find one of these disturbances present with no true aphasia present. These disorders are referred to as associated central disturbances because the site of lesion is within the areas described under central language mechanism, but these are not properly classified as aphasic disturbances in most cases. Accompanying central disturbances may be agnosia, apraxia, alexia, and agraphia. Apraxia is discussed in Chapter 6 because it is a motor speech disorder; agnosia is discussed in Chapter 5 as part of the discussion on the various sensory systems. Alexia and agraphia are introduced here.

Alexia

Alexia is an inability to comprehend the written or printed word as the result of a cerebral lesion. Terms relating to alexia and agraphia (the inability to produce written language normally) are found in Table 11-2. In current usage, alexia is an acquired reading disorder, in contrast to dyslexia, an innate or constitutional inability to learn to read. The childhood disorder is often called developmental dyslexia. Although this distinction in terms is not universal, it is becoming popular. The classic term "word blindness" is rarely used in neurology or speech pathology. When used, it implies difficulty in reading words although letter recognition is more intact. Literal alexia means the inability to recognize letters; verbal alexia indicates that letters are recognized but words are not. Pure alexia is a reading disorder without a writing disorder (agraphia). A variety of terms and types of alexia have been reported, but a limited number of alexic syndromes are widely accepted. The modern understanding of alexia is attributed to Joseph Dejerine (1849-1917), who in 1891 and 1892 described two classic syndromes, **alexia without agraphia** and **alexia with agraphia**.

ALEXIA WITHOUT AGRAPHIA

Alexia without agraphia is also known as **posterior alexia** or **occipital alexia**. The cardinal feature of this uncommon syndrome is loss of the ability to read printed material but retained ability to write both to dictation and spontaneously. Other language functions generally are intact. This alexia occurs suddenly as the result of a left posterior cerebral artery occlusion in a right-handed person. A striking clinical feature is the patient's ability to write lengthy meaningful messages, with a contrasting

TABLE 11-2 **Alexia and Agraphia**	
ASSOCIATED CENTRAL DISTURBANCE	DESCRIPTION OF DISTURBANCE
Agraphia	A disorder of writing caused by cerebral injury; lesion in the left frontal or parietal lobe or in the complex pathways necessary for writing
Alexia	A disorder of reading caused by cerebral injury
Types of Alexia	**Localization**
Alexia with agraphia	Lesion usually in the dominant parietal lobe in the angular gyrus area
Alexia without agraphia	Lesion site is controversial; often two lesions, one in the dominant occipital lobe and the other in the splenium of the corpus callosum (according to Dejerine)
Frontal alexia	Lesion in the dominant frontal lobe in Broca's area and adjacent deep structures; associated with a nonfluent aphasia
Aphasic alexia	Lesions are the same as in the major aphasias

inability to read his or her own writing. The patients generally are able to understand words spelled aloud. Initially patients with pure alexia may show difficulty with letters and words, but letters are easier. With some recovery, the patient is able to read in a letter-by-letter fashion, combining them into syllables and words after saying them. Patients usually are able to regain some reading ability, but reading usually remains quite an effort. The writing seen in the syndrome is not entirely normal, but retained writing capacity is impressive when compared with the minimal reading ability. Often the patient writes better to dictation or spontaneously than when copying. Right homonymous hemianopsia usually is present.

Dejerine[13] found a cerebral infarct in the left occipital lobe and involvement in the splenium of the corpus callosum in a patient with alexia without agraphia. Because the left visual cortex was damaged, all visual information entered the right hemisphere. The right visual cortex perceived the written material but could not transfer it to the left hemisphere because of the callosal lesion. The inferior parietal lobe in the dominant hemisphere, known as the angular gyrus, combined the visual and auditory information necessary in both reading and writing; however, the inferior parietal lobule was disconnected from all visual input. Because the lobule and its connections with the language area were intact, the patient was able to write normally.

Other deficits may be associated with an alexia without agraphia. Patients may have short-term memory problems, a mild anomia, and/or a visual agnosia. A common accompaniment to pure alexia is a deficit in color naming. The patient presents this deficit despite good object naming. Not all cases of pure alexia show defective color identification. Disconnection theory explains this disorder as a loss of pure verbal association similar to that in the reading disorder. The patient recognizes the color but is unable to recall its name because of a disconnection between visual recognition areas and language areas.

ALEXIA WITH AGRAPHIA

Also known as **central alexia** or **parietal-temporal alexia**, alexia with agraphia was classically described as an almost total reading disorder, with limited writing ability, only minimal aphasia, and acalculia (acquired difficulty with calculations). In clinical practice the language symptoms vary more widely than in alexia without agraphia. Some authors separate alexia with agraphia into two different types: the classic syndrome described and the reading and writing disorder discussed below as aphasic alexia. Most accounts of the syndrome relate some aphasia, which is always a fluent aphasia. Gerstmann syndrome is sometimes present. This syndrome is defined when agnosia for the fingers, acalculia, right-left disorientation, agraphia, and alexia are all present. A right homonymous visual field defect frequently is reported but not consistently present.

Deficits in reading letters, words, and musical notes are usually seen. Number reading is disordered, and defects of calculation frequently are observed. Writing disturbance varies in severity but is not severe enough to preclude writing of letters. Patients often cannot copy letters, unlike patients with alexia without agraphia, who copy laboriously and slowly. Also unlike in pure alexia, these patients do not comprehend words spelled aloud.

Dejerine[13] localized the neuropathology in alexia with agraphia to the angular gyrus of the dominant parietal lobe, and this localization has been universally confirmed since 1891. Dejerine surmised that the angular gyrus in the inferior parietal lobule was essential for the recall of written letters and that its destruction results in disturbances in reading and writing in adults.

APHASIC ALEXIA

The most common type of alexia is the reading disturbance that accompanies the major clinical types of aphasia. In **aphasic alexia**, significant aphasic symptoms produce so much disturbance of language that reading is secondarily involved. In aphasiology alexic symptoms in aphasia generally are recognized as belonging in a classification of aphasia, not in an outline of alexia. Reading disturbances in each of the major aphasic syndromes have been previously described.

Psycholinguistic Classifications

In the 1970s British psychologists became interested in reading disorders; literature began to include references to new classifications of reading disorders. The British refer to these disorders as **dyslexias**, even though they are acquired, not developmental, disorders.[8,28] Three types of reading disorder classifications have resulted from psycholinguistic models of patient performance on tasks primarily requiring reading aloud of single words. These disorders are known as deep dyslexia, surface dyslexia, and phonologic alexia. These classifications have become fairly well accepted and the symptoms often are identified in patients.

Deep dyslexia is identified by the presence of semantic errors in reading aloud. Reading errors, such as saying "child" for "girl" or "quiet" for "listen" are common. Derivational errors such as reading "invitation" for "inviting" are present, as are visual confusions. Deep dyslexia implies that the dyslexic reader goes directly to the semantic value of a word from its printed form without appreciating the sound of the word. Deep dyslexia has also been called phonemic, syntactic, or semantic dyslexia.

Surface dyslexia is distinguished by poor ability to use grapheme-to-phoneme conversion rules, although the reader relies heavily on these rules. The errors are phonologically similar to the target, and great sensitivity is paid to spelling regularity. Therefore, although many nonsense words can be pronounced, irregularly spelled words (e.g., yacht) are impossible for the patient to pronounce correctly. There is little sensitivity to meaning; the patient may not recognize that the word does not fit with the context.

Phonologic alexia is characterized by an inability to read nonsense words, with some difficulty noted with low-frequency words.[4] Errors often are visual errors. These patients are assumed to be impaired in the ability to use letter-to-sound conversion rules of the language.

Agraphia

Writing is a complex learned motor act that involves a conversion of oral language symbols into written symbols.

The language symbols to be written are assumed to originate in the posterior language areas in the dominant hemisphere of the brain. These oral symbols are translated into visual symbols in the inferior parietal lobe. The linguistic message is then sent forward to the frontal lobe for motor processing. Lesions in any of these language areas or pathways may produce the writing disorder called **agraphia**. The most common type of agraphia is secondary to aphasia and known as aphasic agraphia. Agraphia also may be seen in the absence of aphasia.

A rare agraphia has been described in which a writing disturbance is present in only the left hand. Patients with lesions of the anterior corpus callosum display this syndrome. The lesion disconnects the right motor cortex in the frontal area from the posterior language areas of the left hemisphere. Writing with the right hand is normal because of intact connections between left motor cortex and the left language areas. The callosal lesion disrupts language messages going to the right motor area, which controls the left hand.

Cognitive-Communicative Disorders

The information presented in Chapter 10 regarding cognition was brief and simplistic in nature. It was intended to give the student an introduction to the topic and to the relatively little we know about the neurologic basis of cognition as well as an appreciation for the rapid expansion of knowledge that occurred at the end of the last century. After digesting this information, compare it with Wernicke's model of the central language mechanism. This should highlight how brain injuries or diseases that involve the right hemisphere or that are more diffuse and involve bilateral cortical and subcortical areas or neural networks could produce a different type of language disorder than that seen with focal left hemisphere damage.

This understanding became critical when SLPs began to be employed more widely in various medical settings, eventually resulting in involvement with a more diverse population of neurologically based communication disorders. This included patients with right hemisphere lesions, traumatic brain injury, and dementia. As previously noted in the discussion of right hemisphere function, the communication disorders that these patients experienced were not truly language based. Rather, all these disorders may lead to neurobehavioral consequences that result in cognitive and communicative problems. This sometimes affects the aspects of language on which aphasia focuses—semantics, syntax, morphology, and phonology—but to a much lesser extent. These disorders more often result in communication problems that affect the accuracy, efficiency, and effectiveness of communication in ways

that differ greatly from focal, left hemisphere damage. These are referred to as **cognitive-communicative disorders**. All or some of the four key aspects of cognition tend to be affected by these disorders, and the resulting communication disorder is clinically quite different from the aphasias previously described. They each have a different neuroanatomic basis and require different approaches to assessment and intervention.

Communication Disorders Related to Right Hemisphere Damage

At the beginning of this chapter, under the section on aphasia, the etiology of brain damage resulting in focal lesions in the language area of the dominant hemisphere was discussed. While learning about deficits seen in patients with right hemisphere (typically nondominant) damage, remember that the right hemisphere is equally vulnerable to these causative factors of reduced blood flow. Thus the same conditions—CVA, focal trauma, neoplasms—are the common causes of focal damage to parts of the right hemisphere.

With right hemisphere lesions in patients for whom that is the nondominant hemisphere, a broad spectrum of deficits are seen. These depend on the site of damage and the expanse of the lesion. The most dramatic deficits are neglect, inattention, denial, visual and spatial perceptual disorders, and constructional disturbances. These may be thought of as nonlinguistic deficits, but as Myers[32] and Tompkins[44] point out, they often have notable influence on communication and result in what Myers terms extralinguistic deficits. These fall in the category of cognitive-communicative deficits rather than aphasia.

If the clinician tests patients with nondominant right hemisphere damage, mild linguistic deficits may be found. Problems that may be noted are difficulty with confrontation naming, word fluency, body part naming, oral sentence reading, writing (especially letter substitutions and omissions), and deficits in auditory comprehension when the input is complex. Although these problems may appropriately be classified as linguistic in nature, a strong argument exists that most of the communication deficits are in reality caused by the nonlinguistic and extralinguistic problems resulting from the brain damage. Attentional problems seem to have a major impact on communication function in patients with damaged right hemispheres.

Take a brief look at some of the major deficits found in some patients with right hemisphere damage.

Keep in mind that great variability exists in the incidence and severity of all these symptoms in the population of persons with right hemisphere damage.

NEGLECT, INATTENTION, AND DENIAL

Neglect is a syndrome in which a patient fails to recognize one side of the body and the environmental space surrounding that side. Patients may use only half of their bodies, even using only one sleeve in their shirts, even though the neglected side of the body is free of paralysis. Neglect of half of the environmental space is not the result of a visual field defect.

The exact neurologic locus of the neglect syndrome with right hemisphere lesions is not exactly known. Chronic parietal lobe damage shows a high correlation with the syndrome. **Unilateral inattention** may be considered a subtle form of the neglect syndrome. Neurologists test for unilateral inattention through a procedure called double simultaneous stimulation, in which all sensory modalities are tested. In tactile testing, corresponding points on the body are touched at the same time with equal intensity. Visual testing involves having the patient fixate on a point on the neurologic examiner's face. The examiner moves his or her fingers into both the right and left peripheral visual fields, and the patient reports where the fingers are seen. Auditory testing is performed by having the examiner stand behind the patient and provide a stimulus of equal intensity to both ears.

Extinction is present when the patient suppresses stimuli from one side. Extinction may occur in all modalities or in a single modality. When extinction is elicited, the degree of inattention can be assessed by increasing the strength of the stimulus on the inattentive side.

Many patients develop a dramatic denial of their neurologic illness; the denial may range from mild to severe. An example of severe denial is the patient's lack of recognition of a hemiplegia. The condition was documented by the Russian neurologist Joseph Babinski (1857-1932), who had a patient with a left-sided hemiplegia and left-sided sensory loss who appeared completely unaware of his neurologic deficit. If the patient's hemiplegic arm was placed on the bed along his left side and the neurologist placed his own arm across the patient's waist, the patient would lift the physician's arm aloft. If he were asked to grasp his left arm with his non-paralyzed right arm, he would grasp the physician's arm. Asked to move his paralyzed arm even though his arm was completely hemiplegic, the patient would emphatically say that he could move his arm. Babinski used the term anosognosia to describe this unawareness. Anosognosia is sometimes used to describe symptoms of denial other than the ones described here, but it probably is best to limit it to the specific denial impairment Babinski described. This example of denial is highly common in right-hemispheric lesions and much less common in left-hemispheric lesions. Anosognosia does not appear to be based on a psychologic mechanism but, rather, a more fundamental neurologic mechanism of gnostic loss.

PROSOPAGNOSIA

Prosopagnosia refers to the inability to recognize familiar faces and their expressions. The patient recognizes individuals by voice rather than visual perception. Bilateral lesions usually are found in the occipital-temporal areas in this disorder. The lesion in the right hemisphere is usually in the right temporal-occipital region. A specific type of color agnosia often accompanies prosopagnosia. The lesions that cause the facial recognition deficit also cause the color agnosia.

VISUAL-PERCEPTUAL DEFICITS

Right hemisphere lesions are associated with deficits in meaningful interpretation and recall of complex visual structures. Deficits in the perception and recall of letters, words, and numbers may produce problems in reading.

SPATIAL ORGANIZATIONAL DEFICITS

As previously noted, constructional disturbances are present with right or left parietal lobe lesions. In most instances right hemisphere lesions tend to cause more frequent and severe constructional deficits, but constructional deficits can also indicate a left hemisphere lesion.

LANGUAGE DISORDERS OF VISUAL-SPATIAL PERCEPTION

Rivers and Love[38] reported on the language performance of patients with right hemisphere lesions when the patients were asked to respond to a series of visual-spatial processing tasks. The language was judged poorer than that of normal control subjects but not as poor as that of the majority of aphasic control subjects with left hemisphere lesions. The patients with right hemisphere lesions showed dysnomia in oral storytelling based on a series of visual stimuli, but the ability to name pictured objects did not differ from healthy subjects. Other investigators have reported mild agrammatism and telegraphic speech plus anomia in a variety of right-hemispheric conditions.

PROSODIC DEFICITS

A common defect in the right hemisphere syndrome is known as **aprosodia**. Prosody, among other things, conveys appropriate emotional affect. Prosody also carries pragmatic information, allowing a listener to discriminate among questions, statements, and explanations. When normal stress or emphasis is disturbed in a sentence, conveying new information becomes difficult.

Ross[40] has reported widely on patients with deficits of both prosodic production and comprehension. Patients often are unable to provide variations in their voices and have a flat emotional tone. Comprehension defects are called affective aprosodia and may include several distinct components. However, these individuals report being able to feel emotions and hear emotions in the voices of others. Ross has developed a set of eight aprosodias and proposed that motor aprosodia is associated with right frontal damage. He has also suggested that sensory aprosodia is associated with right posterior damage. A motor aprosodia on the right is analogous to a motor aphasia in Broca's area, and a sensory aprosodia on the right is analogous to a Wernicke's aphasia on the left.

Many other neurologists have confirmed the presence of prosodic defects in comprehension and expression, but lesion localization for these and other symptoms in Ross' scheme have not been consistently found in the literature. Various lesion sites of left and right hemisphere aprosodia have been associated with lesions in the basal ganglia of the right or left hemispheres and in the anterior temporal lobe. Box 11-2 outlines the signs and symptoms of nonlinguistic and extralinguistic deficits.

Careful and thoughtful consideration of the list of nonlinguistic and extralinguistic deficits in Box 11-2 in the context of discourse and other complex tasks of even routine communication reveals why some patients may have communication disorders that are subtle in nature but devastating to effective, efficient communication interaction. Joanette et al[20] suggest that these deficits may make it difficult for the person to understand fully the context in which communication is taking place; they thus appear to demonstrate a change in attitude when facing a communication situation and are often ineffective because of these factors.

BOX 11-2

Signs and Symptoms of Nonlinguistic and Extralinguistic Deficits

Nonlinguistic Deficits

Difficulty in recognizing and using significant contextual cues

Difficulty integrating these significant cues into an overall pattern

Extralinguistic Deficits

Distinguishing significant from irrelevant information

Integration and interpretation of contextual information

Inhibiting impulsive responses

Grasping figurative and implied meaning

Topic maintenance and efficiency of expression

Appreciation of the communicative situation and listener needs

Recognizing and/or producing emotional responses

Modified from Myers, P. S. (1999). *Right hemisphere damage*. San Diego: Singular.

Dementia

Cummings and Benson[9] adopted the following operational definition of **dementia**: "an acquired persistent impairment of intellectual function with compromise in at least three of the following spheres of mental activity: language, memory, visuospatial skills, emotion or personality, and cognition (abstraction, judgment, executive function, and so forth)" (pp. 1-2). The definition emphasizes that dementia is acquired, is persistent, and does not affect all aspects of intelligence equally. The neurologist and SLP specializing in neurogenic communication disorders should recognize the early features of this syndrome so that the patient and family, if they want, can be proactive to prevent the serious social, economic, and vocational consequences of unrecognized intellectual deterioration.

The incidence and prevalence of dementia are difficult to determine because studies differ vastly depending on how dementia is defined and what particular population is studied. All agree that the incidence of dementia is rising rapidly, with an increasing percentage of the population being affected. This is especially true because most forms of dementia are found in persons older than 65 years, and the number of elderly people in the population is greater than ever before and is expected to rise. The frequency of dementia diagnosis is estimated to be approximately 2% in persons aged 65 to 69 years, 5% in persons aged 75 to 79 years, and 20% for persons between the ages of 85 and 89 years. After age 90, the frequency increases to approximately 30%. The cost of caring for patients with dementia in the United States has been estimated to exceed $30 billion annually.

The causes of dementia are many, and determination of the cause is critical because some dementias can be reversed. Before a diagnosis of dementia of the Alzheimer's type or Pick's disease can be supported, other diseases or disorders that could result in cognitive decline must be ruled out. These are conditions such as ischemic episodes resulting in multiple infarctions, extrapyramidal syndromes (including Huntington's and Parkinson's disease), hydrocephalus, metabolic disorders, toxic disorders, trauma, neoplasms, central nervous system infections, and demyelinating diseases. Even depression can result in cognitive decline and memory loss that mimic the beginning of a dementia such as Alzheimer's. These diseases or conditions, however, have other signs and symptoms of a disease process or a disorder, whereas in the diseases discussing below, such as **Alzheimer's disease**, the dementia is the primary symptom.

CLASSIFICATION OF DEMENTIAS

Cummings and Benson[9] classify the dementias into two basic patterns of neuropsychologic impairment with identified neuroanatomic correlates: cortical and subcortical dementia. A third category of mixed is also noted.

Cortical Dementias
Dementia of the Alzheimer's Type
Alzheimer's disease, or **dementia of the Alzheimer's type (DAT)** afflicts a high percentage of the patients with cortical dementia. Cummings and Benson[9] report that the clinical course of DAT can be divided into three stages, the characteristics of which are fairly agreed on by most experts. These stages and their characteristics are summarized in Table 11-3.

Focal Cortical Dementias
In 1892 Dr. Arnold Pick described atrophy of the frontal lobe with an accompanying dementia in which the patients first presented with psychiatric symptoms and then later developed memory loss, fluent aphasia, and finally a dementia that continued to progress. This syndrome eventually was named after him and is known as Pick's disease. It is quite rare when strict diagnostic criteria are enforced in identification. It has, however, been designated by the National Institute of Neurological Diseases and Stroke as a part of a syndrome complex

TABLE 11-3

Clinical Features of the Different Stages of Dementia of the Alzheimer's Type

STAGE	CHARACTERISTICS
Stage I: Mild	Memory for new learning is defective and remote recall is mildly impaired. Language shows word retrieval problems and some difficulty understanding humor, analogies, and complex implications. The patient may be vague and may not initiate conversation when appropriate. The patient may also show indifference, anxiety, and irritability.
Stage II: Middle	Memory for recent and remote events is more severely affected, and language shows vocabulary diminishment. The patient repeats ideas, forgets topics, has difficulty thinking of words in a category, loses sensitivity to conversational partners, and rarely corrects mistakes. Comprehension is reduced, and language may rely on jargon and paraphasias. The patient becomes increasingly indifferent, irritable, and restless.
Stage III: Late	Memory is severely impaired, as are all intellectual functions. Language is rarely used meaningfully, and some patients are mute or echolalic. Motor function is compromised by limb rigidity and flexion posture.

known as **frontotemporal dementias (FTD)**. The hallmark of FTD is a gradual progressive decline in behavior and/or language. Onset is at a relatively young age (average age of onset is 55 to 60 years). The clear difference between FTD and DAT is that these patients with FTD retain important features of memory, keep track of day-to-day events, and are fairly well oriented in time and space, unlike patients with DAT. Grouped with Pick's disease under the designation of focal cortical dementias is a complex of disorders of which the SLP should be aware. These disorders are categorized under primary progressive aphasia.

Primary Progressive Aphasia

A slowly progressive aphasia without generalized dementia was first described and then further elaborated by Mesalum.[30,31] This syndrome, now called **primary progressive aphasia (PPA)**, is defined as an adult-onset, degenerative language disorder syndrome that selectively affects the language areas of the dominant hemisphere, with preservation of other mental functions as well as the ability to perform normal activities of daily living for at least 2 years. Anomia is often an early sign, but poor auditory comprehension, stuttering, deteriorating verbal memory, and reading and spelling difficulties have been reported. Other intellectual functions remain intact, and psychometric testing reveals overall intelligence quotients within the normal range.

As more cases of PPA began to be identified and discussed in the literature, observations of subtypes of the disorder were documented.[16] A study of 31 patients with PPA with detailed speech and language evaluations identified three clinical variants: nonfluent progressive aphasia (NFPA), semantic dementia (SD), and logopenic progressive aphasia (LPA). Although magnetic resonance imaging (MRI) classified all patients as having left perisylvian region anterior temporal lobe atrophy, further investigation found distinctive patterns. This study and others indicate that the clinical characteristics of nonfluent progressive aphasia are findings of apraxia of speech, agrammatism, and deficits in processing complex syntax. MRI in the patients with NFPA in this study found frontal and insular atrophy in those patients. The cohort with semantic dementia presented with fluent speech and semantic memory deficits as well as reading deficits described as surface dyslexia.

Chan et al[7] studied patients with SD with structural MRI. This imaging showed atrophy in the temporal lobes (predominantly on the left) with inferior greater than superior involvement and anterior temporal lobe atrophy greater than posterior, distinguishing it from Alzheimer's disease. Behavioral and personality changes also are more noticeable in patients with SD than in those with NFPA or LPA. LPA appears to be the least widely accepted variant, but many citations in the literature present this as a true type of PPA. Gorno-Tempini et al[16] described these patients as having slow speech with impaired syntactic comprehension and naming. They showed atrophy in the left posterior temporal cortex and inferior parietal lobule. Figure 11-6 depicts a coronal MRI scan of a patient who was diagnosed with PPA. With the atrophy in the left temporal lobe and the description of nonfluent speech and anomia, the logopenic variant is probably an appropriate diagnosis for this patient. The LPA and the NFPA do overlap in many domains, whereas the SD variant presents the most characteristic neuropsychological pattern.[3]

Neuropathology of the Cortical Dementias

The neuropathology of Alzheimer's disease shows the presence of **neurofibrillary tangles** and **amyloid plaques** in the cytoplasm of nerve cells. These plaques, which begin in the walls of small blood vessels, are thought to result from defective enzymes that cause abnormal production of beta-amyloid protein. The tangles are associated with an abnormal tau protein production and are made up of clumps of these microtubules. These tangles are pronounced in certain granular layers of the inferior temporal lobe, which has connections with the hippocampus.[11] Tangles also tend to accumulate in the amygdala and in the posterior association regions of the cortex. In an individual the two hemispheres may show differences in the density of the tangles. Eventually the tangles are replaced by amyloid. Cortical dementia shows extensive loss of pyramidal neurons in all parts of the brain and a loss of up to 50% of cholinergic neurons from the production areas in the basal nucleus of Meynert and from the septal area. Microscopic examination of the brain tissue of persons with DAT also shows neuritic plaques, which are remains of degenerated nerve fibers.

Subcortical and Mixed Dementias

Subcortical dementias may accompany extrapyramidal syndromes (as in Parkinson's disease and Huntington's chorea), depression, some white matter diseases (such as multiple sclerosis and AIDS-related encephalopathy), and some vascular diseases causing lacunar states. With subcortical dementias cognition slowly and progressively deteriorates. Forgetfulness and alterations of affect are noted. Retrieval in memory is often aided by cues and structure. In mood, the person may appear depressed or apathetic with decreased motivation. The cognitive impairment has been described as one of dilapidation. Patients seem to be unable to synthesize and manipulate information to produce sequential steps to solve a complex problem, though they may correctly perform individual steps. The neurologic examination of these patients is abnormal, with motor, posture, tone, and speech problems noted.

The mixed cortical-subcortical dementias result from such entities as multiple infarcts, toxic and metabolic encephalopathy, trauma, neoplasms, and anoxia. The mixture of characteristics depends on the parts of the brain affected by the disease, trauma, or dementing process.

ROLE OF THE SPEECH-LANGUAGE PATHOLOGIST IN DEMENTIA

The SLP usually is called on to help identify subtle language disorders that may signal intellectual deterioration

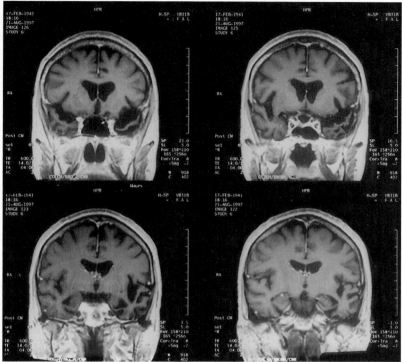

FIGURE **11-6**
Coronal MRI scan of a patient with progressive, nonfluent aphasia. Note the marked atrophy of the left temporal lobe, which is easiest to see in a coronal projection. The temporal lobe atrophy and his symptoms of slow speech and anomia, which were progressive in nature, are consistent with the descriptions of the logopenic variant of PPA. (Reprinted from Bradley W. G., Daroff, R. B., Fenichel, G. M., & Marsden, C. D. (Eds). [2000]. *Neurology in clinical practice. Vol. I* [3rd ed.]. Boston: Butterworth-Heinemann.)

because language is highly sensitive to even mild changes in brain function. The purpose of the assessment by the SLP may be to assist in making the differential diagnosis by trying to determine whether true aphasia, apraxia, or an amnesia is present without language involvement. In Alzheimer's disease, the clinician may be asked to assess the effect of the intellectual deterioration on functional communication and suggest ways that family and other caregivers might improve communication with the patient. In some cases, the SLP may provide a short period of treatment oriented toward training family and other caregivers on how to facilitate and maintain communication with the individual with dementia for as long as possible. In cases of PPA, especially before evidence of much cognitive decline, the SLP works closely with the patient and the family to give them strategies to cope with the changing ability to communicate. Specific treatment targeted at providing alternative communication methods to patients with PPA has been found to show promise if the patients do not have concomitant cognitive deficits.[34]

Acute Confusional States

Several conditions produce confusion, which is characterized by rapid onset over a period of hours or days. The causes of confusion include metabolic imbalance, adverse drug reactions, and alcohol and drug withdrawal reactions. Patients generally are inattentive, incoherent, and irrelevant; they demonstrate fluctuating levels of consciousness. Agitation and hallucinations, usually visual, often are present. Acute confusional states generally respond to primary medical treatment. Confusional states usually are not the result of focal brain lesions; widespread cortical and subcortical neuronal dysfunction generally is present. Confusional symptoms also are seen during the period of posttraumatic amnesia in traumatic head injury.

Symptomatic language impairment is seen in confusional states. The language disturbance may be viewed as a secondary symptom of the confusional state. Halpern et al[19] reported on the language symptoms of patients with confused language in contrast to other language impairments of cerebral involvement. Lesions in these patients were either bilateral or multifocal. Vocabulary and syntax generally were normal. The most striking feature of the language of these confused patients was its irrelevancy and confabulatory nature. Other investigators also have found irrelevant language response and confabulation in dementia, so it is not a pathognomic feature of confused states.

Confabulation is the verbal or written expression of fictitious experiences, generally filling a gap in memory. It is less marked in the presence of aphasia because it is a response in which the language areas must be relatively intact. Confabulation is more often associated with generalized cerebral deficit or dysfunction rather than focal lesions. Some instances in which focal lesions are associated with confabulation are in the Wernicke-Korsakoff amnestic syndrome and in ruptured aneurysms of the anterior communicating artery.

Traumatic Brain Injury

Traumatic brain injury (TBI) is defined by the Brain Injury Association as "a blow or jolt to the head or a penetrating head injury that disrupts the function of the brain." Approximately 1.4 million people in the United States sustain a TBI each year, of which roughly 50,000 are fatal. The primary causes of TBI for nonmilitary situations are falls, motor vehicle accidents, or related incidents and assaults. For military personnel in war zones, blasts are the leading cause of TBI. Risk is higher for men than for women and for persons between the ages of 0 to 4 years and 15 to 19 years.[24] The direct medical costs and the indirect costs in loss of productivity are estimated to be in the billions.

Knowledge about the deficits resulting from TBI has greatly increased over the past 10 years, as have the number of rehabilitation programs and treatment methods devoted to TBI. Patients usually display the language of confusion but often present a more serious and pervasive language deficit, now termed a cognitive-communicative disorder or a cognitive-linguistic disorder.

NEUROPATHOLOGY OF INJURY

The predominant type of injury is an **acceleration-deceleration injury**, in which the head accelerates and then suddenly stops, such as in a motor vehicle accident. Discrete focal lesions may result from direct impact forces. Contusions may be found at the point of direct impact, and evidence of brain damage may be present at the site opposite the point of direct impact. Damage sustained at the site opposite the point of impact is called contrecoup damage. The frontal (frontopolar and orbitofrontal) and temporal (anterior temporal, but not necessarily medial temporal) lobes are the most likely sites of focal cortical contusions.[1]

Frequently in TBI no evidence exists of focal lesions, but diffuse brain injury is present as a result of molecular commotion. The molecular structure of the brain is disrupted after impact as the impact force causes acceleration, rotation, compression, and expansion of the brain within the skull. Brain tissues are compressed, torn apart, and sheared on the bony prominences of the skull, causing **diffuse axonal injury (DAI)** and permanent microscopic alterations of both white and gray matter.

DAI, even severe DAI, may occur without skull fracture or cortical contusion. In nonhuman primate models, DAI has been produced on rapid acceleration of the head with no impact and in cases of mild brain injury in which the nonhuman primate has only transitory alterations in the level of consciousness (e.g., in sports such as football).

The DAI and focal lesions are primary mechanisms of injury in traumatic brain insult. Secondary mechanisms that occur as a result of the initial direct forces also cause further brain damage. These secondary mechanisms of injury include ischemia, hypoxia, edema, hemorrhage, brain shift, and raised intracranial pressure. They all may produce further deleterious effects on brain function.

NEUROBEHAVIORAL EFFECTS

The neurobehavioral sequelae of TBI are usually divided into two classes: focal deficits and diffuse deficits. Focal deficits may be manifested as a specific language deficit or as a paralysis of specific muscles or muscle groups. Disorders such as mutism, dysarthria, palilalia, voice disorder, hearing loss, and visual or auditory perceptual dysfunction may be considered focal deficits. If present they are complicating factors in rehabilitation efforts and their specific treatment may be enormously complicated by the presence of diffuse deficits.

Diffuse deficits are more common and are most often manifested as cognitive disorganization. Ylvisaker and Szekeres[46] note that the cognitive processes of attention, perception, memory, learning, organization, reasoning, problem solving, and judgment are affected. These aspects of cognition and the possible effects of their disruption on behavior and language are outlined in Table 11-4.

ASSESSMENT AND TREATMENT

Although standard aphasia batteries are used in assessing the language impairment in TBI, testing must

TABLE 11-4
Cognitive Impairment after Traumatic Brain Injury: Effect on Behavior and Language

ASPECT OF COGNITION	EFFECT ON BEHAVIOR	EFFECT ON LANGUAGE
Attention Holding objects, events, words, or thoughts in consciousness	Short attention span; distractible, weak concentration	Decreased auditory comprehension, confused or inappropriate language, poor reading comprehension, poor topic maintenance
Perception Recognizing features and relations among features	Weak perception of relevant features; possible specific deficits (including field neglect); poor judgment based on visual or auditory cues; stimulus bound (i.e., focus on part of the whole); spatial disorganization	Difficulty in reading and writing, poor comprehension of facial and intonation cues
Memory and Learning Encoding: recognizing, interpreting, and formulating information, including language, into an internal code (knowledge base, personal interests, and goals affect what is coded) Storage: retaining information over time Retrieval: transferring information from long-term memory to consciousness	Memory problems, inability or inefficiency in learning new material	Difficulty following multistep directions, word-finding problems, difficulty with reading comprehension and spelling, poor integration of new and old information; language may be fragmented, lacking logic, order, specificity, and precision; difficulty with math also seen
Organizing Processes Analyzing, classifying, integrating, sequencing, and identifying relevant features of objects and events; comparing for similarities or differences; integrating into organized descriptions, higher level categories, and sequenced events	Poor organization of tasks and time; difficulty setting and maintaining goals; poor problem-solving, self-direction, self-confidence, and social judgment	Disorganized language (verbal and written), difficulty discerning main ideas and integrating them into broader themes, poor conversational skills (may get lost in details), difficulty outlining material for study, difficulty with math
Reasoning Considering evidence and drawing inferences or conclusions; involves flexible exploration of possibilities (divergent thinking) and use of past experience	Concrete, impulsive, and reactionary; may be easily swayed; vulnerable to propaganda; difficulty discerning cause and effect and consequences of behavior; poor social judgment	Difficulty understanding and expressing abstract concepts; socially inappropriate, lack of tact; difficulty using language to persuade, understand humor, learn academic subjects, and follow complex conversations
Problem Solving and Judgment Problem solving: ideally involves identifying goals, considering relevant information, exploring possible solutions, and selecting the best solutions Judgment: deciding to act or not to act based on consideration of relevant factors, including prediction of consequences	Impulsive, uses trial-and-error approach, difficulty predicting consequences of behavior, shallow reasoning; poor safety and social judgment, inflexible thinking, poor self-direction, poor use of compensatory strategies	Difficulty understanding and expressing steps in problem solving to get a particular outcome; difficulty in math and higher academic tasks, socially inappropriate behavior, lack of tact, difficulty in understanding explanations for behavior

Modified from Szekeres, S. F., Ylvisaker, M., & Holland, A. L. (1985). Cognitive rehabilitation therapy: a framework for intervention. In Ylvisaker, M. (Ed.), *Head injury rehabilitation: children and adolescents*. San Diego: College-Hill Press.

extend beyond these batteries in most cases. As examination of Table 11-4 reveals, the cognitive and communicative deficits of TBI can be quite different from the aphasia of a patient with a vascular lesion. The SLP must attempt to determine which cognitive processes underlying language performance are disrupted, and to what degree, and must also determine if the language impairment has a true aphasic component. Informal or formal testing and observation with assessment scales such as the Rancho Los Amigos Levels of Cognitive Recovery[17] can help the team members identify the patient's best level of cognitive functioning throughout the course of rehabilitation.

The SLP working with TBI patients is a critical part of a rehabilitation team. The most successful rehabilitation of patients with TBI is known to be intensive and long term in nature. Much of what is done to overcome the resulting deficits in attention, memory, reasoning, and problem solving involves training the individual to self-monitor the use of strategies that enable adaptation of his or her external and internal environment to compensate for weaknesses. Follow-up with patients who have had success in vocational and social life after TBI has shown that the ability to incorporate these strategies and adapt them to new challenges seems to be key.[42]

Synopsis of Clinical Information and Applications for the Speech-Language Pathologist

- Aphasia is an acquired disorder of language caused by focal brain damage that can affect any of the four modalities: listening, speaking, reading, and writing.
- The most common etiology of aphasia is CVA, or stroke, which occurs when the arterial distribution to a part or all of the perisylvian language cortex is interrupted. This interruption by a stroke is caused by occlusion of an artery or by hemorrhage resulting from arteriovenous malformation, aneurysm, or trauma.
- Aphasia may also be found after focal lesion caused by trauma, abscess from brain infection, or brain tumor.
- Brain tumors, which primarily arise from neuroglia, are classified according to their origin. Tumors are also graded from I to IV according to the tumor's tendency to spread.
- The most popular aphasia classification system is the Boston classification, which includes Broca's, Wernicke's, conduction, global, anomic, transcortical motor, transcortical sensory, and mixed transcortical aphasias. Each type has a characteristic profile relative to comprehension, fluency, repetition, reading, and writing.
- The aphasias classified well by the Boston system are also relatively consistent with site of lesion, though many questions still exist concerning the traditional localization, especially in conduction aphasia. Anomic aphasia does not localize damage well because storage and retrieval of words seem to be widely diffused in the brain.
- Subcortical damage to parts of the basal ganglia, the thalamus, and the internal capsule has been found to result in particular patterns of communication difficulty consistent with aphasia.
- The SLP is a critical member of the rehabilitation team for persons with aphasia, providing the most complete evaluation and setting treatment goals and plans.
- Some advances have been made in the use of pharmacologic treatment in aphasia, but the drugs studied have always been found to be most effective when combined with behavioral treatment provided by speech pathology.
- Central disturbances associated with aphasia are agnosia, apraxia, alexia, and agraphia. Alexia is a disorder of reading imposed on literate individuals after brain damage. The classic aphasias have associated reading deficits. Two other classifications exist: alexia without agraphia and alexia with agraphia. Psycholinguistic classifications of reading deficits also have been made: deep dyslexia, surface dyslexia, and phonologic alexia.
- Agraphia is a deficit in producing written language.
- Cognitive-communicative disorders are communication disorders related to damage to the nondominant hemisphere or diffuse brain damage. Communication deficits associated with right hemisphere damage, dementia, and TBI are classified as cognitive-communicative disorders.
- The communication deficit associated with right hemisphere damage is primarily related to extralinguistic deficits rather than the true linguistic deficits such as problems with word retrieval, syntax, comprehension, reading, and writing. Attention has a major impact on the communicative effectiveness of these patients.
- Patients with right hemisphere damage have difficulty with distinguishing relevancy, integrating and interpreting context cues, inhibiting impulsive responses, maintaining topic maintenance and efficient expression, grasping figurative language, and producing and responding to emotional responses.

CASE**STUDY**

A 61-year-old man noticed a "stutter" and difficulty expressing himself soon after a stressful situation. His dysfluency became more obvious over the next 2 years and his wife began to notice that he had difficulty with auditory comprehension as well. Audiometric testing revealed only a mild bilateral high-frequency hearing loss. Evaluation at this 2-year mark found normal performance on "bedside" neurologic examination of memory, calculations, general information, and copying of geometric figures. Speech was described as hesitant with occasional literal and verbal paraphasic errors and a marked tendency to add extra syllables to words (palilalia). Comprehension testing found him needing extra repetitions to perform even one-step commands presented verbally, but he could readily follow complex written commands. On the Boston Diagnostic Aphasia examination (Fig. 11-7) he did have some difficulty with reading, but only at the complex paragraph level. Writing was hesitant and contained numerous spelling errors (Fig. 11-8, *A*). Repeat evaluations were done over the next 2 years, showing

a pattern of progressive deterioration of auditory comprehension, speech intelligibility, and writing. Reading comprehension was slower to deteriorate, but by 4 years after onset he could comprehend only some single words written to try to aid communication. His wife reported mild forgetfulness at home, and he showed impaired visual memory and learning on neuropsychologic testing. He remained well groomed and socially appropriate with recognition of examiners who worked with him.

QUESTIONS FOR CONSIDERATION:

1. This patient is an example of what condition discussed in this chapter?
2. Computed tomographic scans of this patient showed generalized cortical atrophy and ventricular enlargement. If more definitive imaging such as MRI had been available, what would it likely have shown as the focus of the atrophy?
3. The long-term retention of the ability to copy geometric figures and draw a clock would speak to the intactness of what part of the brain?

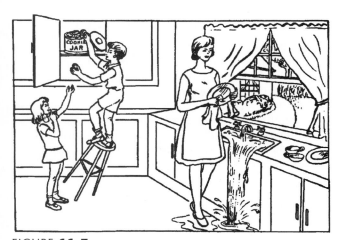

FIGURE **11-7**

Connected-speech elicitation picture (commonly referred to as the cookie theft picture) from the Boston Diagnostic Aphasia Examination. (Reprinted from Goodglass, H., Kaplan, E, & Barresi, B. [2001]. *The assessment of aphasia in related disorders* [3rd ed.]. Philadelphia: Lippincott, Williams & Wilkins, now owned by Pro-Ed, Austin, TX.)

FIGURE **11-8**

Writing samples from four different administrations of the paragraph writing subtest of the Boston Diagnostic Aphasia Exam describing the cookie theft picture (see Fig. 11-7 at left). Samples **A** and **B** were done 2 months apart, approximately 2 years after the first symptoms of difficulty with speech were first noted by the patient. Sample **C** was done 1 year after B and sample D 1 year after C.

REFERENCES

1. Adamovich, B. L. B., & Henderson, J. A. (1990). Traumatic brain injury. In LaPointe, L. L. (Ed.), *Aphasia and related neurogenic language disorders.* New York: Thieme.

2. Alexander, M. P., & Naeser, M. A. (1988). Cortical-subcortical differences in aphasia. In Plum, F. (Ed.), *Language, communication and the brain.* New York: Raven Press.

3. Amici, S., Gorno-Tempini, M. L., Ogar, J. M., Dronkers, N. F., & Miller, B.L. (2006). An overview on primary progressive aphasia. *Behavioral Neurology, 17*, 77-87.

4. Beauvois, M. F., & Derousne, J. (1979). Phonological alexia: Three dissociations. *Journal of Neurology, Neurosurgery and Psychiatry, 42*, 1115-1124.

5. Benson, D. F. (1979). *Aphasia, alexia, and agraphia.* New York: Churchill Livingstone.

6. Bogousslavsky, J., Rehli, F., & Uske, A. (1988). Thalamic infarcts: Clinical syndromes, etiology, and prognosis. *Neurology, 38*, 837-848.

7. Chan, D, Fox NC, Scahill RI, Crum WR, Whitwell JL, Leschziner G, Rossor AM, Stevens JM, Cipolotti L, Rossor MN. (2001). Patterns of temporal lobe atrophy in semantic dementia and Alzheimer's disease. *Annals of Neurology, 49*, 433-442.

8. Coltheart, M., Patterson, K., & Marshall, J. C. (Eds.) (1980). *Deep dyslexia.* London: Routledge and Kegan Paul.

9. Cummings, J. L., & Benson, D. F. (1992). *Dementia: a clinical approach* (2nd ed.). Boston: Butterworth-Heinemann.

10. Damasio, H. (1981). Cerebral localization of the aphasias. In Sarno, M. T. (Ed.), *Acquired aphasia* (pp. 27-50). New York: Academic Press.

11. Davis, A. (1993). *A survey of adult aphasia and related disorders.* Englewood Cliffs, NJ: Prentice-Hall.

12. de Boissezon, X., Peron, P., de Boysson, C., & Demonet, J. F. (2006). Pharmacology of aphasia. *Brain and Language,* (In press. Available online, September 18, 2006).

13. Dejerine, J. (1891). Sur un cas de cecite verbal avec agraphie, suivi d'autopsie. Mémoires de la Société de Biologie *3,* 197-201.

14. Elman, R. J., & Berstein-Ellis, E. (1999). The efficacy of group communication treatment in adults with chronic aphasia. *Journal of Speech, Language and Hearing Research, 42*, 411-419.

15. Goodglass, H., & Kaplan, E. (1983). *The assessment of aphasia and related disorders* (2nd ed.). Philadelphia: Lea & Febiger.

16. Gorno-Tempini, M. L., Dronkers, N. F., Rankin, K. P., Ogar, J. M., Phengrasamy, L., Rosen, H. J., Weiner, M. W., & Miller, B. L. (2004). Cognition and anatomy in three variants of primary progressive aphasia. *Annals of Neurology, 55*, 335-346.

17. Hagen, C., Malkmus, D., & Durham, P. (1979). Levels of cognitive functioning. In *Rehabilitation of the head-injured adult: comprehensive physical management.* Downey, CA: Professional Staff Association of Rancho Los Amigos Hospital.

18. Haines, D. (Ed.) (2006). *Fundamental neuroscience for basic and clinical applications* (3rd ed). Philadelphia: Churchill Livingstone.

19. Halpern, H., Darley, F. L., & Brown, J. R. (1973). Differential language and neurologic characteristics in cerebral involvement. *Journal of Speech and Hearing Disorders, 32*, 162-173.

20. Joanette, Y., Goulet, P., & Hannequin, D. (1990). *Right hemisphere and verbal communication.* New York: Springer-Verlag.

21. Kertesz, A. (1982). *Western aphasia battery.* New York: Harcourt Brace Jovanovich.

22. Kertesz, A., Lau, W. K., & Polk, M. (1993). The structural determinants of recovery in Wernicke's aphasia. *Brain and Language, 44*, 153-164.

23. Kirshner, H. S. (1995). *Handbook of neurological speech and language disorders.* New York: Marcel Dekker.

24. Langlois, J. A., Rutland-Brown, W., & Thomas, K. E. (2004). *Traumatic brain injury in the United States: emergency department visits, hospitalizations and deaths.* Atlanta, GA: Centers for Disease Control and Prevention, National Center for Injury Prevention and Control.

25. LeFaucher, J. P. (2006). Stroke recovery can be enhanced by using repetitive transcranial magnetic stimulation (TMS). *Neurophysiologie Clinique, 36*, 105-115.

26. Lichtheim, L. (1895). On aphasia. *Brain, 7*, 433-484.

27. Luria, A. R., Naydin, V. L., Tsvetkova, L. S., & Vinarskaya, E. N. (1969). Restoration of higher cortical functions following local brain damage. In Vinken, P. J. & Bruyn, G. W. (Eds.), *Handbook of clinical neurology: Vol. 3. Disorders of higher nervous activity.* Amsterdam: North Holland Publishing.

28. Marshall, I., & Newcombe, F. (1973). Patterns of paralexia: a psycholinguistic approach. *Journal of Psycholinguistic Research, 2*, 175-199.

29. Meinzer, M., Djundja, D., Barthel, G., Elbert, T., & Rockstroh, B. (2005). Long-term stability of improved language functions in chronic aphasia after constraint-induced aphasia therapy. *Stroke, 36*, 1462-1466.

30. Mesulam, M. M. (1987). Primary progressive aphasia—differentiation from Alzheimer's disease. *Archives of Neurology, 22*, 533-534.

31. Mesalum, M. M. (2003). Primary progressive aphasia—a language-based dementia. *New England Journal of Medicine, 349*, 1535-1543.

32. Myers, P. S. (1999). *Right hemisphere damage.* San Diego: Singular Publishing Group.

33. Nadeau, S. F., & Rothi, L. G. (2001). Rehabilitation of subcortical aphasia. In Chapey, R. (Ed.), *Language intervention strategies in aphasia and related neurogenic communication disorders* (4th ed.). Philadelphia: Lippincott Williams & Wilkins.

34. Pattee, C., Von Berg, S., & Ghezzi, P. (2006) Effects of alternative communication on the communicative effectiveness of an individual with a progressive language disorder. *International Journal of Rehabilitation Research, 29*, 151-153.

35. Porch, B. E. (1967). *Porch index of communicative ability: Vol. I. Theory and development.* Palo Alto, CA: Consulting Psychologists Press.

36. Porch, B. E. (1971). *Porch index of communicative ability: Vol. II. Administration, scoring and interpretation* (rev. ed.). Palo Alto, CA: Consulting Psychologists Press.

37. Radanovic, M., & Scaff, M. (2003). Speech and language disturbances due to subcortical lesions. *Brain and Language, 84*, 337-352.

38. Rivers, D. L., & Love, R. J. (1980). Language performance on visual processing tasks in right hemisphere cases. *Brain and Language, 10,* 348-366.

39. Rosenbek, J. C., LaPointe, L. L., & Wertz, R. T. (1989). *Aphasia: a clinical approach.* Boston: College Hill Press.

40. Ross, E. (1981). Aprosodia: functional-anatomic organization of the affective components of language in the right hemisphere. *Archives of Neurology, 38,* 561-569.

41. Schuell, H. M. (1965). *Minnesota test for differential diagnosis of aphasia.* Minneapolis: University of Minnesota.

42. Schutz, L. E. (2007). Models of exceptional adaptation in recovery after traumatic brain injury: a case series. *Journal of Head Trauma Rehabilitation, 22,* 48-55.

43. Tanridag, O., & Kirshner, H. S. (1985). Aphasia and agraphia in lesions of the posterior internal capsule and putamen. *Neurology, 35,* 1797-1801.

44. Tompkins, C. A. (1995). *Right hemisphere communication disorders: theory and management.* San Diego: Singular Publishing Group, Inc.

45. Wepman, J. M., & Jones, L. V. (1961). *Studies in aphasia: an approach to testing.* Chicago: Education Industry Service.

46. Ylvisaker, M., & Szekeres, S. F. (1994). Communication disorders associated with closed head injury. In Chapey, R. (Ed.), *Language intervention and strategies in adult aphasia* (3rd ed.). Baltimore: Williams & Wilkins.

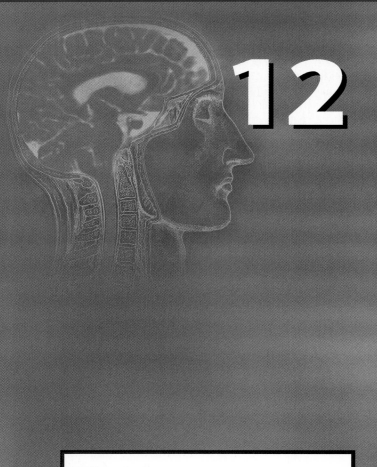

12 Pediatric Disorders of Language

In a child, speech is a new acquisition, and as with most recently evolved faculties it is sensitive. Like an orchard blighted by a late frost, a child loses its speech easily, and he may show a taciturnity or even mutism for a variety of reasons. In such cases there may be no focal lesion of the brain, but only a presumed thinly spread minor cerebral affection…Though vulnerable, speech in the child is also a highly resilient faculty. Hence a considerable restitution of function is always possible and speech may return to normal with little delay.

–Macdonald Critchley, *Aphasiology*, 1970

CHAPTER**OUTLINE**

KEY**TERMS**

acquired childhood aphasia
anencephaly
Asperger's syndrome
attention deficit–hyperactivity disorder
autism
autism spectrum disorder (ASD)
bilingual
callosal dysgenesis
cerebral plasticity
childhood disintegrative disorder
code switching
corpus callosum
developmental dyslexia
developmental language disability
dichotic listening
ear advantage
Landau-Kleffner syndrome
language dominance
language lateralization
mental retardation
minimal cerebral dysfunction
mixed dominance
myelination
myelogenesis
neurolinguistics
pervasive developmental disorder
primary neurulation
Rett syndrome
secondary neurulation
specific language impairment (SLI)

Brain Growth

Acquisition of speech and language is clearly tied to physical development and maturation in the infant and child, yet the exact nature of the interaction of growth and development with emerging speech is unknown. What is known, however, is that the course of speech and language development is a correlate of cerebral maturation and specialization. But a critical question still remains: What indexes of cerebral maturation are of significance to language acquisition? Clearly critical periods occur in the maturation of the brain as well as growth gradients in different brain structures. Can these critical periods be equally applied to the stages of language acquisition?

BRAIN WEIGHT

One obvious index of neurologic development is the change in gross brain weight with age. The most rapid period of brain growth is during the first 2 years of life. The brain more than triples its weight in the first 24 months. At birth, the brain is approximately 25% of its adult weight, and at 26 months it has reached 50% of its full weight. At 1 year, the average age at which the first word appears, the brain is 60% of its adult weight. Thus the brain makes its most rapid growth in the first year of life. By 2.5 years, the brain has reached approximately 75% of its full growth, and at 5 years it is within 90% of its complete maturation. Table 12-1 illustrates this increase in brain weight. It is not until 10 years of age that the brain achieves approximately 95% of its ultimate weight. By approximately 12 years, or puberty, full brain weight is reached.

The late neurolinguist Eric Lenneberg (1921-1975)[27] argued that the accelerated curve of brain growth in the first years of life matched the course of rapid early acquisition of language of the child. He further claimed that primary linguistic skills were achieved by the age of 4 or 5 years and that the ability to acquire language

TABLE 12-1

Language and Brain Growth from Birth to 2 Years

AGE	LANGUAGE MILESTONES	BRAIN WEIGHT (G)
Birth	Crying	335
3 Months	Cooing and crying	516
6 Months	Babbling	660
9 Months	Voicing intoned jargon	750
12 Months	Approximating first words	925
18 Months	Early naming	1024
24 Months	Making two-word combinations	1064
5 Years	Kindergarten age, sentences	1180
12 Years	Fully matured brain weight	1320

diminished sharply after puberty, when accelerating brain growth reached a plateau.

Neurolinguistics

Neurolinguistics is the study of how the brain processes linguistic information—more specifically, the manner and location of this processing.[36] According to Owens,[36] the human brain has three basic functions: regulation, processing, and formulation. Regulation refers to a person's energy level or arousal state and the overall functioning of the brainstem and cerebral cortex. The reticular formation in the brainstem, the main arousal center for brain activity that regulates a person's alertness and awareness of surroundings and multimodality information coming in or going out, helps the brain with processing and formulation.

The main processing center of the brain is located in the posterior cortex. It regulates information in the form of analyzing it, coding it for understanding, and storing it in memory (hippocampal activity). Various sensory stimuli are processed in specific regions of the cortex and, as was stated in Chapter 2, all sensory information, other than olfaction, is processed through the thalamus.

If an individual's arousal level is such that he or she can take in the information in the immediate surroundings (a coma patient cannot process all information; if the brain is unconscious, the arousal center is nonactive), then sensory processing is capable of taking place and the brain analyzes and synthesizes all the sensory input. Then the frontal lobe, the area responsible for formation of ideas, takes over the information that is processed and helps the individual think of, plan, and execute a behavior. This entire process helps the brain pay attention, concentrate on an idea, organize an idea, and then execute it. An individual may plan, organize, and concentrate on a motor movement, but human beings have the capacity to execute that movement or not. A person can think of raising her hand in class, get ready to do so, but because she may be unsure of the question or answer being formulated, she could choose not to raise the hand and not be called upon. If the professor or a peer in the class makes a statement or asks a question, it could trigger her original thought and her brain tells her to raise her hand and participate in the discussion. This highly complex neurolinguistic processing allows human beings to communicate in arguments, conversations, discussions, and debates.

Neurulation

As stated in Chapter 3, the neural tube in the embryo eventually matures into the brain and spinal cord. The neural plate gives rise to the central nervous system. How the neural tube matures into the mature central nervous system is regulated by a process called neurulation. Haines[25] described two types of neurulation. **Primary neurulation** is the process that forms the brain and the spinal cord through the lumbar vertebrae. **Secondary neurulation** is the process by which the caudal neural tube (and eventually the caudal neural plate) gives rise to the sacral and coccygeal vertebrae. Problems with neural development during the primary or secondary neurulation process lead to dysraphic defects (see Fig. 3-30).

Haines[25] described these congenital defects or malformations as dysraphic defects associated with the defective neurulation process (Fig. 12-1). The bone, meninges, muscles, or skin that develops around the neural tissue may fail because of defective neurulation. In the early 1990s, major medical studies in the United States and other countries proved that folic acid, given to pregnant women, reduced the possibility of dysraphic defects in the unborn fetus that were caused by defects in neural tube development. Further research from the United Kingdom during the early 1990s proved that women who were given folic acid during pregnancy had a 70% drop in neural tube defects (dysraphic defects) compared with a control group.[24]

Primary neurulation defects include **anencephaly**, which is a failure of the anterior neural tube to close during maturation. With this condition, the fetus has an unformed brain, the skull may not be present, and facial deformities usually are present. Anencephaly is

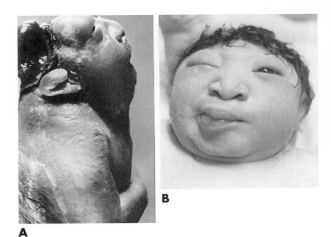

FIGURE 12-1
Anencephaly: lateral (**A**) and frontal (**B**) views. (Reprinted from Haines, D. [2006]. *Fundamental neuroscience* [3rd ed.]. Philadelphia: Churchill Livingstone.)

always fatal. Secondary neurulation defects include spina bifida, which is a defect of the posterior neural tube development (Fig. 12-2). In this condition the posterior neural tube does not close and the posterior spinal cord does not form, resulting in a cleft in the lower spinal cord. Although not typically fatal, spina bifida does cause many growth, maturation, language, and medical problems that usually are quite costly.[10]

DIFFERENTIAL BRAIN GROWTH

Just as the total brain grows at different rates at different ages, so do its different parts, and various brain structures reach their peak growth rates at different times. For instance, brainstem divisions, such as the midbrain, pons, and medulla, grow rapidly prenatally and less rapidly postnatally. The cerebellum develops rapidly from before birth to the age of 1 year. The cerebral hemispheres, important in language development, grow rapidly early, contributing approximately 85% to total brain volume by the sixth fetal month.

The differential growth of the cortex of the cerebral hemispheres is of vital importance for speech and language function because the majority of neural structures for communication are integrated there. Most cortical neurons are in place at birth, but brain growth may be measured through the development of synaptic connections and myelination. One method of establishing a schedule of cortical growth gradients in cerebral maturity is to determine what cortical areas are most developed in myelination at birth. The motor area of the precentral gyrus of the frontal lobe is the first cortical area developed at birth. It is soon followed by the

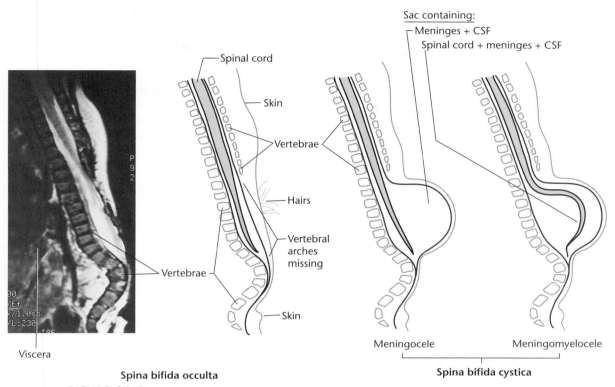

FIGURE 12-2

Spina bifida. (Reprinted from Haines, D. [2006]. *Fundamental neuroscience* [3rd ed.]. Philadelphia: Churchill Livingstone.)

somatosensory area of the postcentral gyrus of the parietal lobe. Next, quite soon after birth, the primary visual receptor area of the occipital cortex matures. The primary auditory area, Heschl's gyrus in the temporal lobe, matures last. The medial surface of the hemispheres shows the final development of the brain.

The cortical association areas lag behind the development of the cortical receptor areas that are present and active at birth. In fact, the major association areas devoted to speech and language mature well into the preschool years and even beyond. The progressive development of Broca's area, the frontal motor area for the face area on the motor strip, and the development of Wernicke's area, the posterior auditory association area, are related to progressive stabilization of the phonologic system. As the phonemic motor planning system matures, the auditory association system increases its ability to process longer and more complex sequences of connected phonemes. The arcuate fasciculus connecting Broca's and Wernicke's areas apparently begins myelination in the first year and continues for some time afterward.

At 1 year the normal child has a vocabulary of one or more word approximations, usually names for objects that have been seen and sometimes touched. This stage of language development requires the ability to mix neural information from the auditory, somesthetic, and visual association areas. The association area of the inferior parietal lobe is where information from the temporal auditory association areas, the occipital visual association area, and the parietal association area combine to provide the neural bases for the feat of naming that the 1-year-old child displays. The rapid growth of vocabulary in the second and third years of life therefore may well be a correlate of the maturation of this significant posterior association area in the parietal lobe, which combines information from surrounding association areas. It no doubt is a master association area, rightly named by Geschwind[21] as the "association area of association areas."

The left hemisphere is destined to serve as the primary neurologic site for speech and language mechanisms in most infants, children, and adults. The left hemisphere shows early structural differences that support later **language dominance**. The sylvian fissure is longer on the left in fetal brains, and the planum temporale on the left is larger in the majority of fetal and newborn brains. Although the temporal lobe appears well differentiated from early life, Broca's area is not differentiated until 18 months, and the corpus callosum is not completely myelinated until age 10 years. The inferior parietal lobe, the master association area, is not fully myelinated until adulthood, often well into the fourth decade.

Differential Brain Growth Anomaly: Callosal Dysgenesis

The corpus callosum is defined under the category of commissural fibers; that is, it interconnects corresponding structure on the left hemisphere with the right hemisphere. The largest bundle of these fibers is called the **corpus callosum** (Fig. 12-3). The corpus callosum consists of a rostrum, genu, body, and splenium (Fig. 12-4). The fibers of the genu interconnect the frontal lobes. Bear[10] described a split brain study; this was done surgically for scientists to understand the importance of the corpus callosum and how the two hemispheres interact. In such a split brain surgical study, the skull is opened and the axons of the corpus callosum are severed. Some hemispheric communication is likely still

possible through the connections in the brainstem. However the majority of the intercerebral communication abilities would no longer exist. From this surgical procedure, surgeons learned that because most of these patients did not display major deficits once the axons were severed, a severe epileptic patient was thought to benefit from the severing of the corpus callosum to reduce or eliminate severe epileptic activity from the right to the left hemispheres, or vice versa.

Callosal dysgenesis is the presence of the dorsal corpus callosum in the absence of a rostral corpus callosum. Children with a particular type of this condition often display developmental delay.[9] Magnetic resonance imaging is capable of detecting such defects of the corpus callosum development. Rubinstein et al[45] suggested that partially formed corpus callosum in children was the result of arrested growth or delayed development of the fetus and therefore the neonatal brain. Understanding the definition of the maturational defect of callosal dysgenesis as it occurs in children will help in the understanding of the important role that the corpus callosum has as a connection of the two cerebral hemispheres. And a developmental delay or other such maturational defect often is the result of the lack of corpus callosum development.

MYELINATION FOR LANGUAGE

Myelination has been considered one of the more significant indexes of brain maturation and is often a prime correlate of speech and language. **Myelination** allows more rapid transmission of neural information along neural fibers and is particularly critical in a cerebral nervous system dependent on several long axon connections between hemispheres, lobes, and cortical and subcortical structures. Lack of maturation of myelin in language association fibers and language centers has frequently been suggested as a cause for developmental delays in language. Immaturity of myelogenesis has not been definitely proved as a demonstrable cause in speech-language delay, but the available data suggest it as a likely factor.

Myelogenesis is a cyclic process in which certain neural regions and systems appear to begin the process early and others much later. In some instances the myelogenetic cycle is short and in other cases much longer. Clear differences in rate of myelogenesis exist between different pathways. Myelination of the cortical end of the auditory projections extends beyond the first year, whereas myelination of the cortical end of the visual projections is complete soon after birth. A similar discrepancy exists between myelination of the auditory geniculotemporal radiations and visual

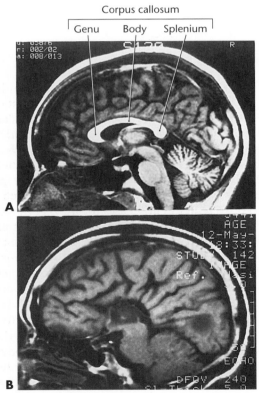

FIGURE 12-3
Corpus callosum through magnetic resonance imagery. Sagittal view of a normal adult (**A**) and one with agenesis of the corpus callosum (**B**). (Reprinted from Haines, D. [2006]. *Fundamental neuroscience* [3rd ed.]. Philadelphia: Churchill Livingstone.)

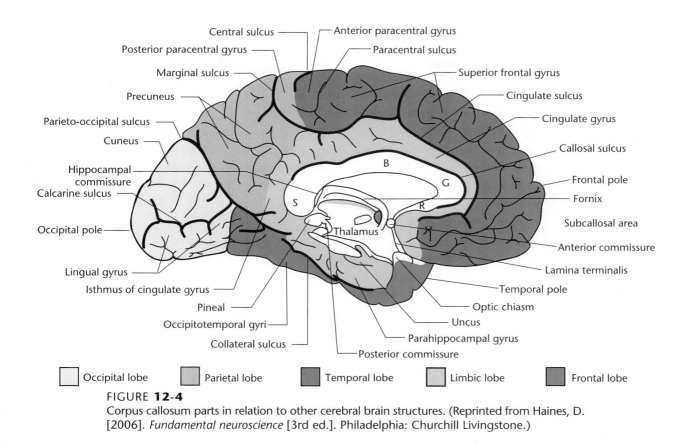

Central sulcus

Anterior paracentral gyrus

Posterior paracentral gyrus

Paracentral sulcus

Marginal sulcus

Superior frontal gyrus

Precuneus

Cingulate sulcus

Parieto-occipital sulcus

Cingulate gyrus

Cuneus

Callosal sulcus

Hippocampal commissure

Frontal pole

Calcarine sulcus

Fornix

Occipital pole

Subcallosal area

Thalamus

Anterior commissure

Lingual gyrus

Lamina terminalis

Isthmus of cingulate gyrus

Temporal pole

Pineal

Optic chiasm

Occipitotemporal gyri

Uncus

Parahippocampal gyrus

Collateral sulcus

Posterior commissure

Occipital lobe Parietal lobe Temporal lobe Limbic lobe Frontal lobe

FIGURE **12-4**

Corpus callosum parts in relation to other cerebral brain structures. (Reprinted from Haines, D. [2006]. *Fundamental neuroscience* [3rd ed.]. Philadelphia: Churchill Livingstone.)

geniculocalcarine radiations. These myelogenetic cycles appear to underlie the early visual maturity and slowly developing auditory maturity of the infant. Myelination cycles can be roughly correlated with the milestones of speech and language development, but because no behavioral way exists of assessing myelogenetic maturation in the living brain of the child with language delay, the concepts have little or no clinical utility for the speech-language pathologist (SLP).

Cerebral Plasticity

Children who have begun to develop language normally and then sustain cerebral injury, particularly to the left hemisphere, show a language disturbance of an aphasic nature. The younger the child, however, the more quickly the language disturbance appears to resolve itself and the child appears to become grossly normal or near normal in language function. This fact is in relatively sharp contrast to the adult who sustains left cerebral injury. In adult brains, resolution of aphasic difficulty after focal injury to the left hemisphere rarely reaches the level of normality of functioning that is possible in the child.

One explanation given for this phenomenon is that the child's brain demonstrates considerable plasticity of function in that undamaged areas are capable of assuming language function. In terms of language function, **cerebral plasticity** is defined as a state or stage in which specific cortical areas are not well established because of the brain's immaturity. The brain is more plastic during the most rapid periods of brain growth, and damage to the left hemisphere before the end of the first year of life is often associated with a shift of language function to the right hemisphere. By contrast, injury to the left hemisphere after this critical period is less likely to be associated with a functional reorganization of the brain. Studies from various neurosurgical centers show that approximately one third of patients with left hemisphere damage before age 1 year continue to have language mediated exclusively by the left hemisphere.[43] In patients in whom left hemisphere dominance for language continues even in the face of damage, it is dependent primarily on the integrity of the frontal and temporal-parietal language areas. This explanation of cerebral plasticity of language mechanisms rests on the concept of a transfer of functional areas from the left hemisphere to uncommitted areas in the right hemisphere.

Another explanation for the rapid recovery of language in children assumes that both hemispheres contain mechanisms for language and that language need not be relearned on the right. If a genetic predisposition exists to develop the mechanisms of the left hemisphere for language, in most healthy infants the mechanisms of the right will be inhibited as the left side develops complex language mechanisms. With damage to the left hemisphere, however, a release of the mechanisms of the right brain is assumed. This explanation also implies that damage to the right hemisphere in the child may be associated with aphasia more frequently than in the adult.

The period of time in which plasticity changes occur is called the critical period. Each area of the cortex has its own critical period; therefore a child's recovery from an injury depends on two factors: where the lesion occurred and the exact critical period for that part of the brain.[25] This critical period has many implications for language functioning in a developing child, which have been previously explained. Axonal and synaptic development are especially vulnerable to perinatal hypoxia, malnutrition, and even environmental toxins such as air pollution, paint, and fumes.[25] When axonal and synaptic development are affected, this vulnerability has adverse consequences on cognitive and language development. Sensory and social deprivation studies have also shown that environmental stimuli can have a significant effect on development during the critical period.[12] According to Castro et al,[12] environmental enrichment programs are considered to be the most effective in overcoming cognitive problems, including the delays in speech and language development often seen in infants with low birth weight.

Ylvisaker[55] and Ewing-Cobbs et al[19] have postulated that the brain-injured child is not as fortunate as some literature has stated. They highlighted the possibility of delayed consequences of brain injury in children.[55] That is, in children, specific brain function may not appear to be altered until the particular part of the injured brain (and its functions) would be expected to mature. Only at the time that a language or cognitive skill would be considered to be developmentally appropriate can the effects of the earlier brain damage be discovered. For example, the child who is injured early in life may show unexpected difficulty with higher level language processing as he or she advances in school. This may have not been evident before the expected ability to handle advanced processing tasks develops. Because of the delayed consequences of the brain injury, the SLP may need to be called back to treat a child who previously had seemed to be progressing well.

This hypothesis of continued cognitive or language deficits in brain-injured children is further supported by Allison,[2] who stated that "the biggest difference between adults and children is not what the effects of brain injury will be but when they will be manifest" (p. 4). Because the child with brain injury has not yet fully developed his or her cognitive and language skills, synapses have not been fully matured, and therefore the long-term effects of a brain injury may not be truly known until later in the child's development, when certain synaptic connections do not take place as a result of a previous injury. Therefore the plasticity theory that children always fully recover from such an injury would not be true. The effects may not be known until later in the child's life. Long-term effects of brain injury in children may not be noticed until later than the earlier researchers predicted. SLPs should be aware of this and advocate for continued monitoring of a brain-injured child's cognitive and language skills.

Development of Language Dominance

An overriding fact of brain functioning is that the cerebral hemispheres demonstrate asymmetry and that language is dominant in one of them. Cerebral dominance appears to be a developing function because, although anatomic differences favor the temporal lobe in the left hemisphere, strong evidence suggests that language is less fixed in the immature brain. Lenneberg[27] advanced the theory that the course of **language lateralization** follows the course of cerebral maturation. He argued that lateralization is completed by puberty, based on the assumption that at birth the two hemispheres have equal potential for the development of language mechanisms and that gradual lateralization is associated with the period of major growth.

Current anatomic evidence suggests that the hemispheres may not have equal potentiality for language and that the left hemisphere is organized differently from the right, with speech mechanisms for language in the left.[24] The planum temporale is larger in adults, newborns, and fetuses (Fig. 12-5).[51]

Research comparing macroscopic aspects (width, height, length, and total volume of the area) of postmortem brains with structural patterns (neuronal density, axonal density, etc.) concluded that the asymmetry could not be explained by neuronal density or glial cell volume.[7] However, the findings pointed to axonal myelination as a possible explanation. Further support was provided by Galuske et al,[20] demonstrating a strong relation of asymmetry of the planum temporale to the organization of the clusters of neurons that characterize the area and the spacing of those clusters. These factors

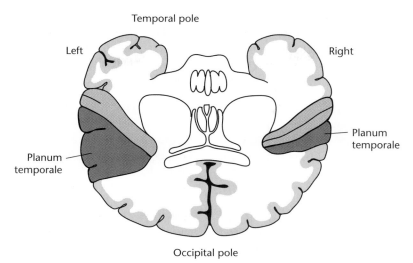

Temporal pole

Left

Right

Planum
temporale

Planum
temporale

Occipital pole

FIGURE **12-5**

Cerebral asymmetry in the planum temporale. Geschwind and Levitsky demonstrated a larger left planum temporale in 65 adult subjects, a larger right planum temporale in 11 subjects, and equal plana temporale in 24 subjects. The drawing shows an exposed upper surface of the temporal lobe with a cut made at the plane of the sylvian fissure. Note a large left planum lying behind the transverse gyrus of Heschl. On the right are two transverse gyri and a small planum. (Modified from Geschwind, N. & Levitsky, W. [1968]. Left-right asymmetries in temporal speech region, *Science, 161,* 186-187. (1979). In Ludlow, C., & Doran-Quine, M. [Eds.], [1979]. *The neurologic bases of language disorders in children: methods and directions for research.* Washington, D.C.: National Institutes of Health Publication 79-440.)

can be referred to as the "intrinsic microcircuitry" of the area, and area 22 of the temporal lobe is indicative of greater complexity of connections. The authors of this study concluded that this higher level of organizational complexity (increasing the area volume) could be partially attributable to use-dependent modifications that occur during development with increasing exposure to human language. As Habib and Robichon[24] point out, however, this conclusion of exposure-dependent increase in volume is incompatible with the fact that the asymmetry is present in the neonate and even the fetus. More likely, they conclude, a genetically predetermined pattern of asymmetry exists that is further reinforced under the influence of specific environmental influences.

Cerebral dominance for language has been long associated with laterality of other functions. As long ago as 1865, Jean Bouillaud (1796-1881) suggested that language dominance and handedness were related in some way. For many years the preferred hand was believed to be contralateral to the cerebral hemisphere dominant for language. This meant that the left cerebral hemisphere was dominant for language in right-handers and the right hemisphere in left-handers. Primarily through the cortical-stimulation studies of Penfield and Roberts,[40] current thinking is that the left

hemisphere is almost always language dominant in right-handers, with approximately 95% of this group left-brained for language. In left-handers, approximately 50% to 70% also show language dominance in the left hemisphere.

Hand preference is a relevant but not totally reliable index in predicting language dominance. Right-handedness is a relatively universal trait and is usually associated with other preferences in laterality. Human beings also tend to prefer one foot, eye, and ear consistently. Degrees of laterality vary. Some people are more strongly right-handed than others, but true ambidexters, those who use either hand equally well, are quite rare.

Inconsistency in lateral preferences also is often seen. A person may write with the right hand, throw a ball with the left hand, and kick a ball with the right foot. This is mixed laterality, or **mixed dominance**. On occasion mixed laterality has been found to be associated with language retardation or developmental dyslexia in children, but the relation between mixed laterality and a disorder of cerebral dominance for language is uncertain.

Most right-handed people demonstrate ear preference, which is considered consistent with a contralateral hemisphere laterality for language in the brain.

This preference can be demonstrated through **dichotic listening** tasks in which simultaneous auditory stimuli are presented to both ears at once. Listeners generally show a consistent lateral preference in recognition of stimuli in one ear over the other ear. This is called an **ear advantage**. Only 80% of right-handers show a distinct right ear advantage, so the relation to cerebral dominance for language is not always clear.

Childhood Language Disorders

To truly understand the origin of language disorders and why a child exhibits disordered linguistic behavior, students should review the neurologic language processing structures in the central nervous system. Likewise, a review of the structures responsible for expressive language and transmitting a processed message from Wernicke's area to Broca's area through the arcuate fasciculus will help the student understand how a message is verbalized through an intricate programming of motor speech structures that allow an individual to verbalize an idea. Owens[36] stated that "Broca's area is responsible for detailing and coordinating the programming for verbalizing the message" (p. 120). Several physiologic systems are triggered by this desire to express a message, including respiration, phonation, resonation, and articulation (Figs. 12-6 and 12-7).

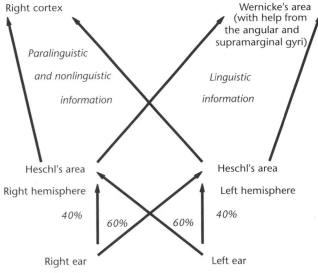

FIGURE 12-6
Linguistic processing structures in the central nervous system. (Redrawn from Owens, R. E. Jr. [2005]. *Language development: An introduction* [6th ed.]. Boston: Allyn and Bacon.)

LANGUAGE DIFFERENCE OR LANGUAGE DISORDER?

An understanding of the difference between a language disorder and a language difference helps the student studying neurologic speech and language disorders in children. The previous discussion on bilingualism should trigger some thoughts for the student studying speech-language pathology or audiology. Is the child whose first language is not English considered disordered in English, delayed in language development in English, or just a child with a difference in his or her language systems and structures? The American Speech-Language-Hearing Association (ASHA)[5,6] and Silverman and Miller[46] describe these differences. A language disorder is defined as impairment in the comprehension and/or production of the language content, form, and/or usage; however, a language difference is "a variation of a symbol system...that reflects and is determined by shared regional, social, or cultural-ethnic factors" (p. 78).[46]

Owens[38] stated that "a dialect within a language as well as a developing bilingualism that is affected by the influence of the first language on learning the second language is not to be considered a disorder but rather a language difference" (p. 98). ASHA has engaged in several position papers in the past 20 years dealing with whether a child from a culturally or linguistically diverse background should be considered disordered or different. The terms English language learner (ELL), "limited English proficiency," or "limited proficiency in both languages"[38] have permeated discussions of language disorders and differences and remain a controversy within the field of speech-language therapy.

Developing cultural sensitivity and competence would help the SLP and audiology student develop a keen awareness of cultures in general and be more prepared to deal with either language differences or disorders. The members of ASHA's Multicultural Issues Board during 2004 introduced readers to the concepts of cultural sensitivity and cultural competence.[30]

BILINGUALISM

Processing of language for an individual who speaks more than one language is unique. **Bilingual** individuals are capable of **code switching**. This is the ability of a bilingual speaker to shift from one language to another within a sentence or within an entire conversation. This usually occurs when both languages are used in the person's home, school, or work environment on a regular basis. According to Owens[36,37] this behavior is neither random nor a deficit. Sprott and Kemper[47] and others indicated that code switching is a phenomenon governed by rules and influenced by the context of the interaction.[36]

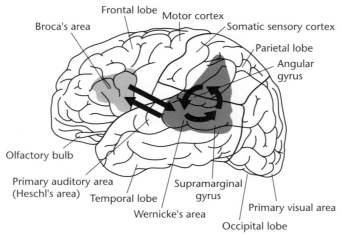

FIGURE **12-7**
Expressive language structures in the central nervous system. (Redrawn from Owens, R. E. Jr.
[2005]. *Language development: An introduction* [6th ed.]. Boston: Allyn and Bacon.)

Code switching is often used as a processing tool to enhance meaning, alert a listener of a change in topic, or express humor attitudes or cultural solidarity.[38]

Neurolinguistically, Ahlsén[1] discussed three types of bilingualism, including compound bilingualism, coordinated bilingualism, and subordinated bilingualism (Table 12-2). Further research has indicated that most

TABLE 12-2 **Types of Bilingualism Distinguished Neurolinguistically**	
TYPE	DESCRIPTION
Compound bilingualism	The first and second languages are learned concurrently before age 6 years; languages are often spoken by one parent
Coordinated bilingualism	The second language is learned before puberty either in the home or another environment (e.g., school)
Subordinated bilingualism	The first language is dominant, and the second language is used as translation; child thinks in the first language and then translates it to the second language for speaking purposes

Modified from Ahlsén, E. (2006). *Introduction to neurolinguistics*. Philadelphia: John Benjamins Publishing Company.

bilingual children do not know each language at exactly the same skill level. Many times, as evidenced by the SLP's experiences in the public schools, the two languages complement each other, with each language used primarily in one setting or another, such as school, work, or play.[1]

Neurolinguists often are interested in the recovery patterns and abilities of bilingual individuals who have a neurologic infarct such as stroke or traumatic brain injury. Parallel recovery of the languages is the most common pattern experienced by these individuals.[1] Minkowski[31] and Ahlsén[1] further postulated that the language used that has the most emotional ties to it is less impaired after infarct and also recovers first. Another hypothesis is that the right hemisphere is more involved in second language (L2) processing than it is with the first language (L1). However, as Dehaene et al,[18] as stated in Ahlsén,[1] explained, "one hypothesis is that the right hemisphere is more involved in L2 processing than in L1 processing...since L2 processing evokes greater activation of the right hemisphere in PET [positron emission tomography] and fMRI [functional magnetic resonance imaging] studies" (p. 122). Paradis[40] and Ahlsén[1] claim that L2 does not cause more right hemisphere activation but that pragmatic factors play an important and greater role in compensation for the poorer proficiency of the speaker of L2.

ACQUIRED CHILDHOOD APHASIA

Acquired childhood aphasia may be identified in a child who has begun to develop language normally and then sustains a language disturbance as the result of cerebral insult. It is usually distinguished from a primary delay or failure to develop language in childhood. A delay or failure to develop language, as opposed to acquired childhood aphasia, usually goes by many names. Neurologists may use the name developmental dysphasia, whereas SLPs typically use developmental language disability. Acquired childhood aphasia is the least common of childhood language problems, but for experts interested in the mechanisms of language development and the brain, it has assumed a pivotal theoretical role.

Onset of acquired childhood aphasia usually is considered to date from infancy through preadolescence, although debate exists regarding its boundaries. The clinical characteristics of the disorder for the most part depend on the same variables of etiology and localization of lesion that are important in adult aphasia, but the age of onset significantly changes the clinical picture for each child. As in the adult, thrombosis, embolism, hemorrhage, and tumor are common causes. Thrombotic stroke appears to be a much more frequent cause than formerly believed.[54]

Earlier literature[14] reported that nonfluent aphasia was overwhelmingly common in acquired aphasia in children, but recently more reports of posterior lesions have been documented in children who exhibit nonfluent expressive speech. The lack of receptive abilities in children with posterior lesions may lead to a gradual loss of expressive speech and may account for the fact that nonfluency was noted in most children as a first sign if they were diagnosed with acquired aphasia.

Although the prognosis in early childhood aphasia caused by unilateral lesions is quite good, complete recovery cannot always be expected. A receptive component usually prolongs recovery. In addition, although language function may appear adequate, it may exceed reading, writing, and numeric skills; writing in particular may show obvious deficiencies. Of course the earlier the onset of the lesion, the better the prognosis; however, this may be complicated by seizures, which slow the recovery. The greatest improvement generally is assumed to occur in children in whom the uninjured hemisphere completely assumes language functions. As children get older, chances of a complete takeover by the uninjured hemisphere are lessened, most likely because brain plasticity decreases with increasing age. Rarely is recovered language, even early in life, equal to that of a normal child of the same age.[54]

Childhood Aphasia with Abnormal Electroencephalographic Findings: Landau-Kleffner Syndrome

An important but small subgroup of patients with acquired aphasia is composed of children whose language disturbance is associated with convulsive seizures and electroencephalographic (EEG) abnormalities, or **Landau-Kleffner syndrome**. Landau-Kleffner is often referred to now as epilepsy-induced aphasia or acquired epileptic aphasia (AEA). The clinical picture in this group is extremely varied. The age of onset of the disorder is generally between 18 months and 13 years. The onset of the language disturbance lasts from a few hours or days to more than 6 months. The defining sign of the disorder is seizure behavior and/or abnormal EEG discharges from one or both of the temporal lobes. The presence of clinical seizures are reported in only 75% to 80% of the children with the syndrome. Seizures may occur before or after the aphasic incident. The child may give the impression of being deaf because the language disturbance usually includes a comprehension disorder. Both expressive and receptive deficits are present, and total mutism may even occur. In some cases the symptoms in AEA resemble those resulting from diffuse damage with traumatic brain injury. These children exhibit executive function problems that include organization, sequencing of ideas, planning, and problem solving. These arise from deficits of memory and problems with attention. The underlying cause of the seizure behavior that affects language is often unknown. The long-term course is unclear, with recovery seen in a minority of cases; many patients have chronic auditory receptive disorders. Anticonvulsant drugs typically are prescribed. A small percentage of cases reported to have acquired epileptic aphasia or Landau-Kleffner syndrome actually experience the seizures secondary to brain damage caused by tumors, stroke or traumatic injury. The term is best used for children whose language disorder cannot be explained by other factors and who show abnormal EEG findings.

Thirteen-year-old F. M. was playing basketball in the school gym when she went at full speed into the wall of the gym after making a lay-up shot. She passed out for approximately 15 minutes. When she regained consciousness, her speech was garbled, she was disoriented, and she experienced naming problems. She was taken to the children's hospital, where she was released in 24 hours after observation. Her parents were told that the above symptoms dissipated within that period. Within a week she began to have mild to severe seizures that were eventually controlled with medication. F. M. was on medication for seizure activity until her twentieth birthday, when all medications were discontinued.

Another seizure occurred just before she turned 22, and she put back on medication. After no seizure activity for 6 months, F. M. decided to stop medication but did not tell her parents or her physician. She had a severe grand mal seizure near her twenty-third birthday. She had three such seizures within 4 days and was sent to a specialist to monitor and examine her seizure activity. The day of that evaluation, F. M. had another severe grand mal seizure. Previous to this one, she had some disorientation, naming problems, and some delusions. But after this last seizure, the physician noted severe expressive and receptive aphasic symptoms similar to acquired aphasia. She was referred to a speech and language clinic, where she was evaluated. Results indicated major problems in thought processing and concentration, emotional lability, difficulty with sentence formation and naming, as well as language symptoms characteristic of both Broca's and Wernicke's aphasia and the repetition difficulties of conduction aphasia. After a year of therapy, F. M. was able to return to college and did very well. Today, she remains on anticonvulsant medication and is a thriving college junior majoring in nursing.

Developmental Language Disability

By far the most prevalent childhood language abnormalities are the developmental language disorders rather than the acquired ones. Children with a **developmental language disability** do not develop language normally. Technically, calling these children aphasic is inappropriate because their language did not develop normally and then become lost or impaired. Terms such as congenital aphasia, developmental aphasia, and dysphasia are not often used by SLPs, who are typically careful not to label children not definitively diagnosed as neurologically or genetically impaired. However, children who do show neurologic signs or possible genetic abnormalities may be labeled as having specific language impairment.

Specific Language Impairment

The term **specific language impairment (SLI)** has been increasing in use in speech-language pathology in recent years. The term has been applied to a subset of children with developmental language disorders, with the implication that many of these children have a consistent history of developmental speech and language delay and have evidence of possible organic involvement.

Professionals who use the term SLI have been particularly concerned with its definition. One critical defining feature of SLI is that the language disorder must not be secondary to a more generalized condition such as peripheral hearing loss, cognitive retardation, a psychiatric disorder (such as childhood schizophrenia), or an acquired neurologic anomaly of the speech mechanism.

SLI generally is defined as a significant expressive and/or receptive language disorder with normal performance in other skills, particularly nonverbal cognition. Of importance is the fact that children with SLI are essentially free of frank neurologic symptoms, in contrast to children with acquired childhood aphasia who often exhibit obvious hemiplegia.

A striking feature of SLI is that it is highly heterogeneous in type and severity as defined by SLPs. Montgomery et al[32] suggest many possible causal factors, including impaired symbolic representational abilities, auditory perceptive processing disabilities at both the speech sound and sentence level, auditory memory problems, problem-solving difficulties (including impaired hypothesis testing and inferential thinking), impaired cognitive styles in linguistic and nonlinguistic thinking, and deficiencies in metalinguistic tasks.

Whether a neurologic basis exists for these behaviors in the child with SLI must be questioned. Lou et al[28] found reduced regional cerebral blood flow in 13 children, 6.5 to 15 years of age, diagnosed with SLI and/or attention deficit disorder. Both cortical and subcortical regions of hypoperfusion were found. Children with dyspraxia of speech showed deficits in the anterior perisylvian area. Children with generalized expressive and receptive disorders showed deficits in both the anterior and posterior perisylvian areas. A single child with a diagnosis of verbal agnosia showed bilateral posterior blood flow problems in both cortical and subcortical areas. Attention deficit–disordered children showed medial frontal hypoperfusion. Six of 11 of these children were language impaired.

Weinberg et al[53] have indicated that information on known lesion sites in adults can be used with children to predict lesion sites from a simple neuropsychologic test given in the office of the pediatric neurologist. Emphasis has also been placed on genetic evidence of loss of certain grammatical features in children with SLI.[23,42]

DIFFERENTIAL DIAGNOSES OF LANGUAGE DISORDERS

Attention Deficit–Hyperactivity Disorder

The lack of evidence of obvious neurologic disturbances in many language-disordered children has led SLPs over the past 40 years to use the concepts of **minimal cerebral**

dysfunction and later, **attention deficit–hyperactivity disorder (ADHD)** as possible explanatory etiologies in children with developmental language disabilities.[3] Some children with language impairment have long been recognized to also display behavioral disorders, perceptual and attention deficits, and minor neurologic deficits, all of which are suggestive of cerebral disorder. Often, however, the neurologic deficits are so mild and subtle that they may be overlooked in the routine pediatric neurologic examination.

The minor neurologic signs most frequently reported are impairments of fine coordination of hands, clumsiness, and mild choreiform or athetoid movements. These have been called soft signs of possible neurologic damage because they are inconsistent and isolated indications of neurologic disturbance, rarely clustering together to present a classic neurologic syndrome allowing reliable lesion lateralization and location.[48] The diagnosis therefore is often made on the basis of behavioral characteristics rather than neurologic signs. For characteristics implying a diagnosis of ADHD, see Box 12-1. As with children with SLI, not all children with ADHD show soft signs or are suspected of having a neurologic disorder.

Neuroimaging and Attention Deficit–Hyperactivity Disorder

Early research reported only nonspecific abnormalities in the scans of children with ADHD. In the late 1990s the most widely used neuroimaging studies that focused on the neuroanatomic structures were computed tomography and magnetic resonance imaging. Several studies done at this time indicated specific (local) abnormalities in a variety of regions in the brain, including the basal ganglia, corpus callosum, and the prefrontal region.[48] The caudate nucleus (basal ganglia)

BOX 12-1

Signs of Attention Deficit–Hyperactivity Disorder

Hyperactivity (hyperkinesis)
Attention disorder
Perseveration
Clumsiness
Emotional lability
Perceptual and cognitive deficits
Memory deficits
Spelling and arithmetic disorders
Speech, language, and hearing disorders
Minor neurologic signs
Nonspecific EEG abnormalities

---

in particular seems to be the most widely found area where abnormalities existed in these children. Some of these studies concluded that the globus pallidus was smaller in the left hemisphere and the caudate nucleus was smaller in the right hemisphere.[48] Finally, one study that used single-photon emission computed tomography techniques with children who were diagnosed with ADHD indicated less brain activity in the left frontal and parietal regions. Because the frontal lobe is the last region to be myelinated, the finding may indicate that this late myelinization could be a possible contributing factor to ADHD.[48]

Positron emission tomography scan studies have demonstrated metabolic abnormalities, especially in the frontal lobe.[48] The premotor and superior frontal cortices were involved and showed a decrease in glucose metabolism both in the adults (more in adult women than in men) who were diagnosed with ADHD in childhood and the children of those adults. The changes in memory and motor skills often seen in children with ADHD may be related to the reduced metabolism in these particularly vulnerable areas. Tannock concluded that gender and age must be considered when working with a diagnosis of ADHD to understand its physiologic and metabolic effects on a child.

Hearing Loss

Hearing impairment of any etiology disturbs or delays language in children and may be one of the most important causes of language delay in children referred to an SLP or pediatric neurologist. A significant hearing loss is not uncommonly associated with brain injury. Many disorders that affect hearing also produce cerebral disorder. Intrauterine infection, hyperbilirubinemia with kernicterus, neonatal anoxia, complications of prematurity, and purulent meningitis are among the well-known causes of hearing loss that also severely affect the nervous system.

Hypoxia and kernicterus are accompanied by a typical high-frequency sensorineural loss with a precipitous drop in the primary speech frequencies (500 to 8000 Hz). If severe, these losses have a significant effect on speech. A profound articulation disorder is present, and in some cases articulatory skills are almost absent.

Cochlear Implants and Language Delay/Disorder and Hearing Loss

Typical consequences of hearing impairment in children with permanent, bilateral hearing loss include significant language development delays and delayed or absent academic achievements.[56] Whether the child has a mild, moderate, or severe loss (and sometimes profound hearing loss), evidence of these delays is found. Despite advances that have occurred in the areas of hearing aid technology, educational techniques specifically for the child with hearing loss, and other intensive interventions (cochlear implants), the academic performance of these children has not changed in the past 30 years.[50,56] Tye-Murray[50] stated that "most children who are profoundly deaf and use hearing aids do not learn the English language well" (p. 638). Bamford and Saunders[8] and Tye-Murray[50] stated that children with hearing problems do not learn grammar as well as hearing children do, which carries over into adulthood when the vocabulary that a hearing-impaired or deaf adult learns is often at the level of an elementary-age child.

Many children are seen in school with delayed or absent pragmatic language skills. As Tye-Murray[50] implied, children with a hearing impairment often do not ask appropriate questions and the initiation, maintenance, and ending of a conversation are three pragmatic concepts that are absent or significantly delayed in children with hearing loss. Most importantly, these children do not know how to repair communication breakdowns and are often embarrassed when this occurs.[50]

As the research cited in Chapter 10 explained, the language delays seen in these children have a neurologic basis; there is distorted or missing auditory input to the auditory cortex and the subsequent connections within the network. Complicating the lack of auditory stimulation to the cortical areas is the fact that these children often do not get practice in using language as much as their hearing counterparts. They cannot listen to their siblings, peers, or parents as models to learn language, including vocabulary. Finally, these children cannot benefit from siblings or parents teaching them social pragmatic skills because they do not have the proper vocabulary to explain situations or the siblings and/or parents do not know American Sign Language well enough.

Yoshinaga-Itano et al[56] investigated the language skills of a large group of children who were identified by 6 months of age as having a hearing loss and compared those results to children who were not identified with a hearing loss until after 6 months of age. Of note, the hearing children had language abilities commensurate with their cognitive skills, but this was not found to be true for children with a diagnosed hearing loss. Furthermore, the study concluded that children with hearing loss identified before or by 6 months of age had a significantly higher receptive and expressive language quotient (over time) than children identified after 6 months. This would support the idea that early intervention with amplification (hearing aids, cochlear implants, etc.) is critical to language and cognitive development.

A child who receives a cochlear implant embarks on a journey in aural rehabilitation that may last for many years.[50] The child's entire family must be involved in the aural rehabilitation process. Siblings, parents, peers, and teachers must constantly allow the child to experience his or her new hearing skills, not only to foster further language and vocabulary development, but also to ensure the development of social pragmatic skills that involve speech, environmental sounds, and the sounds that foster learning in the child's school environment. Despite these advances, controversy still surrounds this issue.

Generalized Cognitive Deficit: Mental Retardation

Cognitive deficits limit language development, and the linguistic skills of the developmentally delayed person are generally poorer than those of the cognitively normal child of equivalent chronologic age. Language development in the majority of developmentally delayed children proceeds on a slower but normal course until early adolescence, when development reaches a plateau. Some have argued that, as in other children, their language development is paced by cerebral maturation. The lack of development of adequate speech and language in **mental retardation** often serves as one of the earliest and most sensitive signs of a degenerative disease of the nervous system for the pediatric neurologist and SLP. Table 12-3 outlines the major language characteristics of children with developmental delay.

Language delay and generalized mental retardation have various causes. Neurologic factors delay or arrest myelinization (maturation), which would inevitably cause brain tissue to remain undeveloped. Certain biologic factors, such as genetic or chromosomal abnormalities, maternal infections in the first trimester of pregnancy, chemical or lead toxicity, metabolic malfunctions, and complications from pregnancy or delivery may also cause mental retardation and a delay of speech and language development. Table 12-4 illustrates causes and consequent syndromes that lead to arrested cognitive and language development.

NEGLECTED AND ABUSED CHILDREN

Parental interactions with the child are often a key factor in the child's overall development of language as well as other behaviors such as social skills, reading, personality development, and interactive skills with peers. This has been documented in many studies in the literature of psychology, speech-language pathology, and education.[17,35,39] Clinicians should be able to recognize some of the signs and salient symptoms of

TABLE 12-3

Language Characteristics of Developmentally Delayed Children

LANGUAGE PARAMETER	CHARACTERISTICS
Phonology	Primitive forms
	Similar to preschoolers no matter the age of the child
Morphology	Preschool developmental characteristics
	Often uses the incorrect form of a free or bound morpheme
Syntax	Short sentence lengths
	Simple sentences lacking complexity
	Lack of clauses and compound sentence structures
Semantics	Concrete thinking; little abstract language comprehension or expression
	Lack of understanding of inferences
	Simple meanings of words noted
Pragmatics	Misunderstands gestures
	Lack of the use of gestures for getting a point across
	Poor turn taking
	Lack of asking for clarification increases miscommunications
	Usually does not initiate topics
Receptive language	Poor comprehension
	Heavily relies on context to understand information presented

Modified from Owens, R.E., Jr. (2004). *Language disorders: a functional approach to assessment and intervention* (4th ed.). Boston: Allyn and Bacon.

TABLE 12-4

Causal Factors of Mental Retardation/ Developmental Delay and the Accompanying Syndromes

CAUSAL FACTORS	SYNDROME OUTCOMES
Chromosomal/genetic	Fragile X
	Down syndrome
Complications of pregnancy/maternal infections	Rubella/German measles
	Syphilis
	Gonorrhea
	AIDS
Chemical/lead toxicity	FAS
	Lead poisoning (eating lead-based paint chips is a common cause)
	Crack cocaine
Metabolic malfunctions	Phenylketonuria
	Poor maternal diet lacking vitamins and minerals
Complications of pregnancy and delivery	Skull malformation/ immaturity of development
	Premature birth
	Lack of prenatal care

Data from Owens, R. E., Jr., Metz, D. E., & Haas, A. (2003). *Introduction to communication disorders: a lifespan perspective* (2nd ed.) (pp. 165-166). Boston: Allyn & Bacon.

child abuse or neglect. Understanding the causes of abuse and neglect and learning about the person who is the abuser will help the SLP deal with these children.

The National Clearinghouse on Child Abuse and Neglect[34] estimated that 900,000 children were abused or neglected in 2003. Because of physical, emotional, or other trauma, these children are at risk for delays in language, communication, and social skills as well as psychologic and emotional harm.[29] According to Lubinski et al,[29] salient signs of physical, sexual, or emotional abuse exist. An understanding of these is helpful for the audiologist and SLP.

Signs of physical abuse include extreme behavior outbursts, self-destructive behaviors, poor academic performance, and language delays. The SLP should be aware of these signs as well as some signs of sexual and emotional abuse.[29] Environmental factors also play a part in the cycle of abuse or neglect. Lubinski et al[29] indicated that these factors may include lack of social support, poverty, and homelessness or poor-quality housing.

For example, many children cry incessantly because of hunger; this type of behavior may lead to neglect or abuse by a frustrated parent or caregiver in families for which poverty is the cause of nutritional deficiencies. Furthermore, the behaviors associated with abuse or neglect and their consequences often lead to developmental milestone delays, which of course include speech and language.

FETAL ALCOHOL SYNDROME AND CRACK-COCAINE ADDICTION

In the last 2 decades of the twentieth century, the incidence and prevalence of babies born with fetal alcohol syndrome or crack-cocaine addiction has plagued public health departments, hospitals, social service agencies, and schools. The problem for these children is that as the developing fetus matures, neurochemical development, production, and function are altered.[39] Many of these babies are born prematurely, with low birth weight, well before central nervous system development is mature. Often these babies undergo spontaneous detoxification as their bodies crave the drug that had been introduced to them by the placenta. At birth, the body goes through natural detoxification, which is a disturbing thing to witness. The seizures, shaking, and muscle destruction that often accompany this period is often severe. Inevitably, these children usually display hyperactivity, poor language development, difficult personalities, difficulty making friends with peers and, as the child grows, poor performance in school. Unfortunately, these delays and the disorders that accompany them are with the child for life and often cannot be rectified by school, therapy, or medications.

Pervasive Developmental Disorders

Recent attention has centered on a group of childhood neuropsychiatric disorders that have become known as **pervasive developmental disorders**. These disorders are diagnostically separated from classic mental retardation syndromes.[13] The pervasive developmental disorders group includes (1) childhood disintegrative disorder, (2) Rett syndrome, (3) Asperger's syndrome, (4) pervasive developmental disorder, not otherwise specified, and (5) autism. Although problems with speech and language may be found, most of the disorders are diagnosed because of more obvious developmental delay and specific behavioral characteristics. Table 12-5 describes the differential diagnosis criteria for onset of the disorder, domains affected, the severity of the disorder, and the delays typically found in these children in the areas of language and cognition.

A **childhood disintegrative disorder** usually is characterized by a period of prolonged normal development, usually 3 to 4 years. This is followed by deterioration in several areas of behavior. Increased motor activity, anxiety, and affective disturbances are present. A general lack of interest in the environment begins, accompanied by a loss of receptive and expressive language functioning. Lost language may return to basic, but not normal, levels of single words and simple sentences. Severe or moderate mental retardation becomes apparent. Although the etiology is not clear, abnormal EEGs are found, as is a history of seizures in many cases. No clear lesion has been identified, however. Recovery of the lost skills is minimal. The incidence appears to be less than that of childhood autism. Males appear to predominate.

TABLE 12-5

Differential Diagnostic Characteristics of Several Disorders along the ASD Continuum

DISORDER TYPE	ONSET TIME	DELAYS FOUND	SEVERITY LEVELS	AFFECTED DOMAINS
Autism	Before age 3 years	General delays may be present, including language, communication, social, and learning difficulties	Spans the spectrum from PDD to high functioning	Social Communication Sensory sensitivity
Childhood disintegration disorder	Typical development until 2 years old, then loss of social skills and language	Often associated with mental retardation; loss of speech	Similar to autism	Usually affects two of the three main domains of autism
Asperger's syndrome	Before or after 3 years of age	Generally no delay in cognitive or language skills but may be disordered as the child develops	Varies by child	Social skills Language-syntax Language-pragmatics
PDD	By age 3 years	Similar to autism; not enough criteria met; child is diagnosed as PDD-NOS (not otherwise specified)	Could differ from autism; not usually described as mild or severe; usually child does not meet autism criteria	Social skills Language Communication Sensory sensitivity

Modified from Wetherby, A. M., & Prizant, B. M. (2000). *Autism spectrum disorders: a transactional developmental perspective.* Baltimore, Md: Brookes.

Rett syndrome, sometimes confused with autism, essentially is marked by a normal prenatal and paranatal development. This is followed by normal psychomotor development for the first 5 months of life. The head circumference at birth is within normal limits. After this period of normality, head growth decreases between 5 and 48 months. Hand skills are lost between 5 and 30 months, along with the development of stereotyped hand wringing and handwashing motions. Awkward gait and trunk movements are also noted. A loss of social interaction occurs early on, but later social interactions improve. Severe impairment in both expressive and receptive language is present. Severe mental retardation is common. Neuropathologic findings are present, but the exact cause is unclear. The disorder appears primarily in females.

Asperger's syndrome is a disorder included in the pervasive developmental disorder class. In some ways it is like autism. Social interaction is markedly impaired, as seen in autism, but differences also exist. Communication and cognitive skills are relatively better than in autism. No significant general delay in language development is found. Most cases are not recognized before 3 years of age; often the children are somewhat precocious in their use of language and seem to be fascinated with letters and numbers. In later life, language in conversation may be one-sided, dealing only with the person's favorite topics. Prosody may be disturbed with a constricted range of intonation. Speech can be described as verbose, tangential, and circumscribed. Early motor ability may be normal compared with the child with autism. Box 12-2 describes the language characteristics of Asperger's syndrome.

BOX 12-2

Language Characteristics of Children with Asperger's Syndrome

Early language milestones may be typical
Concrete and literal thinker
Difficulty with abstract thinking
Often a visual learner
Information may be learned in chunks
Misinterprets idioms, sarcasm, humor
Difficulty with verbal problem solving
May be hyperverbal
Often does not understand the "gestalt," or whole of the situation, and misses the intent
Possible odd prosody; inflection and rate may be different
Pragmatic language is a major concern
Difficulty with theory of mind

Pervasive developmental disorder (not otherwise specified), sometimes referred to as PDD-NOS, is designated as an atypical autism. The category implies a heterogeneous condition with several subgroups. In general, the social impairment is less than is common in childhood autism. The diagnosis is more difficult to make than in other developmental disorders. No period of normality followed by a drastic loss of skills occurs. Although evidence of deficits in relationships with peers and family is present, the degree of social impairment is less than is seen in classic autism.

Autism spectrum disorder (ASD) may include a diagnosis of "autism." The 1996 (revised reprint in 2001) diagnosis from the *Diagnostic and Statistical Manual of Mental Disorders* (DSM IV)[4] lists PDD-NOS (NOS = not otherwise specified) at the mild end and ASD at the severe end of the continuum. This syndrome, in which disturbed communication and delayed development are key signs, has received much attention as of late. Verbal behavior is often severely involved. The child may be mute or echolalic. Other signs of the disorder include obvious disturbance of social relationships, abnormal response to objects, and difficulties in sensory modulation and general motility. Children diagnosed with ASD come from diverse backgrounds.[38] Owens[38] found that slightly more than 50% of these children have IQs lower than 50. Table 12-6 presents a variety of language characteristics of children with ASD. Compare these characteristics with those of the child with Asperger's syndrome (see Box 12-2). Box 12-3 summarizes the pervasive developmental disorders.

The etiology of **autism** is controversial and basically unknown. Some experts believe that it is related to early affective or sensory deprivation. Other experts state that some type of neurologic dysfunction plays a major role in the syndrome. Early brain injury and abnormalities of the cerebral ventricles, brainstem, or cerebellum have been found and cited as possible etiologies. Recent computed tomographic scan studies have revealed cortical lesions in some cases of autism.[15] Some causal factors involved with the diagnosis of PDD-NOS or ASD are listed in Table 12-7.

DEVELOPMENTAL DYSLEXIA

Reading disorders of childhood frequently are associated with inadequate or inappropriate instruction or emotional disorders. However, one form of reading disorder, **developmental dyslexia**, can best be understood in a neurologic context. Known also as congenital word blindness or specific reading disability, developmental dyslexia is the most common disorder of communication found in schoolchildren. It is estimated to occur in

TABLE 12-6
Language Characteristics of the Child with ASD

LANGUAGE PARAMETER	LANGUAGE CHARACTERISTICS
Phonology	Usually disordered
	Degree of disorder varies by child
	Usually the least affected language parameter
Morphology/Syntax	Pronouns and some verbs are quite difficult
	Often uses the incorrect form of a word, especially verbs
	Simple sentence structure, often with incomplete syntax
Pragmatics	Joint attention is disordered
	Topic initiation and maintenance are difficult
	Form and content usually do not match within a context
	Repetitions are frequent and do not add to meaning
	Asks a lot of questions at times irrelevant to the topic at hand
	Very poor eye contact
Semantics	Appears to have word retrieval difficulties
	Often inappropriate answers to questions or statements
Language comprehension skills	Conversational difficulties
	Often appears to not comprehend the task or the gist of a conversation

Modified from Owens R. E., Jr. (2004). *Language disorders: a functional approach to assessment and intervention* (4th ed.). Boston: Allyn & Bacon.

5% to 10% of all schoolchildren and is found at all levels of intelligence, from superior to subnormal. The child with dyslexia has great difficulty in attaching sound and meaning to written words. Oral reading is usually quite difficult. Words with a similar appearance often are confused, and letters that look alike are reversed. Phonemes may be mispronounced in oral reading, and certain phonemes may be omitted or inserted. Reading comprehension is impaired. Disorders of writing are often present, with reversals, poorly formed letters, rotations, repetition, and omission of letters. Written syntax is poor.

Summary of the Differential Diagnosis of PDD

Childhood Disintegrative Disorder

- Prolonged normal development is followed by increased motor activity, anxiety, and affective disturbances.
- Severe or moderate mental retardation and seizures appear in many cases.
- Males are affected in greater numbers than females, and recovery of lost receptive and expressive language function is minimal.

Rett Syndrome

- Normal development is followed by a deceleration of head growth between 5 and 48 months of age.
- Severe mental retardation and impairment of expressive and receptive language.
- Disorder appears primarily in females and is characterized by predictable handwashing and wringing type movements.

Asperger's Syndrome

- Impaired communication and cognitive skills are present; language development progresses at normal levels.
- Fascination with letters and numbers in early language development leads to verbose and tangential speech.
- Later life conversation may be one-sided, focused on specific, favorite topics.

PDD-NOS

- Designated as atypical autism because some, but not all, of the characteristics associated with autism are diagnosed.
- Social impairment is less than those impairments diagnosed as autistic.
- No period of normalcy is diagnosed in the person's affected lingual or social development.

ASD

- Severe verbal and/or social deficits, including abnormal responses to objects, sensory discontinuity, and mute or echolalic characteristics are present.
- Key signs include delayed development and disturbed communication skills in children.
- The diagnosis of "autism" may be included.

TABLE 12-7

Some Controversial Causal Factors of ASD and PDD

FACTOR	DESCRIPTION
Biological factors	Abnormal brain functions as evidenced by neuroimaging
	Newest cause is a genetic link, but whether it is a single gene is controversial
	Unusually high levels of serotonin in some children
	Impaired cortical development
Social/environmental	No evidence of lack of parental interaction as a cause
Processing: visual and auditory	Difficulty analyzing and integrating visual and auditory information
	Auditory sensitivity
	Echolalia caused by difficulty processing information in a timely manner
	Possible link to the limbic system

Adapted from Bernstein, D & Tiegerman, E (1997). *Language & communication disorders in children.* Boston: Allyn & Bacon.

Dyslexia and Neurologic Findings

The reading disorder known as dyslexia is caused by central nervous system dysfunction, much like a learning disability. Left-handedness or ambidexterity, along with mild generalized abnormal EEG patterns, are frequently seen. Often there is a positive family history, with other members of the family having similar problems. Dyslexia occurs more often in males. Some studies show an autosomal dominant mode of inheritance.

Riccio and Hynd[44] and Owens[38] postulated that the left temporal area, the right frontal lobe area, and most likely the subcortical areas connecting the two hemispheres are involved in dyslexia. The fact that several areas are dysfunctional at the onset of dyslexia would explain the vast differences among children who have been diagnosed with this disorder. Along with a reading disability, these children often exhibit a language delay, including auditory comprehension and even difficulties with phonologic processing. These children may also exhibit a mild form of anomia or word finding difficulties usually seen as a result of the comprehension and phonologic deficits.

Clinical Information and Applications for the Speech-Language Pathologist

- Acquisition of speech and language is clearly tied to physical development and maturation.
- The course of speech and language development is a correlate of cerebral maturation and specialization.
- An index of neurologic development is the change in gross brain weight with age.
- Brain weight triples in the first 24 months of life.
- At 10 years old, the brain achieves 95% of its ultimate weight.
- Neurolinguistics is the study of how the brain processes linguistic information.
- The posterior cortex regulates information in the form of analyzing, coding, understanding, and storing information to memory.
- Primary neurulation is the process that forms the brain and spinal cord from the neural tube.
- Secondary neurulation is the process of how the caudal neural tube and plate give rise to the sacral and coccygeal vertebrae.
- Dysraphia is a condition in which the primary neural tube does not close.

- Primary neurulation defects include anencephaly, in which the anterior neural tube does not close during maturation and the fetus develops without a brain.
- Secondary neurulation defects include spina bifida.
- Bilingualism involves code switching.
- Myelinization is one of the more significant indexes of brain maturation and roughly correlates with speech and language development.
- As an infant grows, early reflex motor movements are replaced by more sophisticated motor skills as further myelinization takes place.
- Cerebral plasticity is the concept that a child's brain recovers function more quickly than an adult's because of the young age and the brain's ability to recover quickly.
- Newer theories of plasticity refute this claim, saying that a child's brain may not recover as well as assumed; as maturation continues and tasks become more complex, identification of deficits may simply be delayed.

Clinical Information and Applications for the Speech-Language Pathologist—cont'd

- Cerebral dominance is associated with laterality.
- A language disorder is a delay in the comprehension or production of the language content, form, and/or usage.
- A language difference is a variation of a symbol system that reflects and is determined by shared regional, social, or cultural ethnic factors.
- An SLP should understand the difference between cultural sensitivity (cultural awareness) versus cultural competence when working with linguistically diverse children
- Acquired childhood aphasia is defined by normally developing language before the child sustains a language disturbance or interruption as a result of a cerebral insult.
- Landau-Kleffner syndrome is an acquired aphasia in children associated with EEG abnormalities and seizure activity.
- Epilepsy-induced aphasia is severe seizure activity that induces symptoms similar to acquired aphasic language, as seen in patients with traumatic brain injury.
- Note the difference between a developmental versus acquired language disability
- SLI is a developmental language disorder with a history of language delay and normal nonverbal cognition and other skills.

- ADHD is associated with language disturbance, including memory deficits, perseveration, speech or language delay, and EEG abnormalities.
- Hearing loss in children often causes significant language delays and associated academic achievements
- Hearing aids and cochlear implants are both significant interventions to improve language skills of children. The earlier the intervention, the better chances of developing age-appropriate or near age-appropriate language skills.
- Abused or neglected children often display language delay because of the effects of these actions on the child's overall development and maturation.
- Children born with crack-cocaine addiction or FAS display hyperactivity, language delay, difficult personalities, and pragmatic and social skills.
- ASD includes autism, childhood disintegration disorders, Asperger's syndrome, and PDD-NOS.
- Public schools and private clinics have seen a significant increase in Asperger's patients, characterized by disorder in abstract thinking, abstract language, and auditory learning; concrete thinking; and a lack of pragmatic language skills.
- Developmental dyslexia is difficulty in attaching sound and meaning to words and difficulty associating visual and auditory stimuli.

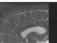

CASE**STUDY**

B. W., a 5-year-old girl, began her kindergarten year at the local elementary school. Her teacher noted that B.W. was quite hyperactive and could not keep up with the children in her classroom during the simplest of activities. She would often sit alone because the other children were sometimes afraid of her outbursts and tantrums. The teacher noted that B.W.'s appearance seemed to be unusual, with widespread eyes and an almost blank, expressionless face most of the time. B.W. was easily distracted by noises or a new person coming into the room. She appeared to have attention difficulties and did not understand the simplest of abstract expressions. She often took things quite literally. The teacher referred her to the school psychologist. Results of testing revealed an IQ score of 72. Speech therapy evaluation further revealed poor sentence structures, often using only two- to three-word phrases; a difficulty with phonics, distractibility, difficulty sharing, and tantrums when she was not permitted to do what she wanted. An individual education plan was written, and B. W. was placed in the self-contained special needs classroom with 2 hours a week in speech and language therapy and 2 hours a week in the elementary learning disability classroom.

QUESTIONS FOR CONSIDERATION:
1. What is the diagnosis for B. W. based on the description above?
2. Based on this child's IQ, would she be classified as a developmentally delayed slow learner or as having mild to moderate mental retardation?

REFERENCES

1. Ahlsén, E. (2006). *Introduction to neurolinguistics.* Philadelphia: John Benjamins Publishing Co.
2. Allison, M. (1992). *The effects of neurologic injury on the maturing brain.* Headlines, October-November, New Medico.
3. American Psychiatric Association. (1987). *Diagnostic and statistical manual of mental disorders III.* Washington, D. C.: Author.
4. American Psychiatric Association. (1999). *Diagnostic and statistical manual of mental disorders, IV.* Washington, D. C.: Author.
5. American Speech-Language-Hearing Association. (2004). *Communication differences vs. language disorder.* http://www.asha.org/NR/rdonlyres/8C3DF431-6762-46A5-BBDO-EC757E75FF6/0/v1IE_cult_comp.pdf. Retrieved May 18, 2007.
6. American Speech-Language-Hearing Association. (2004). *Technical report: cochlear implants.* ASHA Supplement 24.
7. Anderson, B., Southern, B., & Powers, R. E. (1999). Anatomic asymmetries of the posterior superior temporal lobes: a postmortem study. *Neuropsychiatry, Neuropsychology and Behavioral Neurology, 12,* 247-254.
8. Bamford, J., & Saunders, E. (1985). *Hearing impairment, auditory perception, and language disability.* London: Edward Arnold.
9. Barkovich, A. J. (1990). Apparent atypical callosal dysgenesis: analysis of MR findings and their relationship to holoprosencephaly. *American Journal of Neuroradiology, 11,* 333-339.
10. Bear, M. F., Connors, B. W., & Paradiso, M. A. (2007). *Neuroscience: exploring the brain* (3rd ed.). Philadelphia: Lippincott Williams & Wilkins.
11. Brookshire, R. (2003). *Introduction to neurogenic communication disorders* (6th ed.). St. Louis, Mosby.
12. Castro, A. J., Merchut, M. P., Neafsey, E. J., & Wurster, R. D. (2002). *Neuroscience: an outline approach.* St. Louis: Mosby.
13. Coffey, C. E., & Brumback, R. A. (1998). *Textbook of pediatric neuropsychiatry.* Washington, D. C.: American Psychiatric Press.
14. Cohen, M., Campbell, R. E., & Yaghmi, F. (1989). Neuropathological abnormalities in developmental dysphasia. *Annals of Neurology, 25,* 567-570.
15. Cranberg, L. D., Filley, C. M., Hart, E. J., & Alexander, M. P. (1987). Acquired aphasia in children: clinical and CT investigations. *Neurology, 37,* 1165-1172.
16. Dawson, G. (Ed.) (1989). *Autism: nature, diagnosis, and treatment.* New York: Guilford Publications.
17. Demaio, L. (2000). *Parent-child communication program.* Unpublished research.
18. Dehaene, S., Dopoux, E., Mehler, J., Cohen, L., Paulesu, E., Perani, D., et. al. (1997) Anatomical variability in the cortical representation of first and second language. *Neuroreport, 8,* 3809-3815.
19. Ewing-Cobb, L., Levin, H. S., & Fletcher, J. M. (1998). Neuropsychological sequelae after pediatric traumatic brain injury: advances since 1985. In Ylvisaker, M. (Ed.), *Traumatic brain injury rehabilitation children and adults* (2nd Ed.). Boston: Butterworth-Heinemann.
20. Galuske, R.A. W., Schlote, W., Bratzke, H., & Singer, W. (2000). Interhemispheric asymmetries of the modular structure in human temporal cortex. *Science, 289,* 1946-1949.
21. Geschwind, N. (1979). Anatomical foundations of language and dominance. In Ludlow, C. L., & Doran-Quine, M. E. (Eds.), *The neurological basis of language in children: methods and directions for research* (pp. 145-157). Bethesda, MD: National Institutes of Health.
22. Gillis, R. J. (1996). *Traumatic brain injury: rehabilitation for speech-language pathologists.* Boston: Butterworth-Heinemann.
23. Gopnik, M., & Crago, M. (1991). Familial aggregation of a developmental language disorder. *Cognition.* April, 39:1: 1-50.
24. Habib, M., & Robichon, F. (2003). Structural correlates of brain asymmetry: Studies in left-handed and dyslexic individuals. In Hugdahl, K., & Davidson, R. J. (Eds.), *The asymmetrical brain.* Cambridge, MA: MIT Press.
25. Haines, D. E. (2006). *Fundamental neuroscience for basic and clinical applications* (3rd ed.). St. Louis: Elsevier.
26. Lecours, A. R. (1975). Myelogenetic correlates of development of speech and language. In Lenneberg, E., & Lenneberg, E. (Eds.), *Foundations of language development. Vol. I.* New York: Academic Press.
27. Lenneberg, E. (1967). *Biological foundations of language.* New York: Wiley.
28. Lou, H. C., Henderson, L., & Bruhn, P. (1984). Focal cerebral hypoperfusion in children with dysphasia and attention deficit disorder. *Archives of Neurology, 41,* 825-829.
29. Lubinski, R., Golper, L. C., & Frattali, C. (2007). *Professional issues in speech-language pathology* (3rd ed.). Clifton Park, NY: Thomson Delmar Learning.
30. Mahendra, N. J., Ribera, R., Sevcik, R., Adler, R., Cheng, L., Davis-McFarland, E., et al (2004). *Why is yogurt good for you? Because it has live cultures.* Rockville, MD: American Speech-Language-Hearing Association.
31. Minkowski, M. (1963). On aphasia in polyglots. In Halpern, L. (Ed.), *Problems of dynamic neurology.* Jerusalem: Hebrew University.
32. Montgomery, J. W., Windsor, J., & Stark, R. E. (1991). Specific speech and language disorders. In Ober, J. E., & Hynds, G. W. (Eds.), *Neuropsychological foundations of learning disorders.* New York: Academic Press.
33. Murray, L., & Clark, H. (2006). *Neurogenic disorders of language.* Clifton Park, NY: Thompson Delmar Learning.
34. National Clearinghouse on Child Abuse and Neglect. *Diagnostic and statistical manual of mental disorders (DSM-IV) (2000)* (4th ed., rev. ed.). Philadelphia: American Psychiatric Association.
35. Nelson, N. W. (1998). *Childhood language disorders in context: infancy through adolescence* (2nd ed.). Boston: Allyn & Bacon.
36. Owens, R. E., Jr. (2001). *Language development: an introduction* (5th ed.). Needham, MA: Allyn and Bacon.
37. Owens, R. E., Jr. (2005). *Language development: an introduction* (6th ed.). Needham, MA: Allyn and Bacon.

38. Owens, R. E., Jr. (2004). *Language disorders: a functional approach to assessment and intervention* (4th ed.). Boston: Allyn and Bacon.

39. Owens, R.E., Jr., Metz, D. E., & Haas, A. (2003). *Introduction to communication disorders: a lifespan perspective* (2nd ed.). Boston: Allyn Bacon.

40. Paradis, M. (1998). Language and communication in multilinguals. In Stemmer, B., & Whitaker, H. (Eds.), *Handbook of neurolinguistics* (pp. 418-431). San Diego: Academic Press.

41. Penfield, W., & Roberts, L. (1959). *Speech and brain mechanisms.* Princeton: Princeton University Press.

42. Pinker, S. (1994). *The language instinct.* New York: Morrow.

43. Rasmussen, T., & Milner, B. (1977). The role of early left-brain injury in determining lateralization of cerebral speech functions. *Annals of the New York Academy of Sciences, 299,* 355-369.

44. Riccio, C. A., & Hynd, G. W. (1996). Neuroanatomical and neurophysiological aspects of dyslexia. *Topics in Language Disorders, 16,* 1-13.

45. Rubinstein, D., Youngman, V., Hise, J. H., & Damiano, T. R. (1994). Partial development of the corpus callosum. *American Journal of Neuroradiology, 15,* 869-875.

46. Silverman, F. H., & Miller, L. (2006). *Introduction to communication sciences and disorders.* Eau Claire, WI: Thinking Publications.

47. Sprott, R. A., & Kemper, S. (1987). The development of children's code-switching: a study of six bilingual children across two situations. In Pemberton, E. F., Sell, M. A., & Simpson, G. B. (Eds.), (1987) *Working papers in language development.* Lawrence, Kansas, University of Kansas, Child Language Program (pp. 116-134).

48. Tannock, R. (1998). Attention deficit hyperactivity disorder: advances in cognitive, neurobiological, and genetic research. *Journal of Child Psychology and Psychiatry, 39,* 65-99.

49. Tupper, D. (Ed.) (1987). *Soft neurological signs.* Orlando, FL: Grune & Stratton.

50. Tye-Murray, N. (2004). *Foundations of aural rehabilitation: children, adults, and their family members* (2nd ed.). Clifton Park, NY: Delmar Learning.

51. Wada, J. A., Clark, R., & Hamm, A. (1975). Cerebral hemispheric asymmetry in humans. *Archives of Neurology (Chicago), 32,* 239-246.

52. Wetherby, A., & Prizant, B. (2000). *Autism spectrum disorders: a transactional developmental perspective.* Baltimore: P.H. Brookes.

53. Weinberg, W. A., Harper, C. R., & Blumback, R. A. (1995). Neuroanatomic substrate of developmental specific learning disabilities and select behavioral syndromes. *Journal of Child Neurology, 10,* 578-580.

54. Wood, B. T. (1995). Acquired childhood aphasia. Kirshner, H. (Ed.), *Handbook of neurological speech and language disorders.* New York: Marcel Dekker.

55. Ylvisaker, M. (1998). *Traumatic brain injury rehabilitation: children and adolescents* (2nd ed.). Boston: Butterworth-Heinemann.

56. Yoshinaga-Itano, C., Sedey, A., Coulter, D., & Mehl, A. (1998). Language of early- and later-identified children with hearing loss. *Pediatrics, 102,* 1161-1171.

Medical Conditions Related to Communication Disorders

I. Congenital Disorders

A. *Cerebral palsy:* Defect of motor power and coordination related to damage of the immature brain

B. *Congenital hydrocephalus:* Condition marked by excessive accumulation of fluid, dilating the cerebral ventricles, thinning the brain, and causing a separation of cranial bones; caused by a developmental defect of the brain

C. *Craniostenosis:* Contraction of the cranial capacity or narrowing of the sutures by bony overgrowth

D. *Down syndrome:* Syndrome of mental retardation associated with many and variable abnormalities, caused by representation of at least a critical portion of chromosome 21 three times instead of twice in some or all cells

E. *Idiopathic mental retardation:* Mental retardation of unknown cause

F. *Minimal cerebral dysfunction:* Syndrome of neurologic dysfunction in children usually marked by impairment of fine coordination, clumsiness, and choreiform or athetoid movements; learning disorders often associated with this diagnosis

G. *Neurofibromatosis:* Condition in which small, discrete, pigmented skin lesions develop in infancy or early childhood, followed by the development of multiple subcutaneous neurofibromas that may slowly increase in number and size over many years

II. Vascular Disorders

A. *Cerebral embolism:* Obstruction or occlusion of a vessel in the cerebrum by a transported clot or vegetation, a mass of bacteria, or other foreign material

B. *Cerebral hemorrhage:* Bleeding in the brain; a flow of blood, especially if profuse, into the substance of the cerebrum, usually in the region of the internal capsule; caused by rupture of the lenticulostriate artery

C. *Cerebral thrombosis:* Obstruction or occlusion of a vessel in the cerebrum by a fixed clot developing on the arterial wall

D. *Pseudobulbar palsy:* Muscular paralysis from bilateral upper motor neuron lesions of the cranial nerves; often accompanied by signs of dysarthria, dysphagia, and emotional lability with outbursts of uncontrolled crying and laughing

E. *Recurrent cerebral ischemia or transient ischemic attacks:* Temporary disruptions of the blood supply that produce specific neurologic signs; experienced as sudden, transient blurring of vision, weakness, numbness of one side, speech difficulty, vertigo or diplopia, or any combination

F. *Subdural hemorrhage:* Extravascularization of blood between the dural and arachnoid membranes

III. Infections

A. *Acute anterior poliomyelitis:* Inflammation of the anterior cornu of the spinal cord due to an acute infectious disease marked by fever, pains, and gastroenteric disturbances; followed by flaccid paralysis of one or more muscular groups and later by atrophy

B. *Cerebral abscess:* Intracranial abscess or abscess of the brain, specifically of the cerebrum; a collection of pus in a localized area

C. *Encephalitis:* Inflammation of the brain

D. *Jakob-Creutzfeldt disease:* Spastic pseudosclerosis with corticostriatospinal degeneration and subacute presenile dementia; characterized by slowly progressive dementia, myoclonic fasciculations, ataxia, and somnolence with gradual onset; usually fatal within a few months to years

E. *Meningitis:* Inflammation of the membranes of the brain or spinal cord

F. *Neurosyphilis:* Syphilis, an infectious venereal disease caused by a microorganism affecting the nervous system

G. *Sydenham's chorea:* Acute toxic or infective disorder of the nervous system, usually associated with acute rheumatism, occurring in young persons and characterized by involuntary semipurposeful but ineffective movements; movements involve the facial muscles and muscles of the neck and limbs and are intensified by voluntary effort but disappear in sleep

IV. Trauma

A. *Penetrating head injury:* Open head injury, which causes altered consciousness and can produce fairly definitive and chronic aphasias

B. *Closed-head injury:* Injury to the head with no injury to the skull or injury limited to an undisplaced fracture; also known as nonpenetrating head injury; can produce loss of consciousness and often produces diffuse effects

V. Tumors

A. *Astrocytomas (grades 1 and 2) and oligodendrogliomas:* Less-common glial cell tumors, with a better prognosis than glioblastoma multiforme; slow growing; usually treated with surgery and radiation therapy, with an average survival rate of 5 to 6 years after surgery

B. *Glioblastoma multiforme:* Also known as malignant glioma or astrocytoma (grades 3 and 4), the most common primary brain tumor in adults; most frequent sites are frontal and temporal lobes, although tumors may occur anywhere in the brain; infiltrative and rapidly growing, with an average survival rate of approximately 1 year

C. *Meningioma:* Benign tumor arising from the arachnoid cells of the brain; slow growing and usually occurring at the lateral areas and base of the brain; generally does not invade the cerebral cortex; favorable prognosis

VI. Degenerative Diseases

A. *Dementia of the Alzheimer's type:* Progressive mental deterioration with loss of memory, especially for recent events

B. *Parkinson's disease:* Degenerative disease resulting from damage to the dopamine-producing nerve cells of the striatum and the substantia nigra; characterized by rest tremor, rigidity of muscles, paucity of movement, slowness of movement, limited range, limited force of contraction, and failure of gestural expression

C. *Wilson's disease:* Genetic metabolic disorder caused by inadequate processing of dietary intake of copper and characterized by motor symptoms, with a significant dysarthria

D. *Huntington's chorea:* Chronic progressive hereditary disease characterized by irregular, spasmodic, involuntary movements of the limbs or facial muscles; sometimes accompanied by dementia and dysarthria

E. *Friedreich's ataxia:* Hereditary disease characterized by degeneration principally of the cerebellum and dorsal half of the spinal cord; ataxic dysarthria often an accompanying sign

F. *Dystonia musculorum deformans:* Hereditary disease occurring especially in children; characterized by muscular contractions producing peculiar distensions of the spine and hip and bizarre postures

G. *Multiple sclerosis:* Inflammatory disease mainly involving the white matter of the central nervous system; characterized by scattered areas of demyelination causing impairment of transmission of nerve impulses; may cause a variety of symptoms, including paralysis, nystagmus, and dysarthria depending on the lesion sites

VII. Metabolic and Toxic Disorders

A. *Reye's syndrome:* Sudden loss of consciousness in children following the initial stage of an infection, usually resulting in death with cerebral edema (swelling) and marked fatty change in the liver and renal system; surviving children often have motor, cognitive, and speech problems

VIII. Neuromuscular Disorders

A. Progressive muscular atrophies

1. *True bulbar palsy:* Disorder caused by involvement of nuclei of the last four or five cranial nerves and characterized by twitching and atrophy of the tongue, palate, and larynx, drooling, dysarthria, dysphagia, and finally respiratory paralysis; usually a manifestation of amyotrophic lateral sclerosis

2. *Amyotrophic lateral sclerosis:* Disease of the motor tracts of the lateral columns of the spinal cord causing progressive muscular atrophy, increased reflexes, fibrillary twitching, and spastic irritability of muscles

B. Muscular dystrophy

1. *Pseudohypertrophic (Duchenne) type:* Type of muscular dystrophy characterized by bulky calf and forearm muscles and progressive atrophy and weakness of the thigh, hip, and back muscles and shoulder girdle; occurs in the first 3 years of life, usually in boys and rarely in girls

2. *Facioscapulohumeral type:* Type of muscular dystrophy causing atrophy of the muscles of the face, shoulder, girdle, and

upper arms; occurs in either sex, with onset at any age from childhood to late adult life; characterized by prolonged periods of apparent arrest

   3. *Ocular myopathy:* Type of muscular dystrophy affecting external ocular muscles, causing ptosis, diplopia, and occasional total external ophthalmoplegia; sometimes associated with upper facial muscle weakness, dysphagia, and atrophy and weakness of neck, trunk, and limb muscles

C. *Myasthenia gravis:* Disorder characterized by marked weakness and fatigue of muscles, especially those muscles innervated by bulbar nuclei

D. Congenital neuromuscular disorders

   1. *Möbius syndrome:* Congenital disorder characterized by paresis or paralysis of both lateral rectus muscles and all face muscles; sometimes associated with other musculoskeletal anomalies

IX. Other

A. *Epilepsy:* Chronic disorder characterized by paroxysmal attacks of brain dysfunction (seizures) usually associated with some alteration of consciousness; seizures may remain confined to elementary or complex impairment of behavior or may progress to a generalized convulsion

B. *Wernicke-Korsakoff syndrome:* Cerebral disorder characterized by confusion and severe impairment of memory, especially for recent events; patient compensates for memory loss by confabulation; often seen in chronic alcoholics and associated with severe nutritional deficiency

Bedside Neurologic Examination

1. **Mental Status**
   A. Orientation: person, place, time
   B. Memory and information
      1. Three objects at 5 minutes
      2. Presidents back to Kennedy
   C. Language
      1. Spontaneous speech characterization
      2. Confrontation naming
      3. Auditory comprehension (commands, yes/no questions)
      4. Repetition (words, phrases)
      5. Reading (printed commands)
      6. Writing (signature, words, and sentences to dictation)
   D. Calculations
      1. Serial 7s (count by 7s to 100)
      2. Subtract $0.43 from $1.00
   E. Visuospatial ability
      1. Clock drawing
      2. Copying of figures
   F. Insight, judgment
2. **Cranial Nerves**
   A. I: Smell
   B. II: Visual fields, pupillary reactions, optic fundi
   C. III to IV: Extraocular movements
   D. V: Facial sensation
   E. VII: Facial symmetry
   F. VIII: Hearing
   G. IX and X: Articulation, palatal movement, gag reflex
   H. XI: Sternomastoid and trapezius strength
   I. XII: Tongue movement
3. **Motor Examination**
   A. Bulk
   B. Spontaneous movements (fasciculations, tremor, movement disorders)

C. **Strength**
   1. Evaluation of strength on right and left
      a. Deltoid
      b. Biceps
      c. Triceps
      d. Hip flexion
      e. Knee flexion
      f. Ankle dorsiflexion
      g. Ankle plantar flexion
D. **Reflexes**
   1. Evaluation of reflexes on right and left
      a. Biceps
      b. Triceps
      c. Brachioradialis
      d. Ankle
      e. Plantar
      f. Jaw
E. **Stance and Romberg**
F. **Gait**
   1. Spontaneous gait
   2. Tandem gait
   3. Tiptoe gait
   4. Heel gait
G. **Sensory Examination**
   1. Pinprick
   2. Touch
   3. Vibration
   4. Position
   5. Stereognosis, graphesthesia ("cortical" sensory modalities)
H. **Cerebellar**
   1. Finger-nose-finger
   2. Rapid alternating hand movements
   3. Fine finger movements
   4. Heel-knee-shin

Courtesy Howard Kirshner, MD, Department of Neurology, Vanderbilt University School of Medicine, Nashville, TN.

Appendix C

Screening Neurologic Examination for Speech-Language Pathology

I. Mental Status
A. *General behavior and appearance:* Is the patient normal, hyperactive, agitated, quiet, immobile? Neat, slovenly? Is he dressed in accordance with peers, background, and sex?
B. *Stream of talk:* Does the patient respond to conversation normally? Is her speech rapid, incessant, under great pressure? Is she very slow and difficult to draw into spontaneous talk? Is she discursive, able to reach the conversational goal?
C. *Mood and affective responses:* Is the patient euphoric, agitated, inappropriately cheerful, giggling? Or is he silent, weeping, angry? Does his mood swing in a direction appropriate to the subject matter of the conversation? Is he emotionally labile?
D. *Content of thought:* Does the patient have illusions, hallucinations, delusions, or misinterpretations? Is she preoccupied with bodily complaints, fears of cancer or disease, or other phobias? Does she believe that society is maliciously organized to cause her difficulty?
E. *Intellectual capacity:* Is the patient bright, average, dull, obviously demented, mentally retarded?
F. *Sensorium*
   1. *Consciousness:* Note whether the patient is alert, drowsy, or stuporous.
   2. *Attention span:* Note response in cerebral function test.
   3. *Orientation:* Note whether the patient can answer questions about his person, location, and time.
   4. *Memory:* Note recent and remote memory deficits disclosed during history taking.
   5. *Fund of information:* Note in history taking.
   6. *Insight, judgment, and planning:* Note in history taking.
   7. *Calculation:* Note performance on cerebral function test.

II. Speech, Language, and Voice
A. *Dysphonia:* Neuromotor difficulty in producing voice (cranial nerve X)
B. *Dysarthria:* Neuromotor disorder of articulation and voice
   1. Labials (cranial nerve VII)
   2. Velars and velopharyngeal closure (IX and X)
   3. Linguals (XII)
C. *Dysphasia:* Cerebral disorder of understanding and expressing language (give aphasia-screening test)
   1. Fluent (give screening aphasia test)
   2. Nonfluent (give screening aphasia test)
D. *Dyspraxia:* Cerebral disorder of articulation and prosody and/or disorder of oral movement
   1. Dyspraxia of speech
   2. Oral dyspraxia
E. *Dementia:* Cerebral disorder of language or intellectual deficit
   1. Presenile
   2. Senile
F. *Disorganized language:* Cerebral disorder of language or confusion
G. *Dysphagia:* Neuromotor disorder of swallowing (V, VII, IX, X, and XII)

III. Cranial Nerves for Speech and Hearing
A. *Speech* (V, VII, IX, X, XII, and XI)
   1. V: Inspect masseter and temporalis muscle bulk; palpate masseter when the patient bites.
   2. VII: Evaluate forehead wrinkling, eyelid closure, mouth retraction, whistling or puffed out cheeks, wrinkled skin over neck (platysma), and labial articulation.
   3. IX and X: Evaluate phonation, hypernasality, swallowing, gag reflex, and palatal elevation.
   4. XII: Evaluate lingual articulation and midline and lateral tongue protrusion; inspect for atrophy and fasciculations.

Data from DeMeyer, W. (1980). Technique or the neurologic examination. New York: McGraw-Hill.

5. XI: Inspect sternocleidomastoid and trapezius contours; test strength of head movements and shoulder shrugging.

6. Test for pathologic fatigability by requesting 100 repetitive movements (e.g., eye blinks) if the history suggests myopathic or myoneural disorder.

B. *Hearing* (VIII)

1. Evaluate for threshold and acuity, including adequacy of hearing for conversational speech.

2. If history or preceding observation suggests a deficit, perform air-bone conduction audiometric screening.

IV. Motor System

A. *Inspection*

1. Take history, including initial appraisal of the motor system; inspect the patient for postures, general activity level, tremors, and involuntary movements.

2. Observe the size and contour of the muscles, looking for atrophy, hypertrophy, body asymmetry, joint misalignments, fasciculations, tremors, and involuntary movements.

3. Evaluate gait, including free walking, tandem walking, and deep knee bend.

B. *Palpation:* Palpate muscles if they seem atrophic or hypertrophic or if the history suggests they may be tender or in spasm.

C. *Strength*

1. *Upper extremities:* Test biceps.

2. *Lower extremities:* Test knee flexors and foot dorsiflexors if necessary and feasible.

3. *Pattern:* Discern whether any weakness follows a distributional pattern, such as proximal-distal, right-left, or upper extremity–lower extremity.

D. *Muscle tone:* Move the patient's joints to test for spasticity, clonus, or rigidity.

E. *Muscle stretch (deep) reflexes:* Test jaw jerk (cranial nerve V afferent and efferent) as well as other muscle stretch reflexes if necessary and feasible.

F. *Cerebellar system* (gait tested previously)

1. Evaluate finger-to-nose, rebound, and alternating motion rates.

2. Carry out heel-to-knee testing.

V. Sensory Examination

A. Test superficial sensation by light touch with cotton wisp and pinprick on face.

B. Ask if the face feels numb.

C. Test superficial sensation on the tongue surface with swab stick unilaterally and bilaterally, anteriorly and posteriorly.

VI. Cerebral Function

A. When the history or antecedent examination suggests a cerebral lesion, test for finger agnosia and right-left disorientation.

B. Have the patient perform the cognitive, constructional, and performance tasks from standard aphasia or neuropsychological tests.

Glossary

abducens: cranial nerve VI, which supplies motor impulses to abduct the eye.

abduction: movement of a body part away from the midline.

absolute refractory period: the short period of membrane unresponsiveness during the passage of an action potential; another action potential cannot be generated during this time.

acceleration-deceleration injury: type of injury in which the head is accelerated and then suddenly stopped (e.g., motor vehicle accident).

acquired childhood aphasia: language disorder in which cerebral insult halts or disturbs normal language development in a child.

action potential (AP): buildup of electrical current in the neuron.

action tremor: rhythmic, oscillatory, involuntary movement affecting the outstretched upper limbs as well as other parts of the body and the voice. Also known as essential tremor, heredofamilial tremor.

adduction: movement of a body part toward midline.

adequate stimulus: a mechanical, thermal, electrical or chemical stimulus strong enough to change the cell membrane's potential.

adiadochokinesia: inability to perform rapid, alternating muscle movements; see *dysdiadochokinesia*.

afferent: traveling toward a center.

afferent fibers: nerve fibers that carry information toward the cell body; often used to denote sensory fibers.

agnosia: lack of sensory recognition as the result of a lesion in the sensory association areas or association pathways of the brain.

agraphia: acquired disorder of writing caused by brain injury.

akinesia: absence or lack of movements.

alexia: acquired disturbance of reading caused by brain injury.

alexia with agraphia: classic neurologic syndrome of reading disorder in which damage has occurred to the angular gyrus and the surrounding areas.

alexia without agraphia: classic neurologic syndrome of reading disorder, usually caused by a left posterior cerebral artery occlusion in a right-handed person; the resulting infarct produces lesions in the splenium of the corpus callosum and the left occipital lobe.

allocortex: the older, original part of the cerebral cortex.

alpha motor neurons: neurons allowing contraction of extrafusal fibers and that have their final common path in cranial and spinal nerves.

Alzheimer's disease: the most common type of dementia; its most striking feature is progressive deterioration of cognitive functions; language disturbance is a major symptom.

amyloid plaques: axonal endings associated with pathologic deposits of extracellular beta-amyloid. Found in the brain of patients with dementia of the Alzheimer's type.

amyotrophic lateral sclerosis (ALS): a progressive, fatal motor neuron disease usually involving both the upper and lower motor neuron pathways. Also known as Lou Gehrig's disease.

analgesia: loss of the sensation of pain.

anastomosis: a connection between two vessels; an opening created by surgery, trauma, or pathologic condition between two spaces or organs that are normally separate.

anencephaly: absence of the cranial vault at birth with the cerebral hemispheres completely absent or reduced to small masses attached to the base of the skull.

anesthesia: loss of feeling or sensation.

aneurysm: a sac formed by the dilation of the wall of an artery, a vein, or the heart.

angular gyrus: convolution in the left parietal lobe that is critical for language processing.

anion: an ion carrying a negative charge as a result of a surplus of electrons.

anomia: loss of the power to name objects or recognize and recall their names.

anomic aphasia: an acquired disorder of language caused by brain damage in which the primary difficulty is with word retrieval.

anoxia: condition marked by the absence of oxygen supply to organs or tissue.

anterior: for anatomic structures, denoting before, in front of, or the front part of.

anterior horn cell: cell in the ventral portion in an H-shaped body of gray matter in the spinal cord associated with efferent pathways.

anterior spinothalamic tract: the uncrossed fibers of the spinothalamic tract, which carry sensations of light or crude touch.

anterograde: transport of axons from the cell body toward the axon terminal.

aphasia: acquired disorder of language caused by brain damage; may affect comprehension or expression of language in any modality (spoken, written, or gestural language).

aphasic alexia: a disorder of reading caused by brain damage; the reading disorder is part of the overall aphasia syndrome (for example, the reading disorder associated with Wernicke's aphasia).

aphemia: an obsolete term for loss of the power of speech.

apraxia: a disorder of learned movement distinct from paralysis, weakness, and incoordination; results in a disturbance of motor planning.

apraxia of speech (AOS): disorder of programming the muscles of articulation in the absence of paralysis, weakness, and incoordination.

aprosodia: abnormal prosody (stress and intonation pattern in speech), usually resulting from damage to the nondominant hemisphere.

aqueduct of Sylvius: small tube or outlet in the midbrain connecting the third and fourth ventricles.

arachnoid mater: a thin membranous covering (meninges) of the brain and spinal cord that lies between the dura mater and the pia mater

arcuate fasciculus: long subcortical association tract connecting posterior and anterior speech-language areas in the cerebrum.

areflexia: lacking normal reflexive response to an adequate stimulus.

arteriosclerosis: a chronic disease characterized by abnormal thickening and hardening of the arterial walls, with resulting loss of elasticity.

arteriovenous malformation (AVM): congenital morphologic defect resulting in an abnormal cluster of arteries directly connecting to veins; often enlarges over time and is at risk of rupture.

articulatory undershoot: speech production error in which the active articulatory structure (often the tongue) does not reach its target completely. Often a feature of the articulation of persons with hypokinetic dysarthria.

Asperger's syndrome: a developmental disorder characterized by impaired social and occupational skills; normal language (excluding pragmatics) and cognitive development; and restricted, repetitive, and stereotyped patterns of behavior, interests, and activities; often found to show above-average performance in a narrow field against a general background of deficient functioning.

association fiber tracts: the fiber bundles that form connections between and within the association areas of the brain.

astereognosis: loss of the ability to recognize objects through touch alone; caused by brain damage.

astrocyte: a type of glial cell with numerous sheetlike processes extending from its body that are thought to provide nutrients for neurons and may have some information storage function.

asymmetric tonic neck reflex (ATNR): a reflex, normal in the newborn, that consists of extension of the arm and sometimes of the leg on the side to which the head is forcibly turned, with flexion of the contralateral limbs. Considered abnormal if found beyond the eighth or ninth month of age in a term infant.

asymmetry: disproportion or inequality between two corresponding parts around the center of an axis.

asynergia: lack of coordination in agonistic and antagonistic muscles that manifests as a deterioration of smooth, complex movements.

asynergy: lack of coordination of agonistic and antagonistic muscles, particularly associated with cerebellar disorders.

ataxia: defect of posture and gait associated with a disorder of the nervous system; sensory ataxia, associated with dorsal column dysfunction, is distinguished from cerebellar or cerebellar pathway ataxia.

ataxic cerebral palsy: a relatively uncommon type of cerebral palsy resulting from damage to the cerebellum; characterized by hypotonic muscles and an ataxic gait pattern.

ataxic dysarthria: the motor speech disorder associated with damage to the cerebellum and/or its pathways; characterized by irregular articulatory breakdown, prosodic changes, and often a slow rate.

athetoid cerebral palsy: the most common dyskinetic type of cerebral palsy characterized by delayed motor development and involuntary, uncontrolled writhing movements.

athetosis: a neurologic disorder marked by continual, slow movements, especially of the extremities.

atopognosis: loss of the power to locate touch sensation correctly; usually caused by damage to the parietal lobe.

atrophy: decrease in size or wasting of a body part or tissue.

attention deficit–hyperactivity disorder: a condition that usually becomes identifiable in children in the preschool to early childhood years (and may persist into adulthood) in which three types of behavior or primary symptoms may be identified: inattentiveness; impulsiveness with hyperactivity; or a combination of these with inattentiveness, impulsiveness, and hyperactivity prominent.

audition: hearing.

auditory agnosia: inability to recognize the significance of sounds.

auditory brainstem response (ABR): a type of electrophysiologic audiometry in which electrical activity is evoked by brief click stimuli from the eighth cranial nerve and the brainstem; allows inference of hearing and identification of the site of lesion as the cochlea, cranial nerve VIII, or the brainstem.

autism: major developmental disability marked by disturbed stereotyped behavior and language patterns;

echolalic verbal behavior is often present, as are neurologic signs.

autism spectrum disorder (ASD): a group of five pervasive developmental disorders characterized by varying degrees of impairment in communication skills; social interactions; and restricted, repetitive, and stereotyped patterns of behavior; the most commonly occurring disorders of the spectrum are classic autism and Asperger's syndrome. If the specific characteristics for diagnosis of one of these does not fit, the other more common diagnosis is pervasive developmental disorder not otherwise specified. Two rare diagnoses in the spectrum are Rett syndrome and childhood disintegrative disorder.

autoassociator network: network used in simulations of behavior in which every unit in the network is connected to every other unit, with associations stored within a layer of neurons.

autonomic nervous system: a part of the vertebrate nervous system that innervates smooth and cardiac muscle and glandular tissues and governs involuntary actions (e.g., secretion, vasoconstriction, or peristalsis); includes the sympathetic nervous system and the parasympathetic nervous system.

axon: a straight, relatively unbranched process of a nerve cell; literally defined as "the axis."

axonal regeneration: regrowth of damaged axons.

axoplasm: the protoplasm of an axon.

Babinski sign: a reflex movement; when the sole of the foot is tickled, the great toe turns upward instead of downward; normal in infancy but indicates damage to the central nervous system (as in the pyramidal tracts) when occurring later in life. Also known as Babinski, Babinski reflex.

basal ganglia: subcortical structures, part of the extrapyramidal system, associated with motor control of tone and posture.

behavioral neurology: a specialty in neurology emphasizing clinical and research skills in neurodegenerative diseases and neurobehavioral syndromes.

bilateral: related to or having two sides.

bilateral innervation: supply of nerves from both sides of the body.

bilateral symmetry: movements on one side of the body that mirror movements on the opposite side.

bilingual: the ability to understand and converse in more than one language.

bipolar cell: first-order nerve cell of the retina, synapsing with the ganglion cells.

bite reflex: rapid closure of the jaw and a bite response on moderate pressure to the gums; normal in infants up to 9 to 12 months of age.

border zone: the limit of the cerebral area served by either the anterior, middle, or posterior cerebral arteries.

bouton: a synaptic knob; from French, meaning "button."

brain scan: a neurodiagnostic tool using a radioisotope to detect damaged brain tissue.

brainstem: the part of the brain connecting the spinal cord to the forebrain and cerebrum; contains the medulla oblongata, pons, and mesencephalon (midbrain).

branchial: of or relating to gills or to parts of the body derived from the embryonic branchial arches and clefts.

Broca's aphasia: acquired adult language disorder characterized by nonfluent speech and language; usually accompanied by hemiplegia and an anterior lesion of the brain.

Broca's area: major speech-language center in the dominant frontal lobe; important for expression of language.

callosal dysgenesis: defective development of the corpus callosum.

capsular: referring to the internal capsule.

Carl Wernicke: scientific pioneer (1848-1905) who identified an auditory speech center in the temporal lobe associated with comprehension of speech.

cation: a positively charged ion.

caudal: situated in or directly toward the hind part of the body.

central (parietal-temporal) alexia: an acquired disorder of reading and writing caused by brain damage and usually accompanied by some degree of aphasia; also known as alexia with agraphia.

central nervous system (CNS): the brain and the spinal cord structures.

central pattern generator: a term given to a cluster of neurons (afferent, interneurons, and efferent) that, when stimulated, trigger a sequenced series of physical responses. In swallowing, the medullary swallowing center, with the nucleus solitarius and the nucleus ambiguous, is thought to function as a central pattern generator.

cephalic: of or relating to the head; directed toward or situated on, in, or near the head.

cerebellar hemispheres: the two spherical structures comprising the cerebellum.

cerebellum: cauliflower-shaped brain structure located just above the brainstem at the base of the skull.

cerebral palsy: a disability resulting from damage to the brain before, during, or shortly after birth and outwardly manifested by muscular incoordination and often speech disturbances.

cerebral plasticity: the ability of the brain to reorganize neural pathways on the basis of new learning and experiences.

cerebrospinal fluid (CSF): clear, colorless bodily fluid produced by the choroid plexuses and contained within the subarachnoid space circulating around the brain and spinal cord before being absorbed by the arachnoid villi; cushions the central nervous system and provides nutrients.

cerebrovascular accident (CVA): interruption of the blood flow to the brain as a result of occlusive (thrombotic or embolic) or hemorrhagic mechanisms; also known as stroke.

cerebrum: the major portion of the brain, consisting of two hemispheres, that contains the cortex and its underlying white matter as well as the basal ganglia and other basal structures.

childhood apraxia of speech (CAS): a developmental sensorimotor speech disorder characterized by impairment of the ability to program the positioning of the articulators and the sequencing of muscle movements for volitional speech production; also known as developmental apraxia of speech.

childhood disintegrative disorder: a rare, pervasive developmental disorder on the autism spectrum in which communication and social skills develop normally until at least age 2 years (onset usually is between 3 and 4 years) followed by pronounced loss in motor, communication, and social skills.

chorea: disorder characterized by irregular, spasmodic, involuntary movements of the limbs or facial muscles.

choreiform: resembling chorea.

choroid plexus: structures located in certain parts of the ventricle that are composed of fused ependymal and pia mater cells and associated capillaries; makes and secretes cerebrospinal fluid for circulation.

cingulate gyrus: the ridge on the surface of the cerebrum located between the cingulated sulcus and the sulcus of the corpus callosum.

circle of Willis: circle of arteries located at the base of the brain; serves as a vascular mechanism for collateral circulation.

circumlocution: wordy and circuitous description of unrecalled terms.

clinical neurology: medical discipline involving diagnosis and treatment of diseases of the nervous system.

clonus: form of movement marked by contractions and relaxations of a muscle occurring in rapid succession.

cochlear duct: the middle chamber of the cochlea that contains the sensory end organ of hearing, the organ of Corti; also known as the scala media.

code switching: in linguistics, alternating between two or more languages, dialects, or language registers in a single conversation.

cognition: the mental process of knowing, which includes aspects such as awareness, perception, reasoning, memory, and judgment.

cognitive-communicative disorders: communication disorders resulting from the neurobehavioral sequelae of diffuse (as opposed to focal) brain damage, including deficits in information processing, attention, reasoning, and problem-solving and memory.

cogwheel rigidity: increased tone, equalized between agonist and antagonist muscles, with a superimposed cogwheel, ratchetlike resistance; often found in patients with Parkinson's disease.

colliculi: little "hills" or mounds within the brain; the superior and inferior colliculi are found in the midbrain.

computerized tomography (CT): x-ray imaging technique in which the brain is viewed at different depths; the various views are correlated by computer to show structural lesions of the brain.

concentration gradient: ratio of solute and water across a membrane.

conduction aphasia: an adult language disorder in which auditory comprehension is good but exact repetition is poor; the site of the lesion producing the syndrome is in debate, but it may interrupt the arcuate fasciculus.

confabulation: verbal or written expression of fictitious experiences.

confusional state: acute symptoms of mental disorganization and agitation that may accompany head trauma or other medical conditions; the language is often marked by irrelevancy and confabulation.

congenital childhood suprabulbar palsy: a disorder characterized by isolated paralysis or weakness of the oral musculature without major weakness in the trunk or extremities.

constraint-induced therapy (CIT): a treatment method in rehabilitation in which the patient is forced to use the damaged modality to accomplish tasks normally performed with that modality. For example, constraining the nonparalyzed left arm and requiring activities of daily living and therapy tasks to be done with the hemiparetic right arm and hand or, in constraint-induced aphasia therapy, requiring the patient to communicate verbally rather than allowing alternative communication methods or facilitation.

constructional disturbance: the inability to form a construction in space because of a cerebral deficit.

contingent negative variation (CNV): a small negative potential recorded on an electroencephalogram over the front central scalp of some subjects who perform tasks requiring close attention or who have just received a warning stimulus; also known as E wave or expectancy wave.

contralateral: related to the opposite side.

contralateral innervation: the supply of nerve impulses from the opposite side of the body.

convergence: the exciting of a single sensory neuron by incoming impulses from multiple other neurons.

corpus callosum: the largest transversal commissure between the hemispheres; it is approximately 4 inches long.

corpus striatum: subcortical mass of white and gray matter in front of and lateral to the thalamus in each cerebral hemisphere; is used to refer to the putamen, globus pallidus, and caudate nucleus collectively.

cortex: the outer surface layer of the brain (or other organs).

corticonuclear fibers: the fiber bundle pathway in each hemisphere from the motor cortex to the nuclei of the brainstem; depending on the particular nerve, some of the fibers decussate and others travel ipsilaterally.

corticospinal tract: part of the pyramidal system that descends from the cerebral cortex to different levels of the spinal cord; facilitates motor control.

cranial nerve: one of 12 pairs of nerves (fiber bundles surrounded by connective tissue) that exit the brain and pass through the skull to reach the sense organs or muscles of the head and neck with which they are associated.

declarative memory: memory for facts and events.

decussation: crossing over or intersection of parts.

deep dyslexia: an acquired reading disorder resulting from left-hemisphere brain damage and characterized by semantic errors in reading single words.

deglutition: the act of swallowing.

dementia: an organic mental disorder with progressive general intellectual deterioration affecting memory, judgment, and abstract thinking as well as personality changes.

dementia of the Alzheimer's type (DAT): see *Alzheimer's disease.*

dendrite: the short branching processes of a nerve cell; literally means "treelike."

denervation: a cutting of the nerve supply by excision, incision, or blocking.

depolarization: loss of the difference in charge between the inside and outside of the plasma membrane of a muscle or nerve cell caused by a change in permeability and migration of sodium ions to the interior.

dermatome: the lateral wall of a somite from which the dermis is produced.

developmental anarthria: diagnosis involving complete lack of speech as a result of profound paralysis, weakness, and/or incoordination of the musculature of speech.

developmental apraxia of speech: a developmental disorder characterized by impaired ability to execute the appropriate movements of speech voluntarily in the absence of paralysis, weakness, or incoordination of the musculature of speech; also known as childhood apraxia of speech.

developmental dysarthria: speech disorder resulting from damage to the immature nervous system; characterized by weakness, paralysis, and/or incoordination of the speech musculature.

developmental dyslexia: see *dyslexia.*

developmental language disability: congenital difficulty with the production and/or comprehension of language, ranging from mild delay to severe disorder.

developmental motor speech disorders: a group of disorders of speech production resulting from congenital weakness, paralysis, or incoordination of the speech musculature or a congenital disorder of programming the speech musculature. See *developmental dysarthria and childhood apraxia of speech.*

diaphragma sella: a ring-shaped fold of dura mater covering the sella turcica, in which the pituitary gland sits.

dichotic listening: test situation in which simultaneous auditory stimuli are presented to both ears at the same time; ear preference (right or left) is judged by which ear first recognizes the auditory stimulus.

diencephalon: the part of the forebrain between the cerebral hemispheres and the midbrain; includes the thalamus, hypothalamus, the third ventricle, and the epithalamus.

diffuse axonal injury (DAI): extensive tearing of axons as a result of traumatic shearing forces that occur when the head is rapidly accelerated or decelerated, resulting in twisting or rotational force.

diplegia: paralysis of corresponding parts on both sides of the body, with legs more impaired.

diplopia: double vision.

distal: away from the center of the body.

divergence: dissemination of the effect of activity of a single nerve cell through multiple synaptic connections.

dorsal: pertaining to the back; posterior.

dorsal column pathway: major sensory pathway mediating proprioception.

Duchenne muscular dystrophy: a chronic, progressive disease beginning in early childhood that affects the shoulder and pelvic girdles, causing increasing weakness and pseudohypertrophy of the muscles followed by atrophy and the establishment of a peculiar swaying gait.

dura mater: the outermost meningeal layer covering the brain.

dysarthrias: a group of speech production disorders caused by oral-motor weakness, paralysis, or incoordination. May be congenital or acquired.

dysdiadochokinesia: the inability to perform and sustain rapid alternating movements; speech-language pathologists in particular apply this term to a motor deficit in the oral muscles; associated with cerebellar disorder syndromes; also called alternate motion rate.

dysfluency: speech marked by hesitations, prolongations, and/or repetitions that interrupt the natural prosodic flow; also refers to stuttering.

dyskinesia: disorder of movement usually associated with a lesion of the extrapyramidal system.

dyslexia: inability to read despite the ability to see and recognize letters and a history of appropriate instruction.

dysmetria: the inability to gauge the distance, speed, and power of a movement.

dysphagia: difficulty swallowing.

dysprosody: disturbance of stress, timing, and melody of speech.

dystonia: disorder in which the limbs assume distorted static postures as a result of excess tone in selected parts of the body.

ear advantage: demonstrated ear "preference" for certain stimuli. Dichotic listening studies have shown that verbal stimuli are more accurately reported when presented to the right ear than the left ear in persons who are left dominant for language. This is called the "right ear advantage."

ectoderm: the outermost of the three primary germ layers of an embryo

efferent: conducting (fluid or nerve impulses) outward from a given organ or part.

efferent fibers: fibers conducting a neural impulse away from a given neuron; often refers to a motor fiber, though technically it does not necessarily refer to motor impulses.

electroencephalography (EEG): procedure producing a graphic record of electrical activity of the brain as recorded by an electroencephalograph.

embryo: the developing human individual from the time of implantation to the end of the eighth week after conception.

encephalitis: inflammation of the brain.

encephalon: the brain.

encephalopathy: pathology of the brain.

endoderm: the innermost of the three primary germ layers of an embryo that is the source of the epithelium of the digestive tract and its derivatives and of the lower respiratory tract.

endolymph: the watery fluid in the membranous labyrinth of the ear.

enteric: relating to or affecting the intestines.

enteric nervous system: a division of the autonomic nervous system formed by neuronal plexuses in the gastrointestinal tract and directly affecting deglutition and digestion during swallowing.

ependymal cells: glial cells that compose the lining of the ventricles (the ependyma) and the choroid plexuses. The cells function to help make cerebrospinal fluid.

epithalamus: small region of the diencephalon of the brain consisting of the pineal gland, habenular nuclei, and stria medullaris thalami.

equilibrium: the state of being balanced.

essential tremor: organic tremor not associated with any pathologic process.

esthesiometer: instrument used to assess two-point discrimination for tactile sensation.

excess and equal stress: a feature noted in the speech of some persons with dysarthria, especially in ataxic dysarthria, in which normally unstressed words or syllables are stressed equally with other words with the resulting prosody sounding "robotic."

excitatory postsynaptic potential (EPSP): an electrical change (depolarization) in the membrane of a postsynaptic neuron caused by the binding of an excitatory neurotransmitter from a presynaptic cell to a postsynaptic receptor, increasing the likelihood of an action potential being generated in the postsynaptic neuron.

executive functions: capacities, under primary control of the prefrontal cortex, that guide complex behavior over time through planning, decision making, and response control. Common executive abilities include judgment, problem solving, decision making, planning, and pragmatics and depend on cognitive abilities such as attention, perception, memory, and language.

explosive speech: loud, sudden speech attributable to damage to the nervous system.

extensor: a muscle, the contraction of which tends to shorten a limb; antagonist to flexors.

exteroceptors: sense receptors (as of touch, temperature, smell, vision, or hearing) excited by stimuli outside the organism.

extinction: progressive reduction in strength of a conditioned response on withdrawal of the reinforcing stimulus.

extraocular: adjacent to but outside the eyeball.

extrapyramidal system: the basal ganglia and its interconnections.

facilitation: process of making the nerve impulses easier by repeated use of certain axons.

falx cerebri: the larger of the two folds of dura mater separating the hemispheres of the brain that lies between the cerebral hemispheres and contains the sagittal sinuses.

fasciculation: involuntary contractions or twitches in a group of muscle fibers.

fasciculus: a nerve fiber bundle forming a connection between groups of neurons in the central nervous system; also known as a tract.

feedback: in control theory, a process in which some portion of the output signal of a system is passed (fed back) to the input; often used to control the dynamic behavior of the system.

feedforward: system that reacts to changes in its environment, usually to maintain some desired state; exhibits response to a measured disturbance in a predefined way but does not handle novel stimuli.

fetal period: the ninth week after conception until birth.

fissure: a groove on the surface of the brain or spinal cord.

flaccid: flabby, without tone.

flaccid dysarthria: a classification of motor speech disorders associated with damage to the lower motor neuron or some part of the motor unit; marked by certain features depending on the part of the motor unit that is damaged.

flocculus: small, irregular lobe on the undersurface of each hemisphere of the cerebellum that is linked with the corresponding side of the nodulus by a peduncle.

fluency disorders: speech disorders that affect the natural prosody and flow of speech.

fluent/nonfluent: a dichotomous classification of aphasic language on the basis of the type of conversational speech.

focal lesion: an identifiable, circumscribed area of damage or injury.

foramen: an aperture or perforation through a bone or a membranous structure.

forebrain: the anterior of the three primary divisions of the developing vertebrate brain or the corresponding part of the adult brain that especially includes the cerebral hemispheres, the thalamus, and the hypothalamus; in higher vertebrates, is the main control center for sensory and associative information processing, visceral functions, and voluntary motor functions; also called prosencephalon.

fricatives: a consonant sound produced by directing and continuing the restricted breath stream against one or more of the oral surfaces (hard palate, alveolar ridge, teeth, and/or lips); may be voiced or unvoiced. Examples include /f/, /v/, /s/, and /z/.

frontal alexia: reading disorder known as the third alexia; associated with a lesion in the left frontal lobe; often accompanies a Broca's aphasia.

frontal lobe: the anterior division of each cerebral hemisphere having its lower part in the anterior fossa of the skull and bordered behind by the central sulcus.

frontotemporal dementias (FTD): a syndrome complex, designated by the National Institute of Neurological Diseases and Stroke, marked by progressive deterioration in behavior and/or language with retention of important features of memory, unlike other dementias.

functional magnetic resonance imaging (fMRI): the use of magnetic resonance imaging to measure the hemodynamic response related to neural activity in the brain or spinal cord.

funiculi: aggregates of fiber bundles (or tracts) in the nervous system as seen in the spinal cord; also called columns.

gag reflex: reflex contraction of the muscles of the throat especially caused by stimulation (as by touch) of the pharynx.

Galant reflex: a newborn reflex elicited by holding the child face down and stroking along one side of the spine; normal reaction is lateral flexion toward the stimulated side; should disappear by 9 months of age or before.

gamma-aminobutyric acid (GABA): an inhibitory neurotransmitter.

gamma motor neuron: neurons innervating the muscle spindle; allow contraction of intrafusal fibers and increased sensitivity of the fibers to the muscle stretch reflex.

ganglia: nerve cells with common form, function, and connections that are grouped outside the central nervous system.

gasserian ganglion: the large, flattened, sensory root ganglion of the trigeminal nerve that lies within the skull and behind the orbit; also called trigeminal ganglion, semilunar ganglion.

genioglossus: a fan-shaped muscle that arises from the superior mental spine; inserts on the hyoid bone and into the tongue; and advances, retracts, and depresses the tongue.

genu: any structure of angular shape resembling a flexed knee.

Gerstmann syndrome: a cluster of left parietal lobe lesion signs, including finger agnosia, left-right disorientation, acalculia, and agraphia; a developmental form of the syndrome has been described.

glial cells: cellular elements, of which there are several types, that support and expedite the activity of the neurons; glial cells outnumber the neurons 10 to 1; also called neuroglial cells.

glioma: general name for a tumor arising from the supportive tissues of the brain

global aphasia: an acquired disorder of language caused by brain damage and characterized by severe impairment of all language modalities, comprehension, verbal and gestural expression, reading, and writing.

globus pallidus (GPi): a nucleus of the basal ganglia that receives input from the caudate and the putamen and is the main output nucleus.

glottal coup: a rapid, forceful closing and opening of the true vocal folds accompanied by a short, sharp vocalization; used in oral-motor examinations to assess vocal fold movement and strength informally.

Golgi tendon organs: a collection of afferent fibers located in tendons or their processes that respond to tension during muscle contraction.

graceful degradation: an engineering concept adopted in explanations of neural processing in which the loss of one component of a distributed processing network results in a reduced level, but not failure, of performance.

graded potential: short-lived depolarizations or hyper-polarizations of an area of membrane. These changes cause local flows of current (movement of ions) that decrease with distance. When this occurs in a receptor cell, it is called a receptor potential.

gray matter: the grayish substance of brain and spinal cord composed of neuronal and glial cell bodies, unmyelinated nerve fibers, and synapses.

gyrus: an elevation or ridge on the surface of the cerebrum.

helicotrema: the minute opening by which the scala tympani and scala vestibuli communicate at the top of the cochlea of the ear.

hemianopsia: a visual field defect of one half of the eye field.

hemiparalysis: total or partial paralysis of one side of the body that results from disease of or injury to the motor centers of the brain; also called hemiplegia.

hemiplegia: see *hemiparalysis.*

hemorrhage: bleeding; a profuse flow of blood.

Heschl's gyrus: convolution of the temporal lobe that is the cortical center for hearing; runs obliquely outward and forward from the posterior part of the lateral sulcus.

hindbrain: the posterior division of the three primary divisions of the developing vertebrate brain or the corresponding part of the adult brain that includes the cerebellum, pons, and medulla oblongata and that controls the autonomic functions and equilibrium; also called the rhombencephalon.

homeostasis: the physiologic process by which the body's internal systems are maintained at equilibrium despite changes in external conditions.

homunculus: caricature mapping the connections between the area of the motor or sensory cortex and the innervated body part; literally means "little man."

Huntington's chorea: a progressive chorea inherited as an autosomal dominant trait characterized by choreiform movements and mental deterioration leading to dementia; accompanied by atrophy of the caudate nucleus and the loss of certain brain cells with a decrease in the level of several neurotransmitters; usually begins in middle age; also called Huntington's disease.

hyoglossus: extrinsic tongue muscle involved in the retraction and depression of the tongue.

hyperalgesia: increased sensitivity to pain or enhanced intensity of pain sensation.

hyperesthesia: unusual or pathologic sensitivity of the skin or of a particular sense to stimulation.

hyperkinesia: an abnormal, involuntary increase in muscle activity.

hypernasality: the perception of nasal resonance during the production of voiced sounds, particularly vowels.

hyperpolarization: increased production in potential difference across a biologic membrane.

hyperreflexia: a condition in which the deep tendon reflexes are exaggerated.

hypertonia: extreme tension of the muscles.

hypoalgesia: decreased sensitivity to pain.

hypoesthesia: impaired or decreased tactile sensibility; also called hypesthesia.

hypokinesia: diminished muscle movement capacity.

hypokinetic dysarthria: dysarthria caused by basal ganglia disease; most commonly associated with Parkinson's disease.

hyporeflexia: diminished or absent reflexes.

hypothalamus: portion of the brain that composes part of the third ventricle; critical to autonomic and endocrine function, including rage and aggression, regulation of body temperature, and nutrient intake; also exerts neural control over pituitary gland.

hypotonia: muscle flaccidity; a decrease in normal muscle tone when passive movement is performed.

ideational apraxia: disorder of motor planning in which complex motor plans cannot be executed, although individual motor components of the plan can be performed.

ideomotor apraxia: a motor disturbance characterized by the inability to carry out motor acts on command, but some evidence is present that these motor acts can be carried out imitatively or automatically.

inferior: situated below and closer to the feet than another part and especially another similar part of an upright body of a human being.

innervate: to supply with efferent nerve impulses.

input fibers: neural elements that make synaptic connections by synapsing onto the cell body and/or onto dendrites or dendritic spines found on the dendrites.

intention tremor: a slow tremor of the extremities that increases on attempted voluntary movement and is observed in certain diseases of the nervous system (e.g., multiple sclerosis).

internal carotid arteries: the inner branches, right and left, of the carotid artery that supply the brain, eyes, and other internal structures of the head; also called internal carotid.

internuncial: functionally imposed between two or more neurons.

interoceptor: a specialized nerve receptor that receives and responds to stimuli originating from within the body.

interstitial fluid: extracellular fluid.

intervertebral foramina: the openings between the vertebrae of the spinal cord through which the motor and sensory roots exit and unite to form the spinal nerves.

intrinsic neurons (interneurons): nerve cells within the central nervous system that act as a link between sensory and motor neurons.

ipsilateral: on the same side.

irritability: the capacity to respond to stimuli.

ischemia: insufficient blood flow to brain tissue, often leading to cell death in that area.

island of Reil: part of the cerebral cortex forming the floor of the lateral fissure; also known as insula.

kernicterus: a form of infantile jaundice in which a yellow pigment and degenerative lesions are found in areas of the intracranial gray matter.

lacrimal: related to the tears, their secretions, and the organs concerned with them.

Landau-Kleffner syndrome: a pediatric disorder—first described in 1957 by Drs. William M. Landau and Frank R. Kleffner, who identified six children with the disorder—characterized by a gradual or sudden loss of the ability to understand and use spoken language. Abnormal electrical brain waves, documented by an electroencephalogram, are common, as are epileptic seizures; affected children often have hyperactivity; also called acquired epileptic aphasia.

language lateralization: concept that language is not exactly alike between the two hemispheres of the brain.

language dominant: the hemisphere that is the site for the major language areas and connections.

lateral: a position farthest from the medial plane or midline of a body; related to a side.

lateral spinothalamic tract: ascending nerve fibers originating in the spinal cord and terminating in the thalamus.

L-dopa: L-3,4-hydroxyphenylalanine; synthetic dopamine that crosses the blood-brain barrier; often given to Parkinson's patients.

lesion: an area of damage in the body.

ligand-sensitive channel proteins: protein channels in the cell membrane that open and close in response to the presence of certain chemicals or neurotransmitters.

limb apraxia: failure to perform a learned movement; may be ipsilateral or bilateral; also known as ideomotor apraxia.

limbic system: interconnected nuclei in the telencephalon and diencephalon; functions include self-preservation and activities and behaviors, including emotions, sexual behaviors, memory, olfaction sensory processing; composed of the olfactory bulb, hypothalamus, amygdala, hippocampus, insular cortex, and cingulate gyrus.

localization of function: a particular structure in the nervous system assigned to a specific function (e.g., Broca's area is the localized area for language expression).

long-term memory: the part of memory where knowledge is stored permanently and is activated when needed (usually through cues); theoretically unlimited in capacity.

Lou Gehrig's disease: see *amyotrophic lateral sclerosis.*

lower motor neurons: peripheral motor neurons within the spinal cord whose axons terminate in a skeletal muscle; efferent neurons that transmit motor impulses.

magnetic resonance imaging (MRI): neuroimaging procedure in which hydrogen proteins of tissues are aligned with the magnetic field; emits a signal that is recorded in each slice (image).

magnetoencephalography (MEG): magnetic radiography depicting the intracranial fluid spaces after cerebral spinal fluid is extracted and replaced by air or gas.

magnum foramen: opening in the base of the skull through which the spinal cord is continuous with the brain.

masking: the drowning of a weak sound by a louder one.

mastication: the chewing of food.

mechanicoreceptors: Sensory receptor sensitive to mechanical stimulation such as muscles and tendons, sinuses, and hair cells of the inner ear.

medial: toward the midline.

medulla oblongata: also known as the myelencephalon; caudal segment of the brainstem, rostral from the foramen magnum to the pons.

meninges: Membranous coverings of the central nervous system developing from the neural crest and the mesoderm layer.

mental retardation: a developmental delay characterized by impaired learning, social adjustment, and maturational problems in all areas.

mesoderm: the second germ layer apparent during the third week of development of the nervous system; forms the skin (dermis), skeleton, muscles, blood, and blood vessels.

mesencephalon: midbrain.

metacognition: educational process that incorporates knowledge of one's abilities, the demands of the task at hand, and the effective learning strategies needed to achieve success; may be regulated by the individual involved.

microglia: type of glial cell with a primarily scavenger function.

microtubules: part of an axon; help carry out the process of axon transport.

midbrain: the most superior of the three structures making up the brainstem; associated structures found at the midbrain level are the tectum, inferior and superior colliculi, the cerebral peduncles, and the substantia nigra.

minimal cerebral dysfunction: a syndrome of neurologic dysfunction in children usually marked by impairments of fine coordination, clumsiness, and choreiform or athetoid movements; often associated with learning disorders.

mitosis: a type of cell division in which a single cell produces two genetically identical daughter cells; new body cells for growth and repair are produced through mitosis.

mixed dominance: inconsistency in laterality of speech and related motor functions such as hand, foot, and eye dominance in some individuals; sometimes associated with language and learning disorders.

modified feeding: altered intake of food and nutrition; may include tube feedings, specialized diet plans and food consistencies, and solid and liquid restrictions.

monoloudness: no variation in the loudness or volume level; static volume usually attributable to dysarthria caused by phonatory and respiratory weakness.

monoplegia: paralysis of one limb.

Moro reflex: infantile reflex that involves postural responses; rapid lowering of a flexed, supine head of an infant causes abduction and extension followed by flexion, of the arms.

motor association areas: cortical association areas, numbered 44 to 47 in the Brodmann system, that surround the foot of the motor and premotor cortices.

motor endplate: special structural enlargements of the muscle fibers at the synaptic junction.

motor fibers: efferent fibers that go to the muscle and force them to contract.

motor unit: a motor neuron that includes the muscle fibers it innervates.

multiple sclerosis (MS): degenerative disease of the central nervous system with no known cause; some research has linked this disease with a malfunction of the immune system; myelin degenerates but the axon remains intact; the intact axon is probably the reason for periods of remission.

multipolar cell: any cell that contains more than one (usually two) process.

muscle spindle: specialized organ within a muscle; gives muscle length feedback.

muscle tone: the resistance to passive movement or change of muscle length.

muscular dystrophy: genetic, progressive myopathy that includes Duchenne muscular dystrophy and myotonia.

myasthenia gravis: autoimmune disorder in which postsynaptic acetylcholine receptors are blocked, causing muscle weakness and fatigue.

myelin: the fatty substance surrounding some axons that speeds neural transmission; the myelin-covered areas are the white matter of the brain.

myelination: the process of segmental wrapping of myelin around axons; continuous myelin is interrupted by narrow gaps (nodes of Ranvier).

myelogenesis: the cyclic process of laying down of myelin on certain fiber tracts.

myoclonus: rapid, asynchronous movements of the limbs.

necrose: to die.

necrosis: cell death caused by local injury, such as loss of blood supply or disease; nonphysiologic processes; usually occurs in severe trauma.

neocerebellum: the newer parts of the cerebellum phylogenetically provided by the corticopontocerebellar fibers.

neocortex: theoretically, a phylogenetic division of the cerebral cortex; distinguished from the allocortex in lower animals; also called the isocortex.

neologistic jargon aphasia: a temporal lobe syndrome marked by newly coined words and unintelligible utterances.

neoplasm: tumor.

neural integration: complete and harmonious combining of components of the nervous system.

neural tube: embryologically, a hollow structure that gives rise to the central nervous system as the cells mature.

neurofibrillary tangles: tangles of neurofibers common in Alzheimer's disease.

neurofilaments: the fine filaments seen in neurons through an electron microscope.

neurogenesis: the development of neurons from stem cell precursors.

neuroglial cells: see *glial cells*.

neurolinguistics: the study of the relation of communication and language regarding brain function; the manner in which the brain helps produce language and, in turn, communication.

neurology: a branch of science that deals with the normal as well as the diseased or disordered nervous system.

neuron: nerve cell.

neuroplasticity: the capacity of neurons to adapt to a changed environment; in some cases, neuronal areas take over function(s) of damaged neurons.

neurotransmitter: the substance released from an axonal terminal of a presynaptic neuron once the neuron is excited; travels across the synaptic cleft to excite or inhibit the targeted cell; examples are norepinephrine, acetylcholine, or dopamine.

Noam Chomsky: twentieth century linguist who postulated the theory of language controversy as innate versus learned.

nociceptor: a receptor for pain that is stimulated by tissue damage.

Norman Geschwind: early twentieth century pioneer in behavioral neurology.

notochord: a cylindrical group of cells on the dorsal aspect of an embryo; the center of the development of the axial skeleton.

nystagmus: rhythmical horizontal, rotary, or vertical oscillation of the eyeballs.

obligatory: without an alternative path.

occipital lobe: the posterior portion of each hemisphere that forms the posterior-lateral surface of the brain; location of visual cortex; area involved with vision.

olfaction: the sense of smell.

oligodendrocyte: type of glial cell that produces myelin for neurons in the central nervous system.

optic chiasm: the structure located on the floor of the third ventricle composed of crossing optic nerve fibers from the medial (nasal) half of each retina.

optic disk: the head of the optic nerve.

oral apraxia: buccofacial apraxia; inability to program nonspeech oral movements.

organ of Corti: lies against the basilar membrane in the cochlea; contains special sensory receptors for hearing consisting of hair cells and other support cells.

orthograde transneuronal atrophy: process involving the large-scale death of neurons in the central nervous system in response to injury to white matter.

osmotic force: the energy needed to maintain adequate body fluids and set and maintain the proper balance between the volumes of extracellular and intracellular fluids.

palilalia: repeating a word or phrase with increasing rapidity as a result of neurologic damage.

palpate: to examine by feeling and pressing with the palms of the hands and fingers.

parahippocampal gyrus: between the collateral sulcus and the hippocampal sulcus on the inferior surface of each hemisphere; above the cingulated gyrus and below the lingual gyrus.

paralimbic areas: associative areas of the cortex containing structures that form an uninterrupted girdle around the medial and basal aspects of the cerebral hemispheres; areas include the caudal orbitofrontal cortex, insula, temporal pole, parahippocampal gyrus (proper), and cingulate complex.

paralysis: loss of voluntary muscular function.

paraphasia: the substitution of words or sounds in words in such a way as to decrease intelligibility or obscure meaning.

paraplegia: paralysis of both lower extremities and, generally, the lower trunk.

parasympathetic division: pertaining to that division of the autonomic nervous system concerned with the maintenance of the body; its fibers arise from the brain and the sacral part of the spinal cord.

parasympathetic nuclei: part of the autonomic nervous system; preganglionic fibers leave the central nervous system with cranial nerves III, VII, IX, and X and the first three sacral nerves; postganglionic fibers are in the heart, smooth muscles, and glands of the neck and head and the viscera in the thorax, abdomen, and pelvis regions; most of the fibers are in the vagus nerve tract.

paresis: partial paralysis; weakness.

paresthesia: abnormal sensation of burning, tingling, or numbness.

parietal lobe: upper and central portion of each hemisphere between the frontal and occipital lobes and above the temporal lobe.

parkinsonism: a disorder that manifests the symptoms of Parkinson's disease.

Parkinson's disease: a slow, progressive disease characterized by the degeneration of the substantia nigra within the basal ganglia, causing a gradual decrease of the neurotransmitter dopamine; characterized by resting tremor of the hands and feet, hypokinetic dysarthria, and a masklike facial expression.

pathologic tremor: a tremor caused by the structural and functional manifestations of a disease.

pattern-associator network: network used in simulations of behavior that allows transformation of a pattern of activity across its input units into a pattern of activity across its output units.

peduncles: very large mass (like a stalk) of nerve fibers connecting two structures in the nervous system.

perikaryon: the cytoplasmic matrix surrounding a cell body in a neuron.

perilymph: fluid contained in the bony labyrinth of the inner ear.

peripheral nervous system (PNS): Cranial and spinal nerves and their branches.

peristriate cortex: part of the occipital lobe that receives fibers from the optic radiation; the primary receiving area for vision.

perisylvian cortex: an area on the lateral wall of the dominant hemisphere for language that includes the major centers and pathways for language reception and production; see perisylvian zone.

perisylvian zone: the cortex surrounding the sylvian fissure in the dominant temporal lobe; site where the major neurologic components for understanding and producing language are found (e.g., Broca's area, Wernicke's area, the supramarginal and angular gyri).

pervasive developmental disorder: a disorder on the autism spectrum characterized by an impairment in the development of social interaction and social pragmatic skills as well as verbal or nonverbal communication skills and the possibility of stereotyped behaviors and interests.

phasic tone: rapid contraction to a high-intensity stretch (or change in muscle length) assessed by testing tendon reflexes.

phoneme: smallest meaningful unit of sound.

phonologic alexia: the inability to read nonsense words, especially low-frequency words; errors are usually visual errors.

photoreceptors: nerve end organs stimulated by light, as in the rods and cones of the retina.

phrenic nerves: nerves arising from the cervical spinal cord that supply the diaphragm.

pia mater: the innermost layer of the meninges that is vascular in nature.

Pick's disease: a rare and progressive and degenerative form of dementia characterized by cortical atrophy in the frontal and temporal lobes.

Pierre Paul Broca: French physician (1824-1880); localized language areas from two patients who had sustained language and motor speech losses; postulated for the first time that the left hemisphere contained the language center.

plantar: relating to the sole of the foot.

plasticity: the concept that in the immature brain some functional areas are not established and that unestablished areas may assume any one of a variety of functions.

plosives: a class of consonant speech sounds that require a complete closure of the vocal tract followed by a quick release of air and/or acoustic sound energy; they are /p/, /b/, /t/, /d/, /k/, and /g/.

pons: the part of the brainstem that lies between the medulla and the midbrain.

positive support reflex: reflex that is necessary for erect posture; when the balls of the feet (bounced on a flat surface) are stimulated, a contraction of opposing muscle groups fixes the joints of the lower extremities to bear weight.

positron emission tomography (PET): imaging technique that visualizes the functioning brain by showing its activity through blood flow and glucose metabolism.

posterior: directed to or situated in the back; opposite is anterior; also referred to as dorsal.

posterior alexia: see *alexia without agraphia.*

postganglionic: pertaining to nerve fibers in the autonomic nervous system that exit the ganglion.

postsynaptic terminal: what is distal to or beyond a synapse.

postural tone: the resistance striated muscles and tendons offer when stretched by a sustained, low-intensity force by a person or gravity; the recoil capability of the striated muscles and the tendons once they are fully extended by a sustained force.

potential: a relative amount of voltage in an electrical field.

praxis: the normal performance of a motor act.

preganglionic: pertaining to nerve fibers in the autonomic nervous system whose cell body is within the CNS (brainstem or spinal cord) with its axon extending peripherally to synapse on post-ganglionic neurons in the autonomic ganglia.

prematurity: a state of being born after fewer than 37 weeks of gestation (birth weight is no longer considered a critical criterion).

premotor area: area in the frontal lobe in front of the premotor cortex and inferior to the prefrontal cortex; responsible for sensory guidance of movement and control of proximal and trunk muscles.

presynaptic inhibition: inhibitory control of afferent muscle spindles before the synapse occurs.

presynaptic terminal: what is anterior to or before a synapse.

primary auditory receptor cortex: found in the temporal lobe; also known as Heschl's gyrus (areas 41 and 42).

primary motor projection cortex: composed mostly of precentral gyrus; voluntary control of skeletal muscles on the contralateral side of the body contained in the frontal lobe; also called the motor strip.

primary neurulation: a process in which the neural tube forms from the neural plate.

primary olfactory receptor cortex: areas responsible for smell, consisting of anterior olfactory nucleus, olfactory tubercle, piriform cortex, and cortical amygdaloid nucleus; only sensory fibers that do not pass through the thalamus.

primary progressive aphasia (PPA): associated with left hemisphere pathology not necessarily from acute neurologic infarct such as a stroke; may have problems in comprehension, reading, writing, naming; does not improve over time as does aphasia from stroke; deficits continue to be progressive; may be a continuous decline in language abilities over time.

primary somatosensory cortex: areas 1, 2, and 3 on the postcentral gyrus; a primary receptor of general bodily sensation; thalamic radiations carry sensory data from the skin, muscles, tendons, and joints.

primary visual receptor cortex: area 17 in the occipital lobe along the calcarine fissure; receives fibers from the optic tract; also known as the striate area.

procedural memory: stores information from rule-based skills and is accessed through learned behaviors; also known as implicit memory.

projection neurons: the axons that originate outside the telencephalon (thalamocortical fibers) projecting to the cerebral cortex and those that arise from cerebral cortex cells (corticospinal, corticopontine, and corticothalamic) and project to other downward targeted areas.

prone: lying face down.

proprioception: perception mediated by proprioceptors.

proprioceptors: sensory nerve endings that send information regarding body movement and body positioning.

prosencephalon: see *forebrain.*

prosopagnosia: a visual agnosia characterized by the inability to recognize the faces of other people or one's own face in a mirror; associated with agnosia for color, objects, and place.

proximal: toward the midline or center of the body.

pseudobulbar palsy: muscular paralysis from bilateral upper motor neuron lesions of the cranial nerves often accompanied by dysarthria, dysphagia, and emotional lability, such as outbursts of laughing or crying.

pseudohypertrophy: increase in the size of an organ or part not caused by an increase in size or number of the specific functional elements; rather, is caused by an increase in some other fatty or fibrous tissue.

pseudounipolar cell: sensory neurons in the peripheral nervous system that contain a longer dendrite and a smaller axon that connects to the spinal cord.

ptosis: drooping of the eyelid as a result of neurologic damage (paralysis).

putamen: a part of the lenticular nucleus; a structure of the basal ganglia.

pyramidal system: controls voluntary movement of the muscles for speech and all other voluntary muscles; consists of the corticospinal tract, corticobulbar tract, and the corticopontine tract.

quadriplegia: paralysis of all four limbs.

radiograph: see *x-ray.*

reasoning: the process of evaluating information to come to a conclusion.

reflex arc: a pathway leading from the receptor of a sensory stimulus to the motor response; the response is known as an automatic reflex action.

reflexes: subconscious automatic stimulus response mechanisms; in human beings, reflexes are basic defense mechanisms to sensory stimulation.

relative refractory period: momentary state of reduced irritation after a neural response.

regional cerebral blood flow (rCBF): a neuroimaging technique to study somatosensory pathways.

Reissner's membrane: a thin anterior wall of the cochlear duct that separates it from the scala vestibuli.

resting potential: the difference in potential across the membrane of a cell at rest.

resting tremor: a tremor that occurs when the limb is relaxed and supported, as in Parkinson's disease.

reticulospinal tract: nerve fibers that extend from the reticular formation in the brainstem to the spinal cord, contributing to functional contralateral muscle tone; helps with extensor and flexor muscle movements.

retrograde: moving against the direction of flow.

retrograde transneuronal degeneration: pathologic changes that occur across the axon and cell body of neurons as a result of an axonal lesion.

Rett syndrome: a pervasive developmental disorder that affects cerebral gray matter; occurs in females and presents at birth; characterized by autistic behaviors, ataxic movements, and seizures.

rhombencephalon: see *hindbrain.*

Romberg test: a test in which the patient stands with feet together while the examiner notes the amount of body sway with the patient's eyes open and closed; also known as the body sway test.

rooting reflex: a newborn reflex in which a touch to the infant's cheek or upper or lower lip causes the infant to turn toward that stimulus.

rostral: toward the nasal or oral regions; superior in relation to the spinal cord and anterior in relation to the brain.

rubrospinal tracts: fibers from the red nucleus to the spinal cord.

saltatory transmission: the type of neuronal transmission in myelinated fibers compared with the slow transmission in unmyelinated fibers.

scalae: fluid-filled columns that surround the modiolus, the hollow core of the cochlea.

scanning speech: related to ataxic dysarthria; quite slow, with syllable-by-syllable pausing.

Schwann cells: form and maintain myelin in the peripheral nervous system.

secondary association areas: sites in which elaboration of sensation occurs; considered as extensions of the primary sensory receptor areas; also known as sensory association areas or unimodal association areas.

secondary neurulation: process in which the caudal neural tube give rise to the sacral and coccygeal levels of the spinal cord; begins at approximately 3 weeks' gestation.

secretomotor: stimulating secretion.

segmental rolling reflex: the reflex noted when an infant rolls the trunk and pelvis segmentally with rotation of the head or legs.

selective engagement: neural process in which certain neural networks are utilized for optimizing a task while others are limited in participation; primarily manifested in attention with principal cortical area involved thought to be the dorsolateral prefrontal cortex.

sensory fibers: also known as afferent fibers; carry information to the central nervous system about sensations of touch, pain, temperature, and vibrations.

servomechanism control system: a control device for maintaining the operation of another system.

short-term memory: temporary and limited in capacity; related to working memory (the active processing to hold the information); must be continuously acted upon through rehearsal or imaging or information stored here will be lost over time.

Shy-Drager syndrome: condition of unknown etiology characterized by hypotension, constipation, urinary urgency, parkinsonian symptoms, cerebellar incoordination, muscle fasciculations, and leg tremors.

single-photon emission tomography (SPECT): imaging modality that uses the mechanism of the computed tomography scan but instead of detecting x-rays, it detects single photons emitted from an external tracer; radioactive compounds that emit gamma rays are injected into the subject; can scan metabolism and blood flow in the brain.

sodium-potassium pump: related to the physiology of neurons; an ion pump that removes intracellular sodium and concentrates intracellular potassium.

soma: a neuronal cell body; also called the perikaryon.

somatic: pertaining to the structure of the body wall (muscles, skin, and mucous membranes).

somesthetic: pertaining to the senses of pain, temperature, taction, vibration, and position.

somites: Mesodermal tissue that develops into the axial skeleton, dermis, and skeletal muscles.

spastic cerebral palsy: congenital condition with hypertonia, hyperreflexia, and clasp-knife reflex, increased tone, and bilateral central nervous system damage.

spastic dysarthria: strain-strangle, harsh voice quality; imprecise articulation, and hypernasality caused by upper motor neuron bilateral pathology; affects phonation, articulation, respiration, and resonance.

spastic dysphonia (SD): chronic phonation disorder of unknown etiology characterized by a strained voice quality with voice arrests caused by laryngeal adductor spasm; symptoms may occur in some movement disorders; also known as spasmodic dysphonia.

spasticity: syndrome of hypertonus with exaggeration of stretch reflexes as a result of certain neural lesions.

spatial summation: achieving an action potential involving input from multiple cells of different areas of input, usually from the dendrite.

specific language impairment (SLI): a subset condition of children with developmental receptive/expressive language disorders; possible organic involvement; language disorder must not be attributable to a more generalized condition such as hearing loss, autism, or acquired neurologic damage.

speech-language pathology: the study of the diagnosis, treatment, and prevention of communication disorders, including articulation, phonology, voice, fluency, expressive and receptive language, and related disorders.

speech pathology: see *speech-language pathology.*

spina bifida: congenital defect of the spinal cord or the vertebral column.

spinal peripheral nerves: mixed nerves (both sensory and motor) connected to the spinal cord.

spinocerebellar pathway: consists of the dorsal and ventral tracts; arise from the posterior and medial gray matter of the spinal cord; dorsal ascends ipsilaterally but the ventral crosses in the cord; both terminate in the cerebellum and allow proprioceptive impulses from all parts of the body to be integrated in the cerebellum.

splenium: the thickened posterior part of the corpus callosum.

split brain: a condition in which the corpus callosum has been surgically divided so no information transfers between hemispheres.

stereocilia: hair cell processes bent by movement.

stereognosis: recognition of objects through nonvisual and tactile stimulation.

striate cortex: primary visual cortex.

styloglossus: the smallest of the styloid muscles arising from the anterior and lateral surfaces of the styloid process; aids in tongue retraction and swallowing.

subarachnoid space: a space between the dura and pia mater layers filled with cerebrospinal fluid.

subcortical aphasia: aphasia associated with either thalamic or basal ganglia lesions (subcortical structures).

subdural space: region below the dura mater.

sublingual: region below or under the tongue.

substantia nigra: a mass of gray matter extending from the upper border of the pons into the subthalamus.

subthalamus: region composed of subcortical structures of the basal ganglia located below the thalamus.

suckling reflex: infant reflex that occurs when a finger is placed in the infant's mouth and bouts of sucking behavior occur; integrated at birth and develops into jaw movements after 2 to 3 months.

sulcus: groove on the surface of the brain or spinal cord; also known as fissures.

summation: the product of the neural impulses acting on a given synapse.

superior: upper; opposite of inferior or lower.

supine: lying on the back.

supplementary (secondary) motor area (SMA): motor area discovered by Wilder G. Penfield located on the ventral surface of the precentral and postcentral gyri; primary function is controlling sequential movements.

supramarginal gyrus: convolution in the inferior parietal lobe surrounding the posterior end of the sylvian fissure.

surface dyslexia: type of dyslexia distinguished by poor ability to use grapheme-to-phoneme conversion rules.

swallowing reflex: developed after the sucking reflex is integrated into feeding; sucking produces saliva that accumulates in the pharynx, triggering the reflex; may be observed by visible upward movement of the hyoid bone and thyroid cartilage of the larynx.

Sydenham's chorea: involuntary movement disorder following infection; usually occurs in children and adolescents.

symmetric tonic neck reflex: analogous to the asymmetrical tonic reflex but the head is manipulated in flexion and extension in midline rather than turned laterally; the normal execution of this reflex is an extension of the arms and flexion of the legs if the head is extended in midline.

sympathetic division: that division of the autonomic nervous system concerned with preparing the body for fight or flight; its neurons arise in the thoracic and upper lumbar segments of the spinal cord.

synapse: a juncture or connection; the functional contact of one neuron with another.

synaptic cleft: the intervening space before and after a synapse.

synergy: the cooperative action of muscles.

tardive dyskinesia: uncontrolled involuntary movements of the face and tongue; often caused by excessive or long-term treatment with neuroleptic medications.

tectal pathway: projects to the superior colliculi in the brainstem and the thalamus and out to many regions of the cortex; substantially involved in the ability to orient toward and follow a visual stimuli.

tectorial membrane: gelatinous covering of the organ of Corti in the auditory system.

tectum: roof of the midbrain; location of the superior and inferior colliculi.

temporal lobe: bounded superiorly by the lateral fissure and posteriorly by the occipital lobe; the center for auditory processing in the brain.

temporal summation: the additive effect of successive stimuli on one nerve, which collectively can generate a response when the individual stimuli could not.

temporal visual cortex: part of the visual association cortex located within the middle and inferior temporal areas.

tentorium cerebelli: one of two dural folds in the dura mater that help stabilize the brain.

teratology: the study of abnormal embryology.

thalamic reticular nucleus: a layer of cells enveloping the ventral thalamus whose axons are sent back into the thalamus rather than to the cortex; either facilitates or inhibits transmission of other impulses to the cortex.

thalamus: two oval nodes located at the base of the cerebrum; serves as a relay station for all sensory stimulation; consists of gray matter.

thrombus: A stationary blood clot along the wall of a blood vessel.

tinnitus: ringing or buzzing sound heard in the ear.

tongue reflex: typically a part of the suckle-swallow reaction in which the tongue thrusts between the lips; mediated at the medulla; usually disappears by 12 to 18 months of age.

tonic labyrinthine reflex (TLR): associated with changes in tone as a result of changes in head position affecting the orientation of the labyrinths of the inner ear.

tonotopic: pertaining to the spatial arrangement in the auditory system determining where different sound frequencies are perceived, transmitted, or received.

topologic involvement: relation of an anatomic structure to a specific body part or area.

transcortical aphasia: several types of language disturbances whose causes are lesions outside the perisylvian area; repetition is always preserved.

transcranial magnetic stimulation (TMS): a non-invasive method of exciting neurons in the brain; uses weak electric current induced in the brain tissue by rapidly changing magnetic fields.

transient ischemic attack (TIA): a reversible neurologic defect (focal) lasting up to 24 hours; may indicate a risk for a stroke; may be caused by am embolism or obstruction of an artery.

transitory: related to or marked by a transition; not permanent.

traumatic brain injury (TBI): diffuse brain damage that may be caused by an external force (e.g., closed-head injury from a car accident) or a penetrating force (e.g., open-head injury from a bullet wound).

tremor: a purposeless involuntary movement that is oscillatory and rhythmic.

trigeminal ganglia: on the sensory root of cranial nerve V in a cleft within the dura mater; gives off ophthalmic and maxillary nerves and is part of the mandibular nerve branch.

triplegia: paralysis of an upper and a lower extremity and of the face or of both extremities on one side and one on the other.

uncus: the hooked extremity of the hippocampal gyrus.

unilateral: initiated from or affecting structures on only one side of the body.

unilateral inattention: a subtle form of neglect syndrome characterized by the failure to recognize a side of the body and the space around it.

unilateral innervation: indicating that the nerve supply to a particular structure comes from only one side of the body (may be ipsilateral or contralateral), as opposed to bilateral innervation, in which nerve fibers are distributed from both sides of the body.

unilateral upper motor neuron dysarthria: A motor speech disorder primarily caused by unilateral damage to the upper motor neurons that carry impulses to the cranial nerves that innervate the speech musculature; the most affected speech parameter is articulation.

upper motor neurons: Nerves connecting cortical motor areas with cranial and spinal nerves; composed of the direct activation pathway (DAP) and the indirect activation pathway (IAP), the DAP functions for direct voluntary and skilled movements, whereas the IAP functions to control posture, tone, and movements that support voluntary movements.

ventral: towards the belly or abdomen; opposite of dorsal.

ventricular system: cavities that contain cerebrospinal fluid produced by the choroid plexus located in each ventricle; the system consists of lateral ventricles and a third and fourth ventricle; connected by foramen and the aqueduct of Sylvius; found in the deepest areas of the brain.

vertebral artery: supplies the brainstem and cerebellum; from the anterior and posterior spinal arteries to the spinal cord and a branch called the posterior inferior cerebellar artery.

vesicle: a blister or bladder; the intracellular bladder is believed to be filled with neurotransmitter substances.

vestibulospinal tracts: nerve fiber tracts that mediate cerebellar and vestibular influences on the spinal cord; facilitate reflexes and control muscle tone.

visual agnosia: the inability to recognize objects by sight, usually caused by damage to the visual association area of the central nervous system.

volitional: voluntary.

Wernicke's aphasia: an acquired adult language disorder characterized by impaired comprehension, and fluent, paraphasic language; the patient is free of hemiplegia, and the lesion usually is in the temporal lobe.

Wernicke's area: a major speech-language center in the dominant temporal lobe; important for comprehension of language.

white matter: substance of the brain and spinal cord consisting of myelinated fibers and containing no neuronal cell bodies or synapses; in a freshly sectioned brain it glistens white because of the high content of lipid-rich myelin; also called the fimbria.

x-ray: radiograph; film produced by radiographic imaging.

Index

B indicates boxes; f indicates figures; t indicates tables.